A Dictionary of Hearing

D0891279

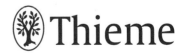

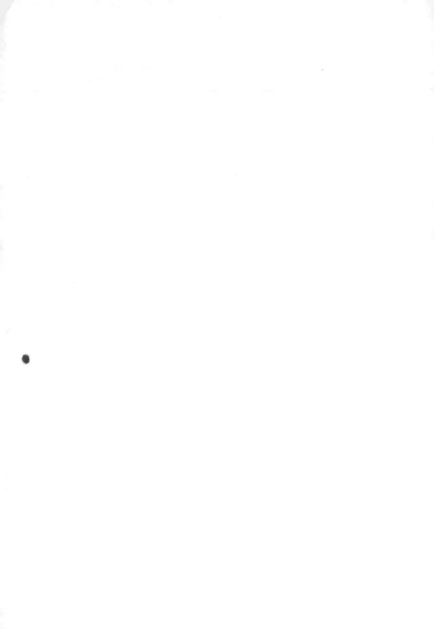

A Dictionary of Hearing

Maryanne Tate Maltby, MEd, MSc, EdD
Senior Lecturer and Pathway Leader in Audiology
Anglia Ruskin University
Cambridge, England

Honorary Audiologist
Addenbrooke's Hospital
Cambridge University Hospitals Foundation Trust
Cambridge, England

Thieme
New York · Stuttgart

Thieme Medical Publishers, Inc.
333 Seventh Ave.
New York, NY 10001

Executive Editor: Timothy Hiscock
Managing Editor: Elizabeth D'Ambrosio
Senior Vice President, Editorial and Electronic Product Development: Cornelia Schulze
International Production Director: Andreas Schabert
Vice President, Finance and Accounts: Sarah Vanderbilt
President: Brian D. Scanlan
Compositor: medionet Publishing Services Ltd.
Printer: Sheridan Books

Library of Congress Cataloging-in-Publication Data
The Library of Congress Cataloging-in-Publication Data is available from the publisher upon request.

Important note: Medical knowledge is ever-changing. As new research and clinical experience broaden our knowledge, changes in treatment and drug therapy may be required. The authors and editors of the material herein have consulted sources believed to be reliable in their efforts to provide information that is complete and in accord with the standards accepted at the time of publication. However, in view of the possibility of human error by the authors, editors, or publisher of the work herein or changes in medical knowledge, neither the authors, editors, nor publisher, nor any other party who has been involved in the preparation of this work, warrants that the information contained herein is in every respect accurate or complete, and they are not responsible for any errors or omissions or for the results obtained from use of such information. Readers are encouraged to confirm the information contained herein with other sources. For example, readers are advised to check the product information sheet included in the package of each drug they plan to administer to be certain that the information contained in this publication is accurate and that changes have not been made in the recommended dose or in the contraindications for administration. This recommendation is of particular importance in connection with new or infrequently used drugs.

Some of the product names, patents, and registered designs referred to in this book are in fact registered trademarks or proprietary names even though specific reference to this fact is not always made in the text. Therefore, the appearance of a name without designation as proprietary is not to be construed as a representation by the publisher that it is in the public domain.

Printed in the United States

5 4 3 2 1

ISBN 978-1-60406-828-3
Also available as an e-book:
eISBN 978-1-60406-829-0

Acknowledgments

This dictionary has been a long-term project, and the assistance of many people is gratefully acknowledged: Professor Robert Maltby, Department of Classics, University of Leeds, England; Jason Galster and Jim Curran, Starkey Ltd., Minneapolis, Minnesota; the Librarians of the Ear Institute and RNID Libraries and of the Wellcome Library, London, England; Daniel Rowan, Department of Audiology, University of Southampton, England; Lisbeth Högvik, the Information Center for Public Diagnoses, Gothenburg University, Sweden; Paul Lamb, Starkey Ltd., United Kingdom; Professor Richard Dowell, Department of Audiology, University of Melbourne, Australia; James LaBranche, HIMSA, Denmark; Professor Richard Seewald, University of Western Ontario, London, Ontario, Canada; and Professor Brian Moore, Department of Psychology, University of Cambridge, England. Thanks also go to Anglia Ruskin University for grant assistance, which was facilitated by Phil Gomersall and Eldre Beukes, who did above and beyond what could be expected of them; Kathryn Lewis; Hugh Crawford; Matthew and Kerry Tate; Clare Kewney; and Barry Downes. To all–and to John Siderov for his encouragement–as well as those that I may have forgotten to mention (for which I can only apologize), I offer my sincere thanks.

About the Author

Maryanne Tate Maltby has been involved in audiology and education of the deaf for more than 40 years. She has degrees in Audiology, Education, and Psychology and is qualified as an audiological scientist, hearing aid audiologist, and teacher of the deaf. She has worked as an audiologist in schools, hospitals, and private industry, and has held lecturing posts in universities (Manchester, Oxford Brookes, and Anglia Ruskin) and private industry in the United Kingdom. She has written several books, including *Principles of Hearing Aid Audiology* (1994 and 2002), *Audiology: An Introduction for Teachers and Other Professionals* (2000), *Occupational Audiometry: Monitoring and Protecting Hearing at Work* (2005), *Adult Aural Rehabilitation* (2009), and *A Supplementary Dictionary of Audiology, Oxford Reference* (2012).

Currently, Dr. Maltby is Senior Lecturer and Pathway Leader in Audiology at Anglia Ruskin University, Cambridge, and Honorary Audiologist at Addenbrooke's Hospital, Cambridge University Hospitals Foundation Trust.

Guide to the Dictionary

The aim of this dictionary is to provide vocabulary found in audiology and hearing-related areas, together with facts about the form and etymology of these words, with pronunciation given for difficult or uncommon words. More than 4,000 entries are presented in alphabetical order, including some basic statistical terms given to assist students when reading academic papers. For the scholar's ease, cross-referencing and the use of abbreviations have been avoided as much as possible. A list of selected acronyms has also been included.

Order of Entries
Entries are listed in alphabetical order based strictly on the standard 26-letter alphabet, with an initial capital letter treated the same as lowercase letter. Word combinations are treated in the same way (i.e., in normal alphabetical sequence).

Pronunciation
The symbols used are given in Table 1. The main stress is indicated by a superior stress mark (') before the stressed syllable. Alternative pronunciations are listed or indicated by the phonetically different part of the word placed in parentheses.

Conventions
The treatment of headwords is comprised of
- Usual spelling
- Acronym
- Part of speech
- Status
- Usual pronunciation
- Alternative plural or singular form
- Etymology

- Onomastic
- Synonym or also known as
- Meaning
- Alternative forms used as other parts of speech

1. Usual spelling. American spellings are used throughout the general text. Accepted alternative spellings are given after a forward slash. Where differing, the British spelling is placed in parentheses after the American spelling.

Table 1 Symbols Used to Describe Pronunciation

Vowels	as in	Consonants	as in
ă	bat	b	bat
ā	fade	ch	cheap
ah	ark	d	den
aw	torn	f	fat
ĕ	bet	g	got
er	fur	h	had
ĭ	bit	j	jelly
ī	hide	k	kill
ŏ	pod	l	lid
ō	toad	m	man
oi	toy	n	no
ow	how	ng	ring
u	book	p	put
ŭ	but	r	rat
ū	food	s	sat
		sh	shed
		t	to
		th	theater
		dh	that
		v	van
		w	will
		y	yes
		z	zoo
		zh	measure

2. Acronym. Where the headword is commonly abbreviated to an acronym, this is given in parentheses directly following the headword, e.g., automatic gain control (AGC). A list of selected acronyms has also been provided.

3. Part of speech. Headwords are described as noun *(n)*, noun phrase *(np)*, verb *(v)*, adjective *(adj)*, adverb *(adv)*, prefix, or suffix (see Table 2).

4. Status. If the word is colloquial or obsolete, this information is given with the part of speech, e.g., boilermaker's deafness *np obs* (see Table 2).

5. Usual pronunciation. A stress mark (') is given before the main stressed syllable, e.g., 'bīta. Accepted alternative pronunciations are given in parentheses, e.g., pēāzōe'lĕktrĭk (pēātzōe'lĕktrĭk).

6. Alternative plural or singular form, e.g., fossa *n pl* fossae.

7. Etymology. The origin of the word is given in brackets, e.g., [Lat *fossa* ditch]. Greek letters have been transliterated, e.g., [Gk *-logia* study of].

Table 2 List of Abbreviations

Abbreviation	Full
abbr	abbreviation
adj	adjective
adv	adverb
colloq	colloquial
e.g.	*exempli gratia:* "for example"
Fr	French
Gk	Greek
i.e.	*id est:* "that is"
Lat	Latin
n	noun
np	noun phrase
obs	obsolete
pl	plural
v	verb

8. Synonyms and also known as.

9. Onomastic. Basic information is included regarding the origin of a word or phrase that is named after a person, e.g., Frenzel glasses/goggles/lenses: Named after Hermann Frenzel (1895–1967), a German otologist, who developed the glasses to measure eye movements in cases of vertigo.

10. Meaning. The meaning of technical terms has been phrased in clear and simple language, e.g., flutter: 1. The first feeling of sound pressure, which is too low in frequency to be heard as a tone. 2. A beating or drumming sensation in the ear, sometimes due to twitching ear muscles or pulsations from blood vessels in the ear.

11. Alternative forms used as other parts of speech, e.g., adenoid: -*adj* adenoidal.

Common Acronyms

A

AAA	American Academy of Audiology
AAO-HNS	American Academy of Otolaryngology–Head and Neck Surgery
AAS	American Auditory Society
AB	Arthur Boothroyd word list
ABC	absolute bone conduction
ABESPA	American Board of Examiners in Speech-Language Pathology and Audiology
ABG	air–bone gap
ABLB	*see* 1. alternate binaural loudness balance; 2. loudness balance test, alternate binaural
AABR	automated auditory brainstem response
ABBT	*see* alternate binaural bithermal caloric test
ABO	American Board of Otolaryngology
ABR	*see* auditory brainstem response
AC or **a.c.**	*see* 1. air conduction; 2. alternating or fluctuating current
ACE	*see* advanced combination encoder
ACh	*see* acetylcholine
AChE	*see* acetylecholinesterase
A/D	analog to digital
AD	*see* Alzheimer disease
ADA	Academy of Dispensing Audiologists
ADD	*see* attention deficit disorder (ADD)/attention deficit hyperactivity disorder (ADHD)
ADHD	*see* attention deficit disorder (ADD)/attention deficit hyperactivity disorder (ADHD)
AEF	auditory evoked field
AEP	auditory evoked potential
AER	auditory evoked response
AERA	averaged evoked response audiometry

AFR	*see* adaptive frequency response
AGC	*see* automatic gain control
AGC-I	automatic gain control–input
AGC-O	automatic gain control–output
AHTL	apparent hearing threshold level
AI	*see* articulation index
AIED	autoimmune inner ear disease
ALD	*see* assistive listening device
ALR	*see* auditory late response
ALSS	*see* Alström syndrome
AM	amplitude modulation
AMFR	*see* amplitude modulation following response
Amg	*see* aminoglycoside
AMLB	alternate monaural loudness balance
ANC	adaptive noise canceler
ANOVA	*see* analysis of variance
ANSD	auditory neuropathy spectrum disorder
ANSI	American National Standards Institute
AOM	acute otitis media
AOR	auditooculogyric reflex
AP	*see* action potential
APD	*see* auditory processing disorder
APHAB	*see* Abbreviated Profile of Hearing Aid Benefit
APR	*see* auropalpebral reflex
APV	assumed protection value
ARA	Academy of Rehabilitative Audiology
ARD	acoustic reflex decay
ARHL	age-related hearing loss
ARO	Association for Research in Otolaryngology
ART	*see* acoustic reflex threshold
ARTS	age-related threshold shift
ASA	1. American Standards Association; 2. adaptive speech algorithm
ASHA	American Speech-Language-Hearing Association
ASL	American sign language
AST	American Tinnitus Association
ATP	*see* adenosine triphosphate
AVC	automatic volume control

B

BAAP	British Association of Physicians
BAAS	British Association of Audiological Scientists
BAAT	British Association of Audiology Technicians
BACDA	British Association of Community Doctors in Audiology
BADGE	Békésy ascending descending gap evaluation
BAEP	brainstem auditory evoked potential
BAER	brainstem auditory evoked response
BAHA	*see* bone-anchored hearing aid
BAOL	British Association of Otolaryngologists
BATOD	British Association of Teachers of the Deaf
BBN	broadband noise
BC	*see* bone conduction
BC-HIS	Board certified in hearing instrument sciences
BCIG	British Cochlear Implant Group
BCL	*see* Békésy comfortable loudness test
BER	brain evoked response
BERA	*see* brainstem evoked response audiometry
BHI	Better Hearing Institute
BiCROS	*see* bilateral contralateral routing of signals
BiFROS	bilateral frontal routing of signals
BILL	*see* bass increase at low levels
BIT	binary digit
BKB	Bamford-Kowal-Bench speech test
BMLD	binaural masking level difference
BOA	*see* behavioral observation audiometry
BOR	*see* branchio-oto-renal syndrome
BOU	*see* branchio-oto-ureteral syndrome
BP	1. bipolar; 2. blood pressure
BPPN	benign paroxysmal positioning nystagmus
BPPV	*see* benign paroxysmal positional vertigo
BRA	brainstem response audiometry
BS	British Standard
BSA	British Society of Audiology
BSAER	brainstem auditory evoked response
BSER	brainstem evoked response
BSERA	brainstem evoked response audiometry
BSHAA	British Society of Hearing Aid Audiologists
BSL	British sign language
BTA	brief tone audiometry

BTE	*see* behind-the-ear hearing aid
BW	1. body-worn; 2. bilateral weakness
BWS	*see* Beckwith-Wiedemann syndrome

C

C	1. compliance; 2. cranial nerve; 3. continuous
CA	1. *see* age, chronologic; 2. compressed analog; 3. central auditory
CAD	central auditory disorder
CAMISHA	computer-aided manufacturing of individual shells for hearing aids
CANS	*see* central auditory nervous system
CAP	1. *see* central auditory processing; 2. *see* compound action potential; 3. compressed analog processing
CAPD	*see* central auditory processing disorder
CAPS	communication assessment procedure for seniors
CAT	computerized axial tomography
CBT	*see* cognitive behavioral therapy
cc	cubic centimeter
CC	1. closed captioning; 2. clinical competence
CCC-A	Certificate in Clinical Competence in Audiology
CCM	contralateral competing message
CCT	California consonant test
CD	1. *see* communication disorder; 2. compact disc
CDL	*see* Cornelia de Lange syndrome
cdp	cubic distortion product
CDP	*see* posturography, computerized dynamic
CEOAE	click evoked otoacoustic emissions
CERA	*see* 1. cortical evoked response audiometry; 2. cardiac evoked response audiometry
CEN	European Committee for Standardization (Comité Européen de Normalisation)
CES	competing environmental sounds (test)
CF	*see* characteristic frequency
CFA	*see* continuous flow adapter
CHI	*see* closed head injury
CIC	1. *see* completely in the canal (hearing aid); 2. commissure of the inferior colliculus
CID	Central Institute for the Deaf
CIS	*see* continuous interleaved sampling process

CM	cochlear microphonic
CMOS	*see* complementary metal oxide semiconductor
CMR	*see* comodulation masking release
CMR	*see* common mode rejection
CMRR	common mode rejection ratio
CMV	*see* cytomegalovirus
CN	1. *see* cranial nerve; 2. cochlear nerve; 3. cochlear nucleus
CNC	consonant-nucleus-consonant
CNE	could not evaluate
CNR	composite noise rating
CNS	*see* central nervous system
CNT	could not test
CNV	*see* contingent negative variation
COCB	crossed olivocochlear bundle
COG	*see* center of gravity
COM	chronic otitis media
COME	chronic otitis media with effusion
COR	*see* 1. conditioned orientation reflex; 2. cervicoocular reflex
CORA	*see* conditioned orientation reflex audiometry
CORFIG	coupler response for flat insertion gain
COSI	Client Orientated Scale of Improvement
COT	critical off-time
COWS	*see* cold-opposite warm-same
CP	*see* cerebral palsy
CPA	*see* cerebellopontine angle
CPHI	communication profile for the hearing impaired
CPR	*see* cochleopalpebral reflex
cps	*see* cycle per second
CROS	*see* contralateral routing of signals
CRP	1. *see* canalith repositioning procedure; 2. corneoretinal potential
CSF	*see* cerebrospinal fluid
CSOM	chronic suppurative otitis media
CST	competing sentence test
CT	*see* computed tomography
CTP	caloric test position
CVA	*see* cerebrovascular accident
CVC	consonant-vowel-consonant
Cz	coronal (C) midline (z) electrode location

D

daPa	*see* decapascal
dB	*see* decibel
dBA	*see* A-weighting
dBHL	*see* decibels hearing level
dBHTL	decibels hearing threshold level
dBnHL	*see* decibels normalized hearing level
dBpeSPL	decibels peak equivalent sound pressure level
dBSL	*see* decibels sensation level
dBSPL	*see* decibels sound pressure level
DC or **d.c.**	*see* direct current
df	*see* degrees of freedom
DIDMOAD	*see* diabetes mellitus optic atrophy and deafness
DL	*see* difference limen
DM	diabetes mellitus
DNA	*see* deoxyribonucleic acid
DPOAE	*see* otoacoustic emissions, distortion product
DSL	*see* desired sensation level
DSP	*see* digital signal processing

E

EA	*see* age, educational
EAS	*see* electric and acoustic stimulation
ECoG or **ECochG**	*see* electrocochleography
EEG	*see* electroencephalography
EM	*see* masking, effective
EN	European standard or norm
ENT	ear, nose, and throat
EOG	*see* electrooculography
ERA	*see* electric or evoked response audiometry
ERB	*see* equivalent rectangular bandwidth

F

F	fast
FAAF	four alternative auditory feature test
FAS	fetal alcohol syndrome
FET	field effect transistor
FFT	*see* fast Fourier transform
FM	*see* frequency modulation

G
GHABP   Glasgow Hearing Aid Benefit Profile

H
HAC   Hearing Aid Council
HAIC   *see* Hearing Aid Industry Conference
HL   *see* hearing level
HLA   human leukocyte antigens
HPL   *see* half-peak level
HPLE   *see* half-peak level elevation
HSC   Health and Safety Commission
HSE   Health and Safety Executive
HTL   hearing threshold level
Hz   hertz

I
I   impulse
ICRA   International Collegium for Rehabilitative Audiology
IEC   international Electrotechnical Commission
IHR   Institute of Hearing Research
ILO   Institute of Laryngology and Otology
IPA   International Phonetic Alphabet
IQ   intelligence quotient
IROS   *see* ipsilateral routing of signals, hearing aid
ISO   International Standards Organization
ISVR   Institute of Sound and Vibration Research
ITC   in-the-canal hearing aid
ITE   in-the-ear hearing aid

J
J   *see* joule
JND   just noticeable difference
K
KEMAR   *see* Knowles electronic manikin for acoustic research
kHz   *see* kilohertz
KID   keratitis, ichthyosis, and deafness syndrome
KSS   Kearns-Sayre syndrome

L

LDL	*see* loudness discomfort level
Leq	*see* equivalent continuous sound pressure level
LEX	noise exposure level
LTSS	*see* long-term average speech spectrum

M

μPa	*see* micropascal
MA	*see* age, mental
MAA	*see* minimum audible angle
MAF	*see* minimum audible field
MAP	*see* minimum audible pressure
MCLL	*see* most comfortable loudness level
MML	*see* minimum masking level
MPO	*see* maximum power output
MRC	Medical Research Council
MRI	Medical Research Institute
MSRS	maximum speech recognition score

N

N	*see* Newton
NAL	National Acoustics Laboratory (of Australia)
NCPA	National Committee of Professionals in Audiology
NDCS	National Deaf Children's Association
nHL	*see* normalized hearing level
NICE	National Institute for Health and Clinical Excellence
NIHL	*see* noise-induced hearing loss
NIL	*see* noise emission level
NIPTS	noise-induced permanent threshold shift noise-induced hearing
NIST	National Institute of Standards and Technology
NOHL	*see* nonorganic hearing loss
NIOSH	National Institute of Occupational Safety and Health
NPL	National Physical Laboratory
NRT	*see* neural response telemetry
NSH	National Study of Hearing

O

OAD	*see* obscure auditory dysfunction
OAE	*see* otoacoustic emissions

ODS	optimum discrimination score
OFI	optic fixation index
OPD	otopalatodigital syndrome
OSHA	Occupational Safety and Health Administration
OSMED	otospondylomegaepiphyseal dysplasia
OSPL90	*see* the output sound pressure level of a hearing aid with an input level of 90 dB

P

Pa	*see* pascal
PAM	*see* postauricular myogenic response
PB	phonemically balanced
PDD	*see* progressive diaphyseal dysplasia
pe SPL	peak-to-peak equivalent sound pressure level
PET	*see* positron emission tomography (PET) scan
POEMS	programmable otoacoustic emission measurement system
POGO	*see* prescription of gain and output
PTA	*see* pure tone audiometry
PTS	*see* permanent threshold shift

Q

QUALY	quality adjusted life year

R

REAG	real ear-aided gain
REAR	*see* real ear-aided response
RECD	*see* real ear to coupler difference
REDD	real ear to dial difference
REIG	*see* real ear insertion gain
REM	real ear measurement
REOG	real ear occluded gain
REOR	real ear occluded response
RESR	real ear saturation response
RETFL	*see* reference equivalent threshold force level
RETSPL	*see* reference equivalent threshold sound pressure level
REUG	real ear-unaided gain
REUR	real ear unaided response
RITE	*see* receiver-in-the-ear
rms	*see* root mean square

RNA	*see* ribonucleic acid
RNID	Royal National Institute for Deaf People
RTG	reference test gain

S

S	slow
SAL	*see* sensorineural acuity level test
SCDS	*see* superior canal dehiscence syndrome
SD	standard deviation
SDTL	speech detection threshold level
SE	standard error
SFOAE	*see* otoacoustic emissions, sustained frequency
SI	Systèm International d'Unité
SIL	*see* sound intensity level
SISI	*see* Short Incremental Sensitivity Index test
SL	*see* sensation level
SLM	*see* sound level meter
SLT	speech and language therapist
SNHL	sensorineural hearing loss
SN	1. sensorineural; 2. speech weighted noise
SNR	*see* S/N signal-to-noise ratio
SOAE	*see* otoacoustic emissions, spontaneous
SPD	*see* spatial processing disorder
SPEAK	*see* spectral peak
SPL	*see* sound pressure level
SPSS	statistical package for social sciences
SRT	*see* speech reception threshold
SRTL	speech recognition threshold level
SSE	*see* sign supported English
SSPL	*see* saturation sound pressure level
SSW	*see* staggered spondaic word test
SVR	*see* slow vertex response

T

T	(telephone) induction loop
TEOAE	*see* otoacoustic emissions, transient evoked (TEOAE)/ transient evoked otoacoustic emissions (TOAE)
THD	*see* total harmonic distortion
TILL	*see* treble increase at low levels
TK	*see* threshold kneepoint/knee point

TMJ   *see* temporomandibular joint
TRT   *see* tinnitus retraining therapy
TTS   *see* temporary threshold shift

U

ULL   *see* uncomfortable loudness level

V

V   *see* volt
VaD   *see* vascular dementia
VCFS   *see* velocardiofacial syndrome
VKH   *see* Vogt-Koyanagi-Harada syndrome
VOR   *see* vestibuloocular reflex
VOT   *see* voice onset time
VRA   *see* visual reinforcement audiometry
VU   *see* volume unit meter

W

W   *see* watt
WDRC   wide dynamic range compression
WHO   World Health Organization

Contents

Contents

a- *prefix* [Gk *a-* without]
Without, against, or opposite.

A-weighting *n*
A standardized frequency weighting response, used to measure sound pressure level. It is based on normal binaural hearing and corresponds to a loudness of 40 phons. The "A" weighting scale reduces the low frequencies (5 dB/octave from 1000 to 250 Hz; 10 dB/octave below 250 Hz) and, to a lesser extent, the high frequencies when compared to a linear or flat scale. The frequencies near 1 kHz are not reduced. It is commonly used in free field hearing tests and for noise measurements in industrial audiometry. Measurements are expressed in terms of dBA, dB'A', or dB(A).

A1/A2
Left/right earlobe location for electrode placement used in evoked response audiometry.

Abbreviated Profile of Hearing Aid Benefit (APHAB)
A questionnaire consisting of four subscales (aversiveness, background noise, ease of communication, reverberation) that is used as a self-reported assessment of hearing aid benefit.

abducens *n/adj* ăbˈdūsĕnz (ăbˈdjūsĕnz) [Lat *abducens* drawing away]
-n Either of the pair of cranial nerve VI that controls the movement of the ipsilateral lateral rectus muscles of the eyes in humans. *-adj* Pertaining to either of the pair of cranial nerve VI.

abduction *n* [Lat *abductio* a drawing away]
The act of leading or drawing away, e.g., away from the midline of the body or away from each other.

aberrant *adj* [Lat *aberrans* straying]
Irregular or abnormal.

abiotrophy *n* ābǐˈōtгɐrfē [Gk *a-* without + Gk *bios* life + Gk *trophe* nourishment]
Progressive loss of function or degeneration.

ablation *n* [Lat *ablatio* a taking away]
Removal usually by surgery or by chemical means of a body part or tissue, e.g., the removal of a large vestibular schwannoma on the auditory nerve.

abruptly falling audiogram *np*
Also: precipitously falling audiogram; *colloq* ski-slope audiogram
An audiometric configuration that is flat or gradual in the low frequencies, but then falls dramatically in the mid to high frequencies.

Abruzzo-Erickson syndrome *np* Named after M.A. Abruzzo and R.P. Erickson, who first described the syndrome in two brothers, their mother, and a maternal uncle in 1977.
A rare genetic condition, thought to be X-linked recessive, in which characteristics include deafness, cleft palate, large protruding ears, coloboma of the eyes (a malformation that leaves a cleft, often in the iris), short stature, and humeroradial synostosis (an abnormality of the elbow joint).

abscess *n* [Lat *abscessus* a draining away]
An enclosed accumulation of purulent material (pus), caused by inflammation.

abscess, subdural *np* [Lat *abscessus* a draining away; Lat *sub* under + Lat *dura* hard matter]
A collection of liquid substance that occurs between the dura mater and the arachnoid mater (the outermost and middle layers of the meninges that covers the central nervous sytem), usually located within the cranium. May result from otitis media and may occur secondary to otitis media.

abscissa *n* ăbˈsĭs *pl* abscissae; abscissas [Lat short for *abscissa linea* a cut-off line]
Horizontal coordinate or x-axis of a graph.

absolute *adj* [Lat *absolutus* perfect, complete]
Accurate or perfect.

absolute latency *np* [Lat *absolutus* perfect, complete; Lat *latere* to lie hidden]
The time interval in milliseconds (ms) from the onset of a sound stimulus to the peak of a wave in evoked audiometry, e. g., wave V in an auditory brainstem response (ABR).

absolute pitch *np*
The ability to identify the pitch of a pure tone in the absence of a reference tone.

absolute refractory period *np*
The recovery time following the firing of a nerve or the excitation of a muscle fiber, in which no impulse can be initiated.

absolute sensitivity *np*
Also: absolute threshold
The minimum amount of energy required in a given stimulus for that stimulus to be detected 50% of the time.

absolute threshold *np*
Also: absolute sensitivity
The minimum amount of energy required in a given stimulus for that stimulus to be detected 50% of the time.

absorb *v* [Lat *absorbere* to swallow up]
To take up a sound instead of transmitting or reflecting it.

absorption *n* [Lat *absorptio* a swallowing up]
The uptake of energy through materials or the uptake of substances through tissues. In acoustics, sound energy can be reduced by being absorbed by the use of certain materials.

absorption coefficient *np*
The ratio of absorbed sound energy to the energy in the original signal, e.g., the coefficient for an open window is 1.00. The value varies with the frequency of the incident sounds.

absorption loss *np*
Loss of sound energy due to dissipation into other forms of energy.

accelerated speech *np* [Lat *accelerare* to speed up]
Time-compressed speech, i.e., recorded speech with increased playback speed.

acceleration *n* [Lat *acceleratio* a speeding up]
Rate of change in velocity over time.

accentuate *v* [Lat *accentuare* to mark, stress]
To emphasize or stress.

acceptable risk *np*
A degree of risk that is generally accepted as being slight or as having benefits that outweigh the risks.

accessory *adj* [Lat *accessorius* additional]
Nonessential, supplementary, or additional.

accessory nerve *np* [Lat *accessorius* additional]
Cranial nerve XI, which conveys motor impulses to the pharynx and muscles of the upper thorax, shoulders, and back. Paralysis of this motor nerve prevents the head from turning away from the affected side and causes the shoulder to droop.

accessory sinuses *np* [Lat *accessorius* additional; Lat *sinus* curve, hollow]
Also: paranasal sinuses
The paired ethmoidal, frontal, maxillary, and sphenoidal air cavities of the nose.

acclimatize (acclimatise) *v* *a*ˈklimatīz [Fr *acclimatiser* to habituate to a new climate]
To become accustomed to a new environment, stimulus or situation, e.g., to change over time as the listener becomes accustomed to a specific auditory stimulus.
Deriv: -*n* acclimatization (acclimatisation)

accommodation *n* [Lat *accommodatio* adaptation]
Adjustment to the environment, differences, or new circumstances.

accredited laboratory *np*
A laboratory that meets the required in-

ternational standards for calibration and has been accredited to supply accurate calibration certificates.

accumulator   *n*   [Lat *accummulator* one who accumulates, collects]
A storage cell for a battery that can be recharged by sending a reverse current through it.

accutane   *n*
A drug given for recalcitrant cystic acne. Maternal ingestion may cause hearing loss and vestibular dysfunction in the fetus.

acetylcholine (ACh)   *n*   asētil'kōlēn
A neurotransmitter found in the brain, spinal cord, and parts of the peripheral nervous system, responsible for muscular contraction.

acetylcholinesterase (AChE)   *n*   asētil'kōle'něsterāz
An enzyme that degrades the neurotransmitter acetylcholine thus terminating the postsynaptic potential.

acetylsalicylic acid   *np*   ăsētil'sălăsilĭk
Also: aspirin
A medicine commonly used to relieve pain and fever. High doses can be ototoxic. Damage is usually temporary but may be permanent, depending on the dosage and duration of use.

achondroplasia   *n*   akŏndra'plāzēa   [Gk *a* without + Gk *khondros* cartilage + Gk *plasis* formation]
A disorder of cartilage formation in the fetus due to a sporadic mutation or an inherited condition. Characteristics include shortended stature with normal-sized skull, protruding forehead, button nose, short fingers and toes, middle and inner ear abnormalities and associated conductive and sensorineural hearing loss.

acouesthesia   *n*   ăkuěs'dhēzēa   [Gk *akouein* to hear + Gk *aisthesis* sensation]
1. An acute sensation of hearing. 2. Pain in the limbs.

acoulalion   *n obs*   ăku'lālēon   [Gk *akouein* to hear + Gk *lalein* to speak]
An early instrument, a speech tube, used for teaching the deaf.

acoumeter/acouometer/acumeter   *n obs*   [Gk *akouein* to hear + Gk *metron* measure]
A predecessor of the audiometer for measuring hearing sensitivity.

acoupedic method   *np*   ăkyu'pēdĭk   [Gk *akouein* to hear + Gk *pais* child]
Acoustic stimulation of residual hearing in children; an aural-oral method for auditory training.

acouphone   *n obs*   [Gk *akouein* to hear + Gk *phone* sound]
An early name for an electrical hearing aid.

acousma/acouasm   *n pl* acousms/acousmata; acouasms   [Gk *akousma* a thing heard]
An illusory auditory perception of nonverbal sounds, e.g., buzzing or ringing. Also known as tinnitus. Commonly referred to as "noises in the head or ears."

acousmatagnosis   *n*   ăkousmatag'nōsĭs   [Gk *akousmata* things heard + Gk *agnosia* lack of knowledge]
Auditory aphasia; the auditory pathways are intact, but there is no understanding of the spoken word.

acousmatamnesia   *n*   ăkusmatămnēzēa   [Gk *akousmata* things heard + Gk *amnesia* forgetfulness]
Auditory amnesia; loss of memory for sounds.

acoustic/acoustical   *adj*   [Gk *akoustikos* pertaining to hearing]
Relating to sound.

acoustic absorption   *np*
The reduction of sound energy through the use of certain materials, generally the energy is converted to heat.

acoustic admittance   *np*
A measure of the ease with which sound passes through a medium or an acoustic system (the reciprocal of impedance). To-

tal admittance is determined by conductance and susceptance. The unit of measurement is the acoustic millimho (mmho). One cc of air has an admittance of one acoustic mmho in reference conditions.

acoustic admittance, static *np*
The greatest amount of acoustic energy absorbed by the middle ear system, i.e., the maximum compliance, shown by the vertical peak of the tympanogram tracing.

acoustic aid *np*
An aid to hearing based on a purely mechanical process, e.g., an ear trumpet.

acoustic attenuation *np*
A decrease in the magnitude, amplitude or intensity of sound, e.g., by absorption or the use of electrical resistors and capacitors (an attenuator).

acoustic axis *np* [Gk *akoustikos* pertaining to hearing; Gk *axis* direction]
The direction of greatest intensity of sound.

acoustic baffle *np*
A device for regulating or diverting the flow of sound waves; commonly used as a shield to reduce unwanted sound transmission, e.g., from the back of a loudspeaker.

acoustic compliance *np*
A measure of the volume displacement of a medium, e.g., air, when exposed to sound waves. The reciprocal of acoustic stiffness, it indicates the ease with which sound passes through a medium or an acoustic system. The term is often used in tympanometry to describe the ease of sound transfer into the middle ear system when the assumption is made that the measurement is dominated by compliant acoustic susceptance. It is generally measured in cubic centimeters of an equivalent volume of air or in milliliters (1 cc = 1 ml).

acoustic conductance *np*
The friction of the system, which determines the absorption of acoustic energy; the reciprocal of acoustic resistance.

acoustic coupler *np*
1. A device to join two parts of an acoustic system. 2. A device of specified shape and volume used in the calibration of an earphone.

acoustic crest *np*
1. A thickened section of the lining of the ampulla in the semicircular canals through which the fibers of the vestibular nerve pass to the hair cells. 2. The highest point of a sound wave.

acoustic ear *np colloq*
A device that can perform a simple daily check of the output of an audiometer.

acoustic feedback *np*
A whistling noise created when sound leaks from a loudspeaker or receiver and is reamplified by the microphone.

acoustic field *np*
An area through which sound waves move unimpeded from their source.

acoustic filter *np*
A device used to alter the acoustic response of an auditory signal as it passes through an amplifier or mechanical apparatus.

acoustic gain *np*
The difference in intensity between the input signal and the output signal of an amplification system, e.g., of a hearing aid, given in decibels.

acoustic immittance *np* [Gk *akoustikos* pertaining to hearing; Lat *immitere* to send in, urge on]
A generic term, relating to the ease or difficulty of the passage of sound through an acoustic system, which includes measurements of impedance to (or admittance of) energy flow.

acoustic impedance *np*
A measure of the opposition to the free flow of sound waves through a medium

or acoustic system (the reciprocal of acoustic admittance). It is determined by the frictional resistance, mass, and stiffness of the medium or system and is influenced by frequency. The unit is the acoustic ohm.

acoustic meatus *np* [Gk *akoustikos* pertaining to hearing; Lat *meatus* passage]
The passage between the pinna and the eardrum.

acoustic nerve *np*
One branch of the cranial nerve VIII (the vestibulocochlear nerve) that carries impulses from the inner ear to the brain. The second branch is the vestibular nerve, concerned with balance information.

acoustic neuroma *np* [Gk *akoustikos* pertaining to hearing; Gk *neuron* nerve + Gk *-oma* denoting tumor, swelling]
Also: acoustic neurinoma/neurilemoma; vestibular schwannoma
A benign tumor that grows from the vestibular branch of the eighth nerve, caused by an overgrowth of the Schwann cells of the myelin sheath. It is therefore more correctly known as a vestibular schwannoma, because it arises from the Schwann cells. Unilateral hearing loss is often the first sign of the condition. Bilateral tumors are very rare, but may be associated with neurofibromatosis.

acoustic ohm *np* Named after George Simon Ohm (1787–1854), a German physicist and professor of experimental physics at the University of Munich, who formulated the law now called Ohm's law.
An acoustic ohm (ac ohm) is a unit of acoustic impedance; it is the ratio of average effective sound pressure to volume velocity. The SI unit of measurement is Pa.s/m3. Ohm's acoustic law was proposed in 1843 by Georg Simon Ohm and later elaborated by Hermann von Helmholtz (1821–1894). It states that perception of a sound by the ear is a function of the number and strength of the harmonics.

acoustic phonetics *np* [Gk *akoustikos* pertaining to hearing; Gk *phone* sound]
The branch of linguistics that deals with the nature and production of speech sounds.

acoustic power *np*
The physical intensity of the sound, which is the square root of the pressure generated by a tone.

acoustic radiation(s) *np*
1. Air-conducted sound leaking from a bone conduction vibrator. 2. Nerve fibers from the medial geniculate body that terminate in the transverse temporal gyri of the temporal lobe.

acoustic reactance *np*
Nonresistive opposition to the flow of sound through a surface, usually due to inertia or stiffness, which produces a phase difference between the force and the resulting motion, without the dissipation of energy.

acoustic reflex *np*
Also: cochlear reflex; cochleostapedial reflex
An involuntary activation of one or both of the middle ear muscles (tensor tympani and/or stapedius muscle) to high intensity acoustic stimulation. Also known as cochleostapedial reflex.

acoustic reflex threshold (ART) *np*
The lowest intensity that will produce the acoustic reflex, which is a middle ear measurement of, predominantly, the stapedius muscle contraction to higher intensity sounds.

acoustic resistance *np*
Opposition or impedance to the flow of sound through a medium or surface.

acoustic shock *np*
A clinical entity that may result from exposure to a sudden, intense, and unanticipated sound from a telephone earpiece or headset. Common symptoms are otalgia, impaired hearing, tinnitus, aural fullness, and fear/dislike of loud sounds.

acoustic susceptance *np*
The ease with which sound or current passes through a system. It is a component of acoustic admittance, which is frequency dependent. It is often subdivided into two further components: compliant acoustic susceptance (the ease of sound flow through a system such as an air-filled tube closed at one end) and mass acoustic susceptance (the ease of sound flow through a system such as an air-filled tube open at both ends).

acoustic trauma *np* [Gk *akoustikos* pertaining to hearing; Gk *trauma* wound]
Damage to the hearing mechanism within the ear from a very loud/intense noise. Symptoms include sudden hearing loss, tinnitus, pain, and hyperacusis.

acoustical suprathreshold asymmetry *np*
Auditory deprivation due to asymmetric auditory stimulation, e.g., monaural aiding with a hearing aid. Results in a reduction in speech recognition ability in that ear.

acoustician *n* [Gk *akoustikos* pertaining to hearing]
An expert in acoustics.

acoustics *n* [Gk *akoustikos* pertaining to hearing]
1. The science of sound. 2. The sound-transmitting qualities of a room or area.

acoustics, earmold (earmould) *np*
The influence of an earmold on a hearing aid's frequency response.

acoustopalpebral/acousticopalpebral reflex *np* ăkŭstōpăl'pēbrĭl [Gk *akoustikos* pertaining to hearing + Lat *palpebra* eyelid]
A rapid eye blink caused by a sudden loud sound.

acoustovestibular *adj* [Gk *akoustikos* pertaining to hearing + Lat *vestibulum* entrance hall]
Pertaining to both the vestibular and cochlear organs.

acquired *adj*
Occurring any time after birth.

acrocephalosyndactyly *n* ăkrōsĕfelō-sĭn'dăktilē [Gk *akron* extremity + Gk *kephale* head + Gk *daktulos* finger or toe]
Also: Apert syndrome
An autosomal dominant inherited condition which involves abnormal growth of the fingers, toes, and head. Parts of the skull close too early resulting in an abnormally shaped head. Characteristics may include wide-set and bulging eyes, crowded teeth, protruding jaw, webbed fingers and toes, low-set ears, preauricular pits, and flat conductive hearing loss. Learning difficulty is common.

acrodysostosis *n* ă'krōdĭsŏstōsĭs [Gk *akron* extremity + Gk *dus* bad + Gk *osteon* bone + Gk *osis* denoting a diseased state]
A rare congenital syndrome in which there are bone deformities, especially in the hands, feet, and nose. Characteristics include unusual facial features, short bones, frequent middle ear infections, hearing problems, and learning difficulties.

acrofacial dysostosis *np* [Gk *akron* extremity + Lat *facies* face; Gk *dus* bad + *osteon* bone + Gk *osis* denoting a diseased state]
A syndrome that is characterized by lack of thumbs and ears and facial features that are similar to those in Treacher Collins syndrome.

acromegaly *n* [Gk *akron* extremity + Gk *megas* great]
A chronic metabolic disorder, in which there is too much growth hormone. It is characterized by dysplasia (abnormal growth) of the skeleton, frequently accompanied by conductive hearing loss due to recurrent otitis media.

acrylic *n/adj*
-*n* A clear plastic material derived from acrylic acid. -*adj* Made from acrylic.

acrylic, hard *np*
A durable nonflexible material, widely used for earmolds, that is easy to manufacture, modify, and clean.

acrylic, light cured *np*
Hard or soft acrylic that has been cured by ultraviolet light to improve its nonallergenic properties. Frequently used for earmolds.

acrylic resin, photo sensitive *np*
Also: optical fabrication
A material used in stereo lithographic apparatuses (SLA) printers to make hearing aid shells and earmolds.

acrylic, soft *np*
An earmold material that is moderately flexible when warm (e.g., when positioned in the ear). This can make it more comfortable and give a better acoustic seal than hard acrylic, although it is less durable and may be susceptible to staining by wax and moisture.

actin *n* [Gk *aktis* ray]
A protein required for muscle contraction and cell motility, e.g., actin filaments in the outer hair cells.

action level *np*
The exposure to noise level at which specified actions must be taken by employers to protect workers, in accordance with occupational health legislation.

action potential *np*
The difference in electrical potential between the excited and unexcited state of a nerve, muscle, or sensory cell, e.g., within the inner hair cells of the cochlea. It is generated by voltage-gated ion channels embedded in a cell's plasma membrane and is passed along the nerve as a self-propagating wave of depolarization.

action potential, compound *np*
1. A synchronous change in the electrical potential of a group of several nerve and muscle fibers. 2. The whole nerve potential of cranial nerve VIII which is the main component in wave I of the auditory brainstem response.

active *adj*
1. Infected. 2. Operative, not merely passive.

active ear protection *np*
Hearing protection (e.g., ear muffs) that provides electronic level-dependent sound protection.

active electrode *np*
An electrode placed on the scalp and used, together with a reference (or indifferent) electrode, in testing auditory evoked potentials.

active filter *np*
A filter that uses reactive elements to produce the required characteristics. Active filters can use operational amplifiers, as well as resistors and capacitors and provide precise filtering, e.g., 1. Active filters used in hearing aids. 2. The non-linear response of the basilar membrane which is partially determined by the mechanical action of the outer hair cells.

active transducer *np*
A transducer, a device that converts input energy into output energy that requires external power to operate, e.g., a battery-powered amplifier in a microphone.

acuity *n* [Lat *acuitas* sharpness]
Sharpness, clearness, or keenness of a sense, e.g., hearing.

acuphen *n* [Gk *akousis* hearing + Gk *phainein* to show]
Also: tinnitus; aural murmurs
A sensation of sound in the head or ears without external origin.

acusis *n* [Gk *akousis* hearing]
Normal hearing.

acusticus *adj* ăk'ŭstĭkŭs [Lat *acousticus* (from Gk *akoustikos* pertaining to hearing)]
Acoustic. 1. Nervus acusticus: acoustic nerve; 2. meatus acusticus: acoustic meatus.

acute *adj* [Lat *acutus* sharp]
1. Of rapid onset, short duration, and with severe symptoms. 2. Having a spe-

cific short duration, e.g., less than 21 days in otitis media. 3. Sensitive, e.g., acute hearing. 4. Description of sounds made toward the front of the mouth.

acyclovir *n* ā'sīkləvēe*r*
An antiviral nucleoside that is commonly used against herpes viruses and that may be used to treat sudden deafness. May also be ototoxic.

adaptation *n*
Decrease in sensitivity or output in response to a continuous signal, e.g., auditory adaptation to a continuous sound.

adaptive *adj*
Being capable of changing.

adaptive compression *np*
A compression circuit in a hearing aid using variable release times, i.e., short release times for intense signals of brief duration and longer release times for intense signals of long duration.

adaptive frequency response *np*
A frequency response that alters, e.g., with changes in the input level.

adaptive procedure or test *np*
Method of testing in which the stimulus level is changed in response to the listener's reactions.

adaptive signal processing *np*
Processing that automatically changes the amplified signal of a hearing instrument in differing sound environments to help improve the sound and the wearer's chances of discriminating speech by altering the signal-to-noise ratio and/or other sound characteristics.

addition cured silicone *np*
A silicone material that sets slowly with virtually no shrinkage, used for ear impressions.

adduction *n* [Lat *adductio* a bringing]
1. The action of bringing to or toward. 2. Toward the midline of the body

adenoid *n* [Gk *adenoides* like a gland]
A mass of lymph gland tissue found in the posterior wall of the nasopharynx

forming the pharyngeal tonsils. Part of the Waldeyer ring of lymphoid tissue. The adenoids are small at birth and grow until puberty when they wither away. Enlarged adenoids may block the Eustachian tube and contribute to otitis media (glue ear).
Deriv: -adj adenoidal

adenoidal facies *np* [Gk *adenoides* like a gland; Lat *facies* face or appearance]
The facial appearance of someone with adenoidal problems, e.g., open-mouth breathing.

adenoidectomy *n* ădenoid'ĕktomē [Gk *adenoides* like a gland + Gk *ektome* a cutting out]
Surgical removal of the adenoids.

adenoma *n* ăd'nōmă(ădĭ'nōma) [Gk *aden* a gland + Gk *-oma* denoting tumor, swelling]
A glandular tumor, generally benign, that may grow in the external auditory canal and middle ear.

adenosine triphosphate *np* ădenōsēn'trīfŏsfāt [Gk *aden* a gland]
A neurochemical found mainly in striated muscle tissue that is important as an energy source for biochemical processes in the body.

adhesions *n* [Lat *adhaerere* to adhere]
Areas where two surfaces that would normally be separate become joined together as a consequence of inflammation and/or the development of scar tissue.

adhesive *adj* [Lat *adhaerere* to adhere]
Sticky, tending to adhere.

adhesive otitis media *np* [Lat *adhaerere* to adhere; Gk *ous* ear + Gk *-ites* denoting disease of; Lat *medius* middle]
An inflammation of the middle ear, characterized by a collection of viscous, glue-like fluid.

adipose *adj* ăd*i*'pōs [Lat *adiposus* fatty]
Connective tissue of fat cells.

aditus *n* [Lat *aditus* entrance]
Entrance.

aditus ad antrum *np* [Lat *aditus ad antrum* entrance to the cave]
Entrance to the mastoid cavity from the attic of the middle ear.

admittance *n*
Ease of energy flow through a vibratory system.

admittance, acoustic *np*
A measure of the ease with which sound passes through a medium or an acoustic system (the reciprocal of impedance). This is calculated as the effective volume velocity through a surface divided by the effective sound pressure averaged over the surface.

advanced combination encoder (ACE) *np*
A speech-processing strategy used in certain cochlear implant systems to analyze and convert the acoustic input signal by defining various parameters of stimulation, e.g., the rate of stimulation and which electrodes are to be stimulated, depending on the energy in the input signal.

adventitious *adj* [Lat *advenire* to arrive]
1. Occuring in an unusual place or manner. 2. Occuring accidentally or spontaneously; not hereditary.

aerotitis/aero-otitis *n* [Gk *aer* air + Gk *ous* ear + Gk *–ites* denoting disease of]
Damage to the middle ear caused by pressure changes while flying in a plane.

affective disorder *np* [Fr *affectif* relating to the emotions (from Lat *afficere* to affect)]
A disorder of mood, e.g., depression, that can adversely affect rehabilitation, including aural rehabilitation.

afferent *adj* [Lat *afferens* leading]
Leading from a sense organ, such as the cochlea, to the brain, e.g., an afferent nerve.

affricate *n* [Lat *affricatus* rubbed]
A speech sound consisting of a stop consonant and a fricative in rapid succession e.g., /ch/.

afterhearing/aftersound *n*
The continuing perception of sound after the stimulus has ceased.

age, chronologic (CA) *np*
The actual age or number of years lived.

age, developmental *np*
The age, based on norms of average child development, which reflects the level of an individual's development.

age, educational (EA) *np*
The age, based on norms of average child development, which reflects the level of an individual's educational achievement. Measured using standardized educational tests.

age, gestational *np* [Lat *gestatio* a carrying in the womb]
The age (in weeks) of a fetus, i.e., the time since conception. More usually calculated from the first day of the mother's last menstrual cycle.

age, mental (MA) *np*
The age, based on norms of average child development, which reflects an individual's intellectual capacity.

ageism/agism *n*
Age discrimination.

agenesis *n* aĵĕnĭsĭs [Gk *a-* not + Gk *genesis* generation, creation]
Incomplete or lack of development of an organ.

ageotropic nystagmus *np* aĵēetrŏpĭk nĭ'stăgmus [Gk *a-* not + Gk *ge* earth + Gk *tropikos* turning; Gk *nystagmos* nodding, drowsiness]
Positioning nystagmus in which the fast-phase of the eye movement is directed away from the ground.

ageusia *n* aĵ'yūsēa [Gk *ageusia* lack of taste (from *a-* not) + Gk *geuein* to taste]
Loss or impairment of the sense of taste.

aggregation *n/v* [Lat *aggregare* to cluster]
-*n* A collection or body mass composed of distinct parts or units, e.g., cells. -*v* To form a body mass consisting of distinct parts or units.

aggregation, familial *n*
The presence of a trait in members of a family, where this is more than could be accounted for by chance.

agnosia *n* ăg'nōsha (ăg'nōzēa) [Gk *agnosia* lack of perception (from *a*- not + Gk *gignoskein* to perceive)]
A loss of the ability to recognize people or objects, e.g., in auditory agnosia the disorder results in lack of recognition of speech or other sounds.
Deriv: -adj anosic

agonist *n* [Gk *agonistes* player, competitor in the games]
1. A muscle that is simultaneously controlled by an opposing contraction in another muscle. 2. A drug that stimulates activity at cell receptors that are normally stimulated by naturally occurring substances.

aid *n/v*
–*n* A hearing instrument or prosthesis. –*v* To give help or assistance, e.g., to improve hearing with a hearing instrument or prosthetic device.

air–bone gap *np*
The difference between air conduction and bone conduction readings on an audiogram, symptomatic of conductive hearing loss.

air cells, mastoid *np* [Gk *mastoeides* breast-shaped]
Air cells in the mastoid (part of the temporal bone) that appear highly irregular but that occur in seven well-defined groups: the zygomatic root, periantrum, subdural, sinodural angle, perisinus, tip, and retrofacial. The mastoid air spaces reduce the mass of the bone in the skull.

air conduction *np*
The normal pathway for hearing in which sound is conducted through the outer and middle ear.

air-dielectric microphone *np*
A condenser microphone that uses air as the dielectric (insulator) between the polarized plates.

ala *n* [Lat *ala* wing]
A wing-like process in the body.
Deriv: -adj alar

ala auris *n* 'ahla 'owrĭs *pl* alæ [Lat *ala* wing; Lat *auris* of the ear]
Also: auricle
The pinna.

Albers-Schönberg disease *np* 'älberz 'shernberg Named after Heinrich Ernst Albers-Schönberg (1865–1921), a German radiologist and professor of radiology at the University of Hamburg, who was a pioneer in radiology.
Also: osteopetrosis; chalk bone disease; marble bone disease
A craniofacial and skeletal disorder with brittle but hardened and thickened bones. Characteristics include enlarged head, learning difficulties, visual problems, and moderate progressive conductive or sensorineural hearing loss due to the increased pressure placed on the nerves by the extra bone.

albinism with blue irides *np* [Lat *albus* white; Gk *iris* rainbow]
An autosomal dominant genetic syndrome of hypopigmentation and deafness, characterized by a white forelock; white spots on the arms, legs, and abdomen; blue eyes; and bilateral profound congenital sensorineural deafness.

Albrecht effect *np* 'älbrĕkt Named after Karl Albrecht (1851–1894), a German anatomist, who first observed this phenomenon.
Also: auditory fatigue; tone decay; auditory adaptation
A reduction in the perception of the loudness of a continuous tone.

alerting device *np*
An assistive device intended to alert a hearing impaired person to a noticeable stimulus, e.g., a flashing light or vibration that occurs when an alarm or doorbell rings.

Alexander aplasia *np* [Gk *a-* not + Gk *plasis* formation] Named after Gustav Alexander (1873–1932), an Austrian neuro-otologist and professor of otology at the University of Vienna.
Congenital defective development of the cochlear duct, which mainly affects the basal turn of the cochlea and results in high-frequency hearing loss.

alexia, auditory *np* [Lat wrongly from Gk *a-* not + Gk *lexis* speech, often confused with Lat *legere* to read; Lat *auditorius* pertaining to hearing]
Acquired or developmental reading problems due to an inability to differentiate sounds, caused by neurological injury or disorder.

Alezzandrini syndrome *np* Named after Arturo Alberto Alezzandrini (b 1932), an Argentinian ophthalmologist, who published an article describing the condition in 1964.
Unilateral visual impairment, characterized by unilateral degenerative retinitis that starts in adolescence or early adulthood. It is followed by unilateral facial depigmentation of sections of skin, and bilateral sensorineural deafness may be present.

algorithm *n* [Arabic *-al* + *Kwārizmī* the man of Kwarizm]
A step-by-step procedure for the solution to a problem by a computer; also a step-by-step protocol for reaching clinical decisions.

aliasing *n* ˈālēₐsĭng [Lat *alias* otherwise]
When different signals become indistinguishable, distorted, or produce artifacts. This results when the signal that is reconstructed from samples is different from the original continuous signal, e.g.,

during analog to digital conversion, due to an inadequate sampling.

aliquorrhea *n* ălĭkwōˈrēₐ [Lat *aliquo* somewhere + Gk *rrhea* flowing away]
Also: hypoliquorrhea
Severe headache especially on sitting or standing accompanied by vertigo and tinnitus. Rare condition caused by spontaneous decrease in spinal fluid.

Allan-Herndon syndrome *np* Named after William Allan (1881–1943) and C. Nash Herndon (1916–1998), American geneticists, who reported the syndrome in 1944.
Also: Allan-Herndon-Dudley syndrome
Rare X-linked disorder of brain development causing intellectual and motor disabilities. Characteristic appearance includes elongated face and large ears. Together with hypotonia, patients suffer from restrictions of the movement of certain joints and an impaired ability to communicate. It occurs exclusively in males.

allele *n* ăˈlēl [Gk *allelos* one another]
One of the two forms of a gene (dominant or recessive) that occur at the same place on an autosome that are responsible for an inherited trait.

allergen *n*
Substance capable of producing allergy, e.g., pollen; dust mites.

allergic rhinitis *np* [Gk *rhis* nose + Gk *-ites* denoting disease of]
Inflammation of the nasal mucous membrane due to allergens, e.g., pollen. May cause mild conductive hearing loss if resultant swelling impairs opening of the Eustachian tube.

allogeneic *adj* ăˈlōjₑnēˈĭk (ăˈlōjₑnāˈĭk) [Gk *allos* different + Gk *genesthai* to become]
Derived from two individuals of the same species that are genetically different.

allograft *n* [Gk *allos* different + Gk *graphion* graft]
A tissue graft from a person, live or de-

ceased, who is genetically unrelated to the donor recipient.

alloplastic *n/adj* [Gk *allos* different + Gk *plastos* formed]
-n A nonbiologic material used as an implanted material. *-adj* Pertaining to a nonbiologic material used for implantation.

alpha rhythm *np* [Gk *alpha* (first letter of alphabet); Gk *rhuthmos* flow]
An electroencephalogram (EEG) reading with a frequency of 8 to 13 Hz, generally of high amplitude, i.e., the normal rhythmic activity of the brain when awake and relaxed.

Alport syndrome *np* Named after Arthur Cecil Alport (1880–1959), a South African physician, who first recognized deafness as part of the syndrome.
Also: Dickinson syndrome; deafness nephropathy
An inherited syndrome that is characterized by progressive kidney disease, sensorineural hearing loss, and visual difficulties. Mostly affects males.

Alström syndrome (ALSS) *np* Named after Carl Henry Alström (1907–1993), a Swedish psychiatrist, who first described the syndrome in two interrelated families in Sweden in 1959.
An autosomal recessive disorder caused by a genetic mutation. Characteristics include progressive blindness, nystagmus, sensorineural hearing loss, childhood obesity, and diabetes mellitus.

alternate binaural bithermal caloric test (ABBT) *np*
A common test of vestibular function that involves caloric stimulation of each ear with alternating warm and cool water or air.

alternate binaural loudness balance (ABLB) *np*
A method of assessing the loudness growth of a unilaterally impaired ear by comparing it with the loudness growth of the normal ear.

alternating current *np*
Electric current that regularly reverses its direction of flow.

alternative communication *np*
1. A method of communication that supplements or replaces speech. 2. A manual method of communication.

alternobaric vertigo *np* [Lat *alter* other + Gk *baros* pressure; Lat *vertigo* whirling, dizziness]
Dizziness that may occur during flying or diving when the Eustachian tubes do not ventilate equally.

alveolar *adj* ăl'vē*ol*a [Lat *alveolus* a little channel or hollow]
1. Pertaining to a small cavity or hollow, e.g., air sacs in the lungs; the sockets of the teeth. 2. Formed with the tongue positioned against the alveolar ridge behind the teeth, as in the production of the speech sounds /t/, /d/, and /n/.
Deriv: *-n* alveolus (*pl* alveoli)

alveopalatal *adj* ăl'vē*o*păl*ā*t*al* [Lat *alveolus* a little channel or hollow + Lat *palatum* palate]
Formed with the front of the tongue positioned toward the alveolar ridge behind the teeth, as in the production of the speech sounds "sh" and "j."

Alzheimer disease *np* Named after Alois Alzheimer (1864–1915), a German neurologist, who first studied the disease and published his work on the condition in 1907.
A type of degenerative brain disease leading to dementia characterized by loss of immediate memory and disorientation in time and space. Linked to depleted levels of the neurotransmitter acetylcholine in the brain.

ambient *adj* [Lat *ambiens* going round]
Background or surrounding.

ambient pressure *np*
Atmospheric pressure.

amblyacousia *n* [Gk *amblys* blunt + Gk *akousis* sense of hearing]
Dull hearing, loss of hearing acuity.

amikacin *n* ămĭ'kāsĭn
An ototoxic aminoglycoside antibiotic used to treat bacterial infections. May be used against gentamicin-resistant bacteria.

amimia *n* 'āmĭmēₐ [Gk -*a* without + Gk *mimos* mime or gesture]
Loss of the ability to communicate using gesture or sign due to neurologic injury or disease.

amino acids *np*
Molecules that group together to form proteins.

aminoglycoside (amg) *n*
The mycin group of antibiotics, e.g., gentamycin, tobramycin, amikacin, kanamycin, streptomycin, and neomycin, most of which have known ototoxic properties. Bilateral severe to profound hearing loss is associated with aminoglycoside ototoxicity, which may occur within a few days or weeks after administration.

amorphosynthesis *n* āmawfō'sĭnthēsĭs [Gk *amorphos* shapeless + Gk *sunthesis* a putting together]
Unawareness of one side of body. Inability to integrate hearing, vision, and touch on that side. Most commonly affects the right side of the body. May be a sign of a parietal lobe lesion on the opposite side.

ampclusion *n* [amp from *amplification* + Lat *occludere* to close]
Occlusion experienced when the ear is blocked during hearing aid use or audiometric testing.

ampere *n* Named after André-Marie Ampère (1775–1836), a French mathematician and physicist, who is noted for his work on electromagnetism.
The unit of current, equal to that generated when a one volt potential difference is applied over a resistance of one ohm.

ampicillin *n*
A semisynthetic antibiotic based on penicillin.

amplification *n* [Lat *amplificatio* an enlarging]
1. The action of increasing sound intensity. 2. A hearing instrument or assistive listening device.

amplification, dichotic/split-band *np* [Lat *amplificatio* an enlarging; Gk *dikhos* separate + Gk *ous* ear]
An amplification system in which the right ear receives a high-frequency response in an attempt to fully utilize the right-ear speech-processing advantage, while the left ear receives a flat frequency response.

amplification, group *np*
An amplification device made to be used for more than one listener, e.g., in a classroom.

amplification, linear *np* [Lat *amplificatio* an enlarging; Lat *linea* a line]
Amplification in which the gain remains constant for all input levels up to maximum output.

amplification, nonlinear *np* [Lat *amplificatio* an enlarging; Lat *non* not + Lat *linea* a line]
Amplification in which the gain is not the same with all input levels.

amplification, personal *np*
An amplification device made to be worn by an individual.

amplification, selective *np*
An amplification device providing a restricted frequency response suited to the wearer's hearing loss.

amplification, sound field *np*
An amplification device used to improve the signal-to-noise ratio in a room or area, e.g., a public address system or a classroom soundfield system.

amplifier *n*
A device for increasing the strength of a signal.
Deriv: -v amplify

amplifier class *np*
A division of types of amplifier based on the output stage: A (single-ended), B (push–pull), and D (pulse-width modulated).

amplifier, differential *np*
An amplifier used to reject common electrical activity, e.g., in evoked response audiometry—electrical noise that is common to both electrodes is canceled out.

amplitude *n* [Lat *amplitudo* abundance]
Maximum displacement of a vibratory movement from its mean position to its extreme; the magnitude of an acoustic or electrical signal, measured from a peak to the baseline.

amplitude modulation following response (AMFR) *np* [Lat *amplitudo* abundance]
Also: auditory steady state response; envelope following response
An auditory evoked potential that follows the envelope of the eliciting signal and is an objective measure of frequency specific threshold testing and/temporal processing in the auditory nervous system.

amplitude ratio *np* [Lat *amplificatio* an enlarging; Lat *ratio* a reason or ratio]
1. The ratio of the amplitude of wave V to wave I, in brainstem evoked respose audiometry. 2. The ratio of the amplitude of the summating potential to the action potential, in electrocochleography.

ampulla *n* ăm'pulₐ *pl* ampullae [Lat *ampulla* pot (with a central swelling)]
A swelling at the base of a canal, especially at the base of the semicircular canals where they join the utricle.

ampullofugal *adj* ămpŭlō'fyugₐl [Lat *ampulla* pot (with a central swelling) + Lat *fugare* to flee]

The flow of endolymph and the deflection of kinocilia away from the ampulla and utricle.

ampullopetal *adj* ămpulō'pētal [Lat *ampulla* pot (with a central swelling) + Lat *petere* to make for]
The flow of endolymph and the deflection of kinocilia toward the ampulla and utricle.

amusia *n* ā'myūzēₐ [Gk *-a* without + Gk *mousa* muse]
A congenital or acquired disorder specific to the musical domain, characterized by an inability to recognize and produce musical sounds and to process pitch and rhythm. Musical memory and recognition, and the ability to sing and to tap to music may be affected.

amygdala *n* ă'mĭgdₐlₐ *pl* amygdalae [Gk *amygdale* almond]
An almond-shaped mass of gray matter found in the temporal lobe of the brain. It forms part of the limbic system and is concerned with motivation and the processing and memory of emotional reactions.

amygdaloid *adj* ă'mĭgdₐloid [Gk *amygdale* almond + Gk *eidos* shape]
Almond shaped or tonsil-like.

amyloidosis *n* ămĭloi'dōsĭs [Gk *amulos* starch + Gk *eidos* shape + Gk *-osis* denoting a diseased state]
Also: Muckle-Wells syndrome
Syndrome in which a starch-like substance known as amyloid is deposited in the kidneys and other tissues. Symptoms and signs include a recurrent rash, limb pain, renal failure, and progressive sensorineural deafness. The organ of Corti may be absent and the cochlear nerve atrophied.

anacousia *n* ānₐ'kyūsēₐ [Gk *a-* not + Gk *akousis* sense of hearing]
Also: anakusis
Total lack of hearing.

analgesia *n* [Gk *an-* without + Gk *algos* pain]
Insensibility to pain without loss of consciousness.

analgesic *n/adj*
–*n* A substance producing pain relief, e.g., aspirin and paracetamol. Can be ototoxic.
–*adj* Producing analgesia.

analog (analogue) *n/adj* [Gk *analogos* proportionate]
–*n* 1. An identical pattern. 2. A continuously varying voltage used to represent a continuously varying waveform. *-adj* Identical.
Deriv: -adj analogous

analog-to-digital converter *np*
Device for converting a continuously varying electrical signal to a series of discrete numerical values.

analysis of variance (ANOVA) *np* [Gk *analusis* a solving]
A statistical procedure used to test the hypothesis that the means among two or more groups are equal, where the sampled populations are normally distributed.

analysis time *np*
The period in which the signal is measured or averaged following signal onset.

analytic speechreading *np*
A method of speechreading that emphasizes the recognition of individual speech sounds through the use of vision.

anastomosis *n* ănăsta′mōsĭs [Gk *anastomosis* making a connection between]
Interconnection of adjacent parts, organs, or spaces.

anatomic frequency scale *np* [Gk *anatome* a cutting up]
A modified logarithmic scale that presents audiometric frequencies so that they accord with their spatial distribution along the cochlear duct.

anatomy *n* [Gk *anatome* a cutting up]
Study of the form and structure of the human body.

Anderson-Fabry disease *np* Named after William Anderson (1842–1900), an English surgeon and professor of surgery and anatomy at the Royal College of Surgeons, and Johannes Fabry (1860–1930), a German dermatologist, who both described the condition in 1898.
A group of inherited metabolic disorders caused by a lack or malfunction of lysomal enzyme, needed to break down glycosaminoglycans, a long chain of sugar needed for connective tissue, e.g., bone and cartilage. After a period of normal growth, characteristics develop including abnormal facial features, abnormal bone size and shape, progressive cellular damage, organ dysfunction, and learning difficulty. Abnormal bone size and shape may compress nerves and press on organs, leading to associated disorders, e.g., hearing loss.

anechoic *adj* [Gk *an-* without + Gk *ekho* echo]
Without echo, totally "dead" to sound.

anechoic chamber *np*
A soundproof room built such that there are no reflected sound waves, i.e., sounds within the room are rapidly absorbed.

anemia (anaemia) *n* [Gk *an-* without + Gk *haima* blood]
A deficiency of hemoglobin (present in red blood cells), which may result in pallor, shortness of breath, and lack of energy.

anencephaly *n* ănĕn′sĕfalē [Gk *an* without + Gk *enkephalos* brain]
A congenital disorder in which the cerebral and cerebellar hemispheres of the brain are missing. Frequently accompanied by malformation of the outer, middle, and inner ear, as well as the temporal bones.

aneneia *n* ă′nĕnēa [Modern combination of Gk *eneos* deaf and dumb + Gk *aneos* deaf and dumb]
Lack of or underdeveloped speech due to deafness.

anesthetic (anaesthetic) *n/adj* [Gk *an-* without + Gk *aisthesis* sensation]
-*n* An agent that induces lack of feeling, either locally or generally. -*adj* Without feeling.

aneurysm (aneurism) *n* ănyū'rĭzum [Gk *aneurusma* dilation]
A dilation of a blood vessel that may be a potential site for a hemorrhage.

angiofibroma *n* [Gk *angeion* vessel + Lat *fibra* fiber, entrails + Gk *-oma* denoting tumor, swelling]
An uncommon benign tumor of fibrous tissue in which there are numerous blood vessels. Usually occurs in adolescent males. Typically starts over the nose and can spread locally causing bone damage. Symptoms include repeated nose bleeds, difficulty breathing, and hearing loss.

angioma *n* ănjēō'mă [Gk *angeion* vessel + Gk *-oma* denoting tumor, swelling]
A tumor of blood or lymph cells.

angiotitis *n* ăn'jēōtītĭs [Gk *angeion* vessel + Gk *ous* ear + Gk *-ites* denoting disease of]
Inflammation of the blood vessels in the ear.

angle *n*
The space where two lines or planes meet, a corner, e.g., a vestibular schwannoma may progress into the cerebellopontine angle.

angle of incidence/angle of reflection *np*
The angle formed when an incoming wave or line falls on (is incident to) or reflects from a surface. Measured from an imaginary line perpendicular to the surface. The angle of incidence is equal to the angle of reflection.

angular acceleration *np*
Head rotation; a term used in balance testing.

anion *n* 'ănĭon [Gk *anion* going up]
A negatively charged ion.

ankyloglossia *n* ăngkelō'glŏsēa [Gk *ankulos* twisted + Gk *glossa* a tongue]
Also: colloq tongue tie
The condition in which the movement of the tongue is restricted by a lingual frenulum that is too short. Surgical intervention may be required if it interferes with speech or feeding.

ankylosis *n* ăngke'lōsĭs [Gk *ankulosis* a twisting]
An abnormal fusion of a joint by growth of bony tissue or by shortening of the connecting fibrous tissue, e.g., stapedial ankylosis.

ankylotia *n* ăngke'lōshēa [Gk *ankulos* twisted + Gk *ous* ear]
Also: atresia
Closure of the external auditory canal.

annoyance level *np*
The level at which sound begins to become disturbing or aggravating.

annular *adj* [Lat *annularis* ring-like]
Ring-like.

annular cartilage *np*
Also: annulus tympanicus
The ring of cartilage that holds the eardrum in place.

annular otosclerosis *np*
Calcification of only the annular ligament of the stapes footplate.

annular stapedial ligament *np*
The ring of cartilage holding the stapes footplate in the oval window.

annular (tympanic) ligament *np*
The ring of cartilage holding the eardrum in place.

anode *np* [Gk *anodos* the way up]
The terminal through which electric current flows into a device. In an electrolytic cell this is the positively charged electrode; in a primary cell, it is the negative terminal.

anomaly *n* [Gk *anomolos* irregular]
An irregularity or deviation from normal: in structure or function.

anomia *n* ă'nōmē*a* [Gk *a-* without + Gk *nomos* a name]
Difficulty in recalling words.

anosmia *n* ăn'ŏzmē*a* [Gk *a-* without + Gk *osme* smell]
Loss of sense of smell.

anotia *n* ăn'ōshē*a* [Gk *an-* without + Gk *ous* ear]
Congenital absence of the pinna.

anotus *n* ăn'ōt*u*s [Gk *an-* without + Gk *ous* ear]
A person (or fetus) without external ears.

anoxia *n* ăn'ŏksī*a* [Gk *an-* without + Gk *oxus* sharp]
A condition in which the body tissues receive inadequate oxygen.

antagonist *adj* [Gk *antagonistes* an opponent]
1. One muscle of a pair, i.e., agonist and antagonist. When one contracts, the other relaxes. The antagonist counteracts the movement of the agonist and allows return to the original position. 2. A drug that inhibits the action of another drug or a body chemical.

antenatal *adj* ăn'tēnāt*a*l [Lat *ante* before + Lat *natus* birth]
Occurring before birth.

anterior *adj* [Lat *anterior* in front]
Forward or at the front.

anterior semicircular canal *np*
Also: superior semicircular canal
One of the three semicircular canals; a vertical canal that is parallel to the posterior semicircular canal. Joins the utricle at one end and combines with the posterior semicircular canal at the other before joining the utricle as a common canal. Involved in sensing movement in the vertical plane.

anterograde *adj* [Lat *anterior* in front + Lat *gradus* step]
1. In the forward direction. 2. Toward the axon tip. 3. Affecting time immediately following an event, e.g., anterograde amnesia.

anthracycline *n* ănthra'sīklēn
One of a group of anti-neoplastic antibiotics that is used in cancer chemotherapy. Uncommonly may be ototoxic.

anthropocentricism/anthropocentrism
n ănthr*a*pō'sĕntrĭs*i*zm/sĕntrizm [Gk *anthropos* man + Gk *kentron* center]
The belief that everything centers around man.

anti- *prefix* [Gk *anti* opposite]
1. The opposite, opposing. 2. Serving to prevent, cure, or alleviate a condition or state.

anti-aliasing *adj*
Reducing the distortion that occurs if the frequency of the signal being sampled when converting an analog to digital signal exceeds half the sampling rate.

antibiotic *adj/n* [Gk *anti* opposite + Gk *biotikos* pertaining to life]
-adj Able to destroy or inhibit the growth of microorganisms. *–n* Substance able to destroy or inhibit the growth of microorganisms.

antibody *n*
One of any of the proteins in the body that fights disease. Each antibody reacts to the introduction of a specific antigen.

anticholinergic *n* ăntēkōl*i*'nergĭk
A class of medications that block the neurotransmitter acetylcholine.

antigen *n*
A foreign substance that when introduced into a living body stimulates the production of an antibody.

antihelix/anthelix *n* [Gk *anti* opposite + Gk *helix* spiral]
The ridge on the pinna that mirrors the shape of the helix.

antihistamine *n*
An antiinflammatory drug that inhibits the allergic reaction of histamine in the body. Also used to prevent motion sickness.

antilobium *n* [Gk *anti* opposite + Gk *lobos* lobe, pod]
Also: tragus
A small cartilaginous prominence anterior of the external opening to the ear canal.

antinode *n* [Gk *anti* opposite + Lat *nodus* knot]
A region of maximum amplitude between nodes on a standing wave.

antiphasic *adj* [Gk *anti* opposite + Gk *phasis* appearance]
Pertaining to two similar waveforms, but one inverted in comparison to the other.

antipsychotic drugs *np* [Gk *anti* against + Gk *psukhe* soul or mind]
Medications such as chlozapine, risperidone, and quetiapine, for treatment of the positive symptoms of psychosis, e.g., auditory hallucinations. Side effects may include sedative effects, motor disorders, and agitation.

antisepsis *n* [Gk *anti* against + Gk *sepsis* rotting]
The prevention of infection from microorganisms by inhibiting their growth and multiplication.

antitragicus *n* [Gk *anti* opposite + Gk *tragos* goat]
The small vestigial muscle attached to the antitragus.

antitragus *n* [Gk *anti* opposite + Gk *tragos* goat]
The inferior termination of the antihelix, opposite to the tragus.

Antley-Bixler syndrome *np* Named after R.M. Antley and D. Bixler, who first described the syndrome as "trapezoidocephaly" in 1975.
Also: Bixler syndrome; Harper dwarf; trapezoidocephaly
An autosomal recessive syndrome characterized by bone and cartilage malformations. Signs and symptoms include short stature, delayed psychomotor development, heart murmurs, microtia, cleft lip, hypoplastic pinna, etc.

antrotympanic *adj* ăntrōtǐm'pănǐk [Gk *antron* or Lat *antrum* cave + Gk *tumpanos* drum]
Pertaining to the tympanic or mastoid antrum and the middle ear cavity.

antrotympanitis *n* [Gk *antron* or Lat *antrum* cave + Gk *tumpanos* drum + *-ites* denoting disease of]
Inflammation of the middle ear and mastoid antrum.

antrum *n* [Gk *antron*; Lat *antrum* cave]
A hollow space or a cavity that is not completely closed.

antrum auris *np* [Gk *antron* or Lat *antrum* cave; Lat *auris* of the ear]
The external auditory meatus or canal.

antrum, mastoid/antrum tympanicum *np* [Gk *antron* or Lat *antrum* cave; Gk *mastoeides* breast-shaped]
Also: tympanic antrum
The cavity in the petrous portion of the temporal bone that links the mastoid air cells with the epitympanic recess or upper part of the middle ear.

anvil *n colloq*
Also: incus
The middle bone of the ossicular chain, the incus, which early anatomists thought to be shaped like an anvil.

aperiodic *adj* āpiarǐŏdǐk [Gk *a-* without + Gk *periodos* regularity]
Not occurring regularly; not periodic.

Apert syndrome *np* Named after Eugène Charles Apert (1868–1940), a French pediatrician, who first documented the syndrome in 1906.
Also: acrocephalosyndactyly
A condition that involves abnormal growth of the fingers, toes, and head in which the eyes appear wide-set and bulging, the teeth are crowded, the jaw protrudes, and fingers and toes may be webbed. Flat conductive hearing loss and learning difficulty are common.

aperture *n* [Lat *aperire* to open]
An opening or cleft.

apex *n* [Lat *apex* a peak]
The peak or uppermost extremity.
Deriv: –adj apical

Apgar score *np* Named after Virginia Apgar (1909–1974), an American anestheologist and professor of anesthesiology at Colombia University College of Physicians and Surgeons, who developed this test, which was the first test to assess the health of neonates, in 1952. The letters have been formed into an acronym to summarize the criteria used in the test: Appearance, Pulse, Grimace, Activity, Respiration.
A measure of the physical status of a newborn baby, obtained by adding points for color, heart rate, respiration, muscle tone, and response to stimulation, where 10 is the best possible score.

aphasia *n* ă'fāzēa [Gk *aphasia* speechlessness]
Loss or lack of the ability to comprehend or generate speech usually as a result of brain infection or damage.
Deriv: –adj aphasic

aphemesthesia *n* ăfēmĕs'thēzēa [Gk *a-* not + Gk *phemi* I speak + Gk *aesthesis* perception]
An inability to understand the meaning of words when spoken (word deafness) or written (word blindness).

aphemia *n* ă'fēmēa [Gk *a-* not + Gk *phemi* I speak]
Speech where short, unaccented vowels or initial phonemes are omitted.

aphonia *n* ă'fōnēa [Gk *aphonos* voiceless]
Loss of voice, an inability to speak except in whispers. May be due to disease, injury, or psychological trauma.

aplasia *n* ă'plāzēa [Gk *a-* without + Gk *plasis* formation]
Lack of development of an organ or tissue.

apnea (apnoea) *n* 'ăpnēa (ăpnōa) [Gk *apnous* breathless]
A temporary halt in breathing, e.g., during sleep.

apoplectiform *adj* ăpō'plĕktēfawm [Gk *apoplexia* disablement by stroke + Lat *forma* form]
Having the form of a very sudden and severe attack of vertigo caused by an excess of blood or serum into the brain.

apoplexy *n obs* ăpō'plĕksē [Gk *apoplexia* disablement by stroke]
An excess of blood or serum into the brain; a vascular stroke.

apoptosis *n* ăpŏp'tōsīs [Gk *apoptosis* falling off]
The natural programmed death of a cell.

apraxia *n* ă'prăksēa [Gk *apraxia* inaction]
Inability to execute purposeful movements.

aprosexia *n* āpro'sĕksēa [Gk *a-* without + Gk *prosexia* attention]
An abnormal inability to sustain attention.

aqueduct *n* [Lat *aqua* water + Lat *ducere* to lead]
A small canal.

aqueduct, Fallopian *np* Named after Gabriel Fallopius (1523–1562), an Italian anatomist and professor of anatomy at Padua, who is regarded as the founder of modern anatomy. He introduced the terms "cochlea" and "labyrinth."
A small canal, in the petrous part of the temporal bone, containing the facial nerve. Runs from the internal auditory canal to the stylomastoid foramen.

aqueduct, vestibular *np*
A bony canal linking the vestibule to the cranial cavity.

aqueous *adj* [Lat *aqua* water]
Related to water.

arachnoid *adj* ă'răknoid [Gk *arakhnoides* like a cobweb (from Gk *arakhne* spider)]
Covered with cobweb-like fibers.

arachnoid cyst *np* [Gk *arakhnoides* like a cobweb (from Gk *arakhne* spider); Gk *kustis* bladder]
A collection of arachnoid cells and collagen containing cerebrospinal fluid found

on the surface of the brain; the skull base or on one of the membranes that cover the brain and spinal cord.

arachnoid membrane *np* [Gk *arakhnoides* like a cobweb (from Gk *arakhne* spider); Lat *membrana* a covering]
The middle layer of the meninges.

arcuate fasciculus *np* [Lat *arcuare* to curve; Lat *fasciculus* little bundle]
An area of white matter that connects the Broca area with the Wernicke area. Responsible for intelligible speech.

arcus senilis *np* ˈahkus sĕˈnīlĭs [Lat *arcus* a bow; Lat *senilis* pertaining to an old person]
Deposit of fat that appears as a white ring around the eardrum and is indicative of aging. Occurs also in the cornea of the eye, but both are not necessarily found in the same individual.

area ratio (areal ratio) *np*
The relation between two magnitudes in respect of area; the main way the middle ear overcomes the impedance mismatch between air and the cochlear fluids.

areflexia *n* ārĕˈflĕksēa [Gk *a-* without + Lat *reflexia* bending back]
Lack of reflexes.

armamentarium *n* ahmă̆mĕnˈteɑrēum [Lat *armamentarium* equipment]
The equipment and methods of a medical practitioner.

Armendares syndrome *np* ahmĕnˈdeɑrēs
Named after Salvador Armendares Sagrera (1925–2010), a Spanish-born Mexican geneticist, who reported the condition in 1974.
A congenital syndrome. Characteristics include abnormally small head, cranial asymmetry, small face, short nose, scanty eyebrows, drooping eyelids, retinitis pigmentosa, and ear malformations.

Arnold-Chiari syndrome/malformation *np* Named after Hans Chiari (1851–1916), a professor of obstetrics in Vienna, who described the malformations in 1891. Julius Arnold (1835–1915), a professor of anatomy at the University of Heidelberg, further contributed to the description.
Also: cerebellomedullary malformation syndrome; Chiari malformation
A malformation, most commonly congenital, of the cerebellum and brainstem. May cause symptoms such as muscle weakness, balance problems, head and neck pain, dizziness, hearing loss, and tinnitus.

Arnold nerve *np* Named after Phillip Friedrich Arnold (1803–1890), a professor of anatomy and physiology at the University of Heidelberg, whose primary area of research was the vagus nerve. He first described the auricular branch of this nerve.
Also: Alderman nerve
The auricular branch (also known as the mastoid branch) of the vagus nerve (cranial nerve X) that innervates the external auditory meatus (ear canal). May cause a cough reflex when stimulated, e.g., when inserting an otoblock while taking an impression.

arousal *n*
An increase in activity.

array, microphone *np*
A group of microphones used to achieve improved directionality.

arsacetin *n* ahsăˈsētĭn
An ototoxic arsenic derivative formerly used in the treatment of syphilis and parasitic infections.

arteriole *n* ˈahteɑrēōl [Lat *arteriolus* small artery]
A minute artery.

arteriosclerosis *n* ˈahteɑrēōsklerōsĭs [Gk *arteria* artery + Gk *skleroun* to harden]
A general term for hardening of the arteries. Abnormal thickening and hardening of the walls of the arteries due to deposit of fatty material that calcifies and may eventually block the arteries. Occurs mainly in old age.

artery *n* [Gk *arteria* artery]
A blood vessel carrying blood away from the heart to the various parts of the body.

arthritis *n* [Gk *arthron* a joint + Gk *-ites* denoting disease of]
Inflammation of the joints.

arthroophthalmopathy, hereditary progressive *np* ahthrōŏfthăl'mŏpạthē [Gk *arthron* a joint + Gk *ophthalmos* eye + Gk *patheia* suffering]
Also: Stickler syndrome
A progressive genetic disorder that affects the connective tissues, characterized by flattened facial appearance caused by underdeveloped bones in the middle of the face, eye abnormalities including retinal detachment, joint problems, and progressive hearing loss that is usually conductive. Cleft palate, a large tongue, and small lower jaw are also common.

articulate *v* [Lat *articulare* to divide into joints or parts]
1. To speak distinctly 2. To become united or connected by, or as if by, a joint.
Deriv: -n aticulation

articulation curve *np* [Lat *articulare* to divide into joints or parts]
A graph that shows the percentage of words a listener can identify at increasing loudness levels.

articulation index *np* [Lat *articulare* to divide into joints or parts]
Also: audibility index (AI); speech intelligibility index
A means of quantifying the amount of the speech signal available to the listener depending on the extent of their hearing loss. The speech signal is weighted according to the importance of each frequency band to speech intelligibility.

articulator *n* [Lat *articulare* to divide into joints or parts]
A structure, e.g., tongue, teeth, lips, used to produce speech sounds.

artifact (artefact) *n* [Lat *ars* art or skill + Lat *factum* made]
An artificial product or unwanted signal.

artifact (artefact), blooming *np*
An inaccurate frequency response that occurs when tonal signals fail to activate frequency dependent compression.

artificial *adj* [Lat *ars* art or skill + Lat *factum* made]
Not natural.

artificial ear *np*
Also: acoustic coupler
A device with a microphone and cavity intended to replicate the impedance of the human ear; used for calibrating earphones.

artificial mastoid *np*
A device intended to replicate the mechanical characteristics of the human mastoid; used for calibrating bone vibrators.

arytenoids *n* a'rĭtĕnoids [Gk *arutainoides* funnel-shaped (from Gk *arutaina* funnel)]
Muscle and cartilage in the larynx that control the vocal folds.

ascending method *np*
An audiometric method that determines hearing thresholds, measured by varying the signal from inaudible to audible.

aseptic *adj* [Gk *a-* without + Gk *sepsis* rotting]
Sterile.

aspartate *n* ăs'pahtāt [Gk *asparagos* asparagus (Aspargine was isolated from asparagus. Aspartate can be synthesized from asparagine and a base.)]
A nonessential amino acid that may act as a neurotransmitter in the cochlear nucleus and other parts of the hearing system.

Asperger syndrome *np* ăsper'ger Named after Hans Asperger (1906–1980), an Austrian pediatrician, who described the condition in 1944.
A disorder in which the person has some autistic behaviors, e.g., lack of social

skills, despite having normal intelligence. Characteristics include uncoordinated movement, nonverbal communication deficits, egocentric social inability, repetitive routines, and preoccupation in limited interests, often with a particular aptitude, e.g., memory of facts. May have unusual intolerance to sound.

aspergillus *n* ăsperjˈĭlus
A fungus that can affect the external ear canal. Sometimes also infects the lungs and middle ear.

asphyxia *n* ăsˈfĭksēa [Gk *a*- without + Gk *sphuxis* pulse]
Suffocation.

aspirate *v* ăspĭˈrāt [Lat *aspiratus* breathed]
1. To add breath to a sound. 2. To remove by suction.

aspirin *n*
Also: acetylsalicylic acid
Salicylic acid. A drug that reduces pain and blood clotting. Can be ototoxic, causing a temporary threshold shift and/or tinnitus.

assay *n/v*
-*n* An experiment or analysis. -*v* To measure, test, or analyze.

assimilation *n*
1. The changing of one speech sound by another adjacent to it. 2. The development of a child's ability to understand; a term coined by Jean Piaget (1896–1980, biologist).

assistive listening device (ALD) *np*
Equipment used by persons with hearing loss to overcome specific difficulties caused by being unable to hear, e.g., flashing lights to alert to the ringing of a doorbell, an induction loop system in a classroom, wireless systems for listening to television.

association *n* [Lat *associare* to join]
1. A combination of traits (at least one of genetic origin) in a population. 2. A body of people with a common purpose.

assonance *n* [Lat *assonare* to sound in accompaniment]
The repetition of vowel sounds in two or more words or syllables to create internal rhyming, e.g., you are blue.

astasia *n* asˈtāzēa [Gk *a*- not + Gk *stasis* standing]
A disorder of motor coordination that results in an inability to stand.

asthenia *n* ăsˈthēnēa [Gk *asthenes* weak]
A lack of strength.

astrocytoma *n* astrōˈsītōma [Gk *astron* star + Gk *kutos* vessel + Gk -*oma* denoting tumor, swelling]
A locally invasive tumor occurring in the central nervous system, but most commonly in the cerebral hemispheres. Early symptoms may include headaches on one side.

asymmetrical *adj* āsĭˈmĕtrĭkal [Gk *a*- not + Gk *summetros* equal]
Not symmetrical or balanced; different on each side.

asymmetrical hearing loss *np*
A different degree of hearing loss in each ear.

asymptomatic *adj* [Gk *a*- without + Gk *sumptoma* chance, symptom]
Having no symptoms.

ataxia *n* aˈtăksēa [Gk *a*- without + Gk *taxis* order]
A lack of muscle coordination.

ataxia-hypogonadism syndrome *n* [Gk *a*- without + Gk *taxis* order + Gk *hupo* under + Gk *gone* generation, seed]
Also: Richards-Rundle syndrome
An autosomal recessive syndrome affecting the nervous system and characterized by ataxia, muscle wasting, severe learning difficulties or dementia, and progressive sensorineural hearing loss.

atelectasis *n* ăteˈlĕktasis [Gk *ateles* imperfect + Gk *ektasis* extension]
1. Collapse or imperfect dilation, e.g., collapse of the utricle and ampulla walls. 2. Lack of air in a cavity, e.g., the middle ear.

atelolalia *n* ăt̆elō'lălēa [Gk *ateles* imperfect + Gk *lalia* speech]
Poor speech development due to a central (neurologic) disorder.

atherosclerosis *n* ăther̄ōskle'rŏsĭs [Gk *ather* ear of corn, gruel or porridge + Gk *sklerosis* hardening]
A form of arteriosclerosis with degeneration of the walls of the arteries.

athetosis *n* ăthe'tōsĭs [Gk *athetos* without position + Gk *-osis* denoting a diseased state]
A type of cerebral palsy characterized by continual slow involuntary movements of the extremities.
Deriv: -adj athetoid

Atkin syndrome *np* Named after Joan F. Atkin, who, together with Katherine Flaitz, Shivanand Patil, and Wilbur Smith, American medical specialists, reported the syndrome in 1984.
Also: Atkin-Flaitz-Patil-Smith syndrome
Congenital X-linked syndrome. Characteristics include mild to moderate learning difficulties; abnormally small eyes; cloudy cornea; cleft lip; webbed neck; malformed ears, hands, feet, and heart; and cerebral cysts.

atmosphere *n* [Gk *atmos* vapor + Gk *sphaira* globe]
The gaseous envelope around a celestial body, particularly used to refer to the air around the earth.
Deriv: –adj atmospheric

atonia/atony *n* ā'tōnēa/'ātonē
Without normal muscle tone.

atonic *adj* [Gk *a-* without + Gk *tonos* tension]
Having no accent or stress.

atopic *adj* ā'tŏpĭk [Gk *atopos* out of place, unusual]
Due to an allergic reaction, particularly hypersensitivity without predisposition to any particular type of allergic reaction or in a part of the body not in contact with the allergen.

atopic dermatitis *np* [Gk *atopos* out of place, unusual; Gk *derma* skin + Gk *-ites* denoting disease of]
A chronic eczema characterized by itchy, inflamed skin that in some families is genetically linked with congenital nonprogressive sensorineural hearing loss.

atoxyl *np*
An ototoxic drug used mainly in the treatment of syphilis and parasitic infections.

atresia *n* atrē'zēa [Gk *a-* without + Gk *tresis* perforation]
Abnormal closure or occlusion of a natural passage of the body, e.g., atresia of the external auditory meatus is closure or absence of the ear canal.
Deriv: –adj atretic

atrium *n* ā'trēum *pl* atria, atriums [Lat *atrium* open-roofed central court]
Also: hypotympanum
1. A cavity affording entrance to another structure. 2. The part of the middle ear below the malleus.
Deriv: –adj atrial

atrophy *n* ă'trofē [Gk *a-* without + Gk *trophe* nourishment]
Wasting away of body tissue. Decrease in size of cell, tissue, or organ.
Deriv: –adj atrophic

attack time *np*
The time taken for a compression circuit to respond to an increase in input level.

attention deficit disorder (ADD)/attention deficit hyperactivity disorder (ADHD) *np*
A disorder that includes certain behavioral symptoms, e.g., hyperactivity, distractibility, and impulsiveness.

attenuation *n*
Reduction or weakening, the reduction in intensity of a signal.
Deriv: –v. attenuate

attenuator *n*
Device for reducing signal amplitude in calibrated steps; used in an audiometer

as a means for varying level of signal presentation.

attic *n*
Also: epitympanic recess; epitympanum
The upper part of the middle ear cavity above the eardrum, which contains the head of the malleus and the body of the incus.

atticitis *n* ătĭk'ītĭs
Inflammation of the attic.

atticoantral *adj* ătĭ'kōăntrɐl [attic + Gk *antron* or Lat *antrum* cave]
Relating to the attic and mastoid antrum of the middle ear.

atticoantrotomy *n* ătĭ'kōăn'trŏtōmē [attic + Gk *antron* or Lat *antrum* cave + Gk *-tomia* excision, cutting]
Surgery that exposes the epitympanic recess (attic) and mastoid antrum.

atticotomy *n* ătĭ'kŏtōmē [attic + Gk *-tomia* excision, cutting]
Incision into the tympanic attic.

atypical *adj*
Not usual.

audibility index *np* [Lat *audire* to hear; Lat *index* index finger, pointer]
Also: articulation index; speech intelligibility index
A means of quantifying the amount of the speech signal available to the listener.

audible *adj* [Lat *audire* to hear]
Capable of being heard.

audible frequency range *np*
The range of frequencies that can be heard. In a young person this is from approximately 20 Hz to 20,000 Hz.

audicle *n obs* [Lat *audire* to hear]
Early name for hearing aid.

audile *adj* [Lat *audire* to hear]
Pertaining to hearing.

auding *n* [Lat *audire* to hear]
The process of listening to and understanding spoken language.

audio- *prefix* [Lat *audire* to hear]
Pertaining to hearing.

audioanalgesia *n* [Lat *audire* to hear + Gk *an-* not + Gk *algein* to feel pain]
Giving apparent relief from pain using a sound stimulus, often white noise or music.

audiofrequency *n*
A frequency within the range of human hearing, which is generally accepted to be 20 Hz to 20 kHz.

audiogenic *adj* [Lat *audire* to hear + Gk *–genes* born from]
Caused by intense and/or high frequency sound.

audiogram *n* [Lat *audire* to hear + Gk *gramma* thing written] The first "audeogram" illustrating hearing loss (later termed *hearing level*) relative to normal hearing was presented in 1922 by Harvey Fletcher (1884–1981), an American physicist; R.L. Wegel, an American physicist; and Edmund Prince Fowler (1872–1966), an American otolaryngologist who is best known for his discovery of loudness recruitment. Fowler considered that the audiogram should be used to indicate the percentage of residual hearing and, therefore, placed the "100% of normal" line at the top of the graph. In 1926, Fletcher concluded that a physical scale of sound intensity was a better way to express degree of hearing loss and changed the 100% of normal to become 0 dBHL, causing the audiogram to be "upside down."
Graph showing a person's hearing levels at different frequencies.

audiogram, abruptly/precipitously falling *np*
An audiometric configuration in which the hearing loss is within normal limits in the low frequencies, but then falls dramatically in the mid/high frequencies.

audiogram, corner *np*
An audiogram configuration of profound deafness. Hearing thresholds are only measurable in the low frequencies and these may be vibrotactile rather than true hearing.

audiogram, flat *np*
An audiogram showing hearing threshold levels that do not vary by more than 5-10 dB per octave.

audiograms, serial *np*
A series of audiograms usually obtained at regular intervals, e.g., as part of a hearing conservation program.

audiogram, shadow *np*
A configuration of thresholds in the test ear that mirrors that of the nontest ear. Usually due to lack of masking and crossover from the nontest ear.

audiogram, speech *np*
A graph that shows how an individual's ability to discriminate speech varies with intensity. The audiogram has two axes: The horizontal axis indicates the intensity in decibels and the vertical axis indicates the speech recognition score given as the percentage of correct words or phonemes.

audiogram, trough/U-shaped *np*
Also: cookie bite audiogram; saddle curve
An audiogram configuration in which the mid frequency thresholds are markedly poorer than those in the high and the low frequencies.

audiograph *n* [Lat *audire* to hear + Gk *graphos* writing]
An early term for audiogram.

audiogravic illusion *np*
False localization of a sound resulting from an error in the perception of body position.

audiogyral illusion *np* [Lat *audire* to hear + Gk *guros* a circle]
An error in auditory perception resulting from rapid rotation of the body without visual cues.

audio input *np*
Also: direct input
Connection to a hearing aid or other listening device that allows direct input of an audio signal, e.g., from media players.

audiologic *adj*
Concerned with assessing and managing hearing and balance disorders.
Deriv: audiological

audiologist *n*
A person who identifies, assesses, and manages hearing and/or balance disorders.

audiology *n*
The study of hearing and balance.

audiometer *n* awdē'ŏmet*er* [Lat *audire* to hear + Gk *metron* a measure]
An instrument used in the assessment of hearing sensitivity by either air conduction, bone conduction, or speech.

audiometric *adj* awdēō'mĕtrĭk
Pertaining to audiometry.

audiometric booth *n*
A sound-treated enclosure used when testing hearing.

audiometric configuration *np*
The shape of the audiogram, i.e., flat, trough, etc.

audiometric descriptor *np*
A word or phrase used to describe the hearing levels depicted on a person's audiogram, i.e., the degree, configuration, and type; e.g., a moderate flat conductive hearing loss.

audiometric frequencies *np*
The frequencies tested in pure tone audiometric testing.

audiometric simulator *np*
A computer program used for training purposes that simulates a patient's responses to sound.

audiometric (test) booth *np*
A sound-treated test enclosure designed to reduce levels of ambient noise and promote hearing test accuracy.

audiometric zero *np*
The reference equivalent sound pressure level (RETSPL) used as the average normal air conduction threshold on the audiogram, or the reference equivalent

threshold force level (RETFL) in the case of bone conduction.

audiometrist (audiometrician) *n* awdē'ŏmĕtrĭst (awdēō'metrĭshɑn)
An audiology technician, who may conduct hearing tests and assist with hearing aid fittings and repairs.

audiometry *n* awdē'ŏmĕtrē
A procedure for determining an individual's hearing ability using an audiometer.

audiometry, Békésy *np* awdē'ŏmĕtrē, bākāshē ('bākashē)
Automated audiometry used to assess hearing in which continuous and interrupted tones are presented. The patient presses a signal button when tones are heard and releases the button when no tones are heard. The intensity of the tone decreases as long as the button is depressed and increases when it is released. The audiogram is usually displayed as a zigzag trace.

audiometry, industrial *np*
Audiometric testing undertaken to monitor the effects of high noise levels in a workspace.

audiometry, play *np*
A method of pediatric hearing testing in which the auditory stimuli are paired with an operant task (e.g., dropping a block in a bucket) that requires the active cooperation of the child.

audiometry, pure tone *np*
A procedure using pure tones to establish an individual's hearing threshold levels.

audiometry, screening *np*
The use of quick tests to identify individuals who require further diagnostic testing.

audiometry, speech *np*
A method of assessing an individual's hearing for speech. Lists of spondaic or phonetically balanced (PB) words or sentences are presented at varying intensities. A score is given for correct reproduction of the target words or phonemes.

The resulting scores are often presented on a speech audiogram.

audioprosthetist/audioprosthologist *n*
[Lat *audire* to hear + Gk *prosthesis* an addition]
Also: hearing aid dispenser/hearing aid audiologist
A person who prescribes and dispenses hearing aids.

audioreflexometry *n*
A method of estimating hearing thresholds by observation of involuntary responses to sound.

audiovisual *adj* [Lat *audire* to hear + Lat *videre* to see]
Using auditory and visual information.

audiphone *n obs* [Lat *audire* to hear + Gk *phone* a sound]
An early device for conveying sound to the auditory nerves through the bones in the head.

audition *n*
The faculty of hearing.

auditive *adj*
Auditory. Pertaining to hearing.

auditognosis *n* awdĭtŏg'nōsĭs [Lat *audire* to hear + Gk *gnosis* recognition]
The sense by which sounds are known, understood, and interpreted.

audito-oculogyric reflex *np* [Lat *audire* to hear + Lat *oculus* eye + Gk *guros* a circle]
Rapid turning of the eyes toward a sudden sound source.

auditory *adj* [Lat *auditorius* pertaining to hearing]
Pertaining to hearing.

auditory after-effect *np*
Continuance of hearing when the stimulus has ceased.

auditory area *np*
The primary auditory cortex, i.e., the part of the brain in which auditory information is processed.

auditory boundaries, natural *np*
The sound discrimination ability that is present at birth.

auditory brainstem response (ABR) *np*
An auditory evoked potential that originates between the cochlea and the brainstem. It is extracted from ongoing electrical activity and is recorded via scalp electrodes. ABR can be used in the assessment of hearing thresholds and for site of lesion identification through the analysis of the presence and or absence of a series of waves.

auditory capsule *np*
Also: auditory cartilage
The cartilage in the embryo that becomes the external ear.

auditory cohesion *np*
The act of drawing together and interpreting abstract information that has been heard.

auditory cortex *np* [Lat *auditorius* pertaining to hearing; Lat *cortex* bark of a tree, outer layer]
The part of the temporal lobe of the brain concerned with hearing.

auditory deprivation *np*
A lack of sound stimuli over time.

auditory dyssynchrony *np* [Lat *auditorius* pertaining to hearing; Gk *-dus* bad + Gk *sunkhronia* happening in the right order]
Also: auditory neuropathy
Hearing loss due to a neural disorder.

auditory evoked gamma band field/potentials *np*
Transient neural activity from the cortex, in the high-frequency gamma band (approximately 40 Hz), in response to auditory stimulation. Small waves are superimposed on middle and late latency evoked potentials.

auditory fatigue *np*
Also: Albrecht effect; tone decay; auditory adaptation

A decrease in auditory sensitivity that occurs from constant stimulation by a signal at a level above hearing threshold.

auditory feedback *np*
The hearing of one's own voice, which is important for monitoring vocalizations.

auditory filter *np*
One of a set of band-pass filters or tuning curves used to represent the pattern of vibration on the basilar membrane. The human auditory system consists of a number of overlapping auditory filters or tuning curves, each having a center frequency to which it is normally finely tuned, i.e., it responds only to a small range of frequencies. The auditory filters are less highly tuned to high-frequency sounds. As frequency increases, the bandwidth of the filter increases: The wider the bandwidth, the less finely tuned is the filter.

auditory fusion *np*
A phenomenon, related to temporal processing, which shows whether consecutive sounds are described as one or two events. It may be tested using pure tones presented in pairs with changing intervals between the tones. The auditory fusion threshold is the interval at which the two tones start being heard as one.

auditory hallucinations *np*
Also: paracusia
Sounds heard without auditory stimulus that appear real to the person hearing them that are usually linked with mental or neurologic illness.

auditory late response (ALR) *np*
Also: long latency auditory evoked potential (LLAEP)
An evoked potential originating from the cortex recorded with a vertex negative peak at approximately 90 ms after the signal and a vertex positive peak at approximately 180 ms.

auditory meatus *np* [Lat *auditorius* pertaining to hearing; Lat *meatus* passage]
An auditory canal. 1. The external auditory meatus is the ear canal. 2. The internal auditory meatus is the canal that carries the auditory nerve.

auditory memory *np*
The ability to recall auditory stimuli.

auditory nerve *np*
One branch of the eighth cranial nerve (the vestibulocochlear nerve) that carries impulses from the inner ear to the brain. The second branch is the vestibular nerve, concerned with balance information.

auditory neuropathy *np* [Lat *auditorius* pertaining to hearing; Gk *neuron* nerve + Gk *patheia* suffering]
Also: auditory dyssynchrony
Hearing loss due to a neural disorder.

auditory-oral communication approach *np* [Lat *auditorius* pertaining to hearing + Lat *os* mouth]
A way of teaching deaf children through listening and talking, making full use of the child's residual hearing through appropriate hearing aids or cochlear implants; the approach may be natural or structured.

auditory pathways *np*
1. Specifically, the nerves that carry signals from the cochlea to the auditory cortex. 2. Generally, includes the outer, middle, and inner ear, neural pathways, and the brain.

auditory perception *np*
The ability to perceive sound.

auditory placode *np* [Gk *plax* flat + Gk *-odes* expressing the nature of a thing]
Embryonic cells that develop into the inner ear.

auditory plate *np*
The bony roof of the external ear canal.

auditory point *np*
The lowest point of the notch between the tragus and the rim of the concha.

auditory processing disorder (APD) *np*
Also: King-Kopetzky syndrome; central auditory processing disorder; *obs* obscure auditory dysfunction
An impairment of neural function that does not solely result from a deficit in general attention, language, or other cognitive processes. It may be characterized by difficulty in understanding speech, especially in background noise, and poor recognition, discrimination, separation, grouping, localization, or ordering of nonspeech sounds.

auditory radiations *np*
Also: acoustic radiations
Nerve fibers from the medial geniculate body to the primary auditory cortex.

auditory receptor *np*
Hair cell.

auditory resolution *np*
The ability to distinguish between sounds with different temporal, frequency, and amplitude characteristics.

auditory teeth (of Huschke) *np* Named after Emil Huschke (1797–1858), a German anatomist and professor of anatomy and physiology at the University of Jena, who first used the term "auditory teeth" to describe these projections.
Toothlike projections along the vestibular lip (an overhang from the limbus) of the cochlea.

auditory training unit/device *np*
Also: auditory trainer; audiotherapy device
Any form of equipment specially designed to provide high quality amplified auditory signals to (especially) children with hearing loss.

auditory tube *np*
Also: Eustachian tube
The tube joining the middle ear tympanic cavity to the nasopharynx. Opened during swallowing, it functions to maintain middle ear pressure equal to external atmospheric pressure and to drain the middle ear. If the Eustachian tube is

blocked so that middle ear pressure becomes negative in relation to atmospheric pressure a conductive hearing loss can occur.

aural *adj* [Lat *auris* ear]
Relating to the ear or hearing.
Deriv: –adv aurally

aural reflex *np*
Involuntary response to a sound stimulus.

aural speculum *np*
Funnel used in otoscopy for looking down the ear canal.

auralism *n* [Lat *auris* ear]
System of teaching the deaf using an oral approach.

aural-oral approach *np* [Lat *auris* ear + Lat *os* mouth]
A method of teaching and habilitation based on auditory and speechreading cues and in which signing has no place.

auricle *n* ˈawrĭkəl (ŏrˈĭkəl) [Lat *auricula* external ear, ear lobe]
Also: pinna; ala auris; *colloq* the ear
1. The external part of the ear that projects from the side of the head around the opening of the ear canal. 2. *obs* A kind of ear-trumpet for the deaf.

auricular *adj* [Lat *auricularis* pertaining to the ear]
Pertaining to the ear.

auriform *adj* [Lat *auris* ear + Lat *forma* shape]
Ear-shaped.

aurilave *n* [Lat *auris* ear + Lat *lavare* to wash]
Instrument for cleaning the ear and auditory meatus, consisting of a sponge on a handle.

auripuncture *n* [Lat *auris* ear + Lat *pungere* to puncture]
Surgical opening of the eardrum.

auriscalp *n obs* [Lat *auris* ear + Lat *scalpere* to scratch]
An ear-pick or surgical probe for the ear.

auriscope *n* [Lat *auris* ear + Gk *skopos* observing, observer]
Also: otoscope
An instrument for visual examination of the ear canal and eardrum.

aurist *n obs*
An otologist.

auristics *n*
Treatment of ear diseases.

aurometer *n obs* [Lat *auris* ear + Gk *metron* measure]
Early name for audiometer.

auropalpebral reflex *np* awrōpălpˈēbrəl [Lat *auris* ear + Lat *palpebra* eyelid]
Also: acoustopalpebral reflex; cochleoorbicular reflex; cochleopalpebral reflex; startle reflex
A rapid eye blink caused by sudden loud sound.

auscultation *n* ˈawskŭltˈāshun [Lat *auscultare* to listen]
The act of listening with an ear or stethoscope.

autism *n* [Gk *autos* self]
A disorder characterized by restricted and repetitive behavior and impaired social interaction, in particular self-absorption and an inability to relate to others.
Deriv: –adj autistic

autogenic/autogenous *adj* [Gk *autogenes* self-produced]
Also: functional
Self-generated.

autoimmune deafness *np*
Also: autoimmune inner ear disease (AIED)
Sensorineural hearing loss that occurs when antibodies are directed at the inner ear. Hearing loss may be sudden or progressive and is usually bilateral. Other symptoms may include episodic dizzy light-headedness, tinnitus, and a feeling of pressure in the ear. Autoimmune deafness may be a feature of other autoimmune disease or triggered by trauma or infection.

autoimmunity *n* [Gk *autos* self + Lat *immunis* exempt, immune]
A condition directed against a person's own body tissues.

autologous *adj* aw'tŏlog*u*s [Gk *autos* self + Gk *logos* reason]
Transferred from one's own body, e.g., autologous cartilage grafts used in the middle ear.

automatic *adj* [Gk *automatos* self-acting]
Self-acting.

automatic gain control (AGC) *np*
Also: obs automatic volume control (AVC)
The method by which the volume of hearing aids may be automatically controlled without the need for the wearer to adjust the device.

automatic speech recognition *np*
Recognition of speech by a computer system.

autonomic *adj* [Gk *automatos* self-acting]
Not under voluntary control, e.g., the autonomic nervous system.

autophony *n* aw'tŏfonē [Gk *autos* self + Gk *phone* sound]
Louder than normal perception of one's own voice while speaking, or of other self-generated noises. Sometimes associated with patulous Eustachian tube or semicircular canal dehiscence.
Deriv: –adj autophonic

autosome *n* 'awtosōm [Gk *autos* self + Gk *soma* body]
A chromosome that is not a sex chromosome. There are 23 pairs of chromosomes in a human body cell and 22 of these are autosomes.
Deriv: –adj autosomal

auxiliary aid *np* [Lat *auxiliarius* additional or helping]
Equipment used by persons with hearing loss to overcome specific difficulties caused by being unable to hear, e.g., flashing lights to alert to the ringing of a doorbell, an induction loop system in a classroom, wireless systems for listening to television.

average *adj*
A measure of what is central or typical in a set of scores.

average (long-term) speech spectrum *np*
Also: colloq the speech banana
The intensity range of speech, averaged over a specified time scale, normally expressed in dBHL. It is sometimes drawn on the audiogram.

avulsed *v* [Lat *avellere* to tear away]
Forcibly torn away.

axial *adj* [Lat *axis* axis, pivot]
1. Situated on or along an axis; a direction in human anatomy. 2. Forming an axis or pivot.

axial skeleton *np*
The bones of the head and trunk.

axion *n*
The brain and spinal cord.

axon *n* [Gk *axon* axis, pivot]
The long single filament of a nerve cell that carries the outgoing nerve impulses.

azimuth *n* 'ăzim*u*th [Arabic *as-sumut* the directions, points of the compass]
A horizontal circular direction measured in degrees, e.g., 0° would be directly in front of a listener and 180° would be directly behind.

azithromycin *n*
A macrolide antibiotic that may be used to treat middle ear infections and other bacterial infections. Occasionally ototoxic.

azygos (azygous) *adj* a'zīg*u*s [Gk *azygos* unyoked, not a pair]
Not in a pair.

B

B-weighting scale *np obs*
The filtering network on a sound level meter that corresponds to an equal loudness contour at 70 phons and approximates to loud speech.

babble *n*
1. Competing speech noise consisting of several speakers. 2. Preverbal language that consists of strings of sounds in a consonant-vowel-consonant-vowel (CVCV) structure, e.g., mama, baba.

Babinski reflex/sign *np* Named after Joseph F. Babinski (1857–1932), a French neurologist, who described this reflex in 1896.
Stimulation of the sole of the foot causing extension and fanning of the toes. This is a normal response in infants, but one that should not be present in older children and adults. An abnormal response is a sign of neurologic disorder.

baby talk *np*
Also: motherese
A variation in speech commonly implemented by adults when talking to babies and toddlers that may include differences in intonation as well as shortened and simplified words and sentences.

back end noise *np*
Hearing aid circuit noise from the amplifier or receiver.

back vowel *np*
A vowel sound produced by arching the tongue in the back of the mouth.

background noise *np*
Also: ambient noise
Extraneous noise. Any noise other than the desired signal.

back up *v*
To copy a document or program in case the original is lost or corrupted.
Deriv: –n/-adj backup

backward masking *np*
Masking of a sound signal that appears to happen fractionally before the louder masking sound has been presented, possibly due to some confusion of the signal with the masker.

bacteriocidal *adj* băk'tiarēōsīdal [Gk *bakterion* little rod, cane + Lat *caedo* kill]
Capable of destroying bacteria.

bacteriostatic *adj* [Gk *bakterion* little rod, cane + Gk *statikos* causing to stand]
Capable of inhibiting the growth and reproduction of bacteria, e.g., ear wax is bacteriostatic.

bacterium *n pl* bacteria [Gk *bakterion* little rod, cane]
A primitive microorganism; most are unicellular. Found widely distributed, e.g., in soil, air, and water. The cause of many diseases, sometimes through the production of toxins.

baffle *n*
A device for regulating or diverting the flow of sound waves. Commonly used as a shield to reduce unwanted sound transmission, e.g., from the back of a loudspeaker.

baffle effect *np*
Reduction of low frequency sound by diffraction, caused by a shield formed by the body and/or head.

Bakke horn *np* 'băka Named after Nils Bakke, a Norwegian acoustic engineer, who worked for Erik Hoeyer AS in the 1970s, which was the Norwegian distributor for Danavox who produced and distributed this invention for a number of years.
A horn-shaped plastic tube that is glued directly into an earmold to extend high-frequency sounds. The horn has a diameter of 3 mm at the end opening into the ear, tapering to 2 mm at the tubing end.

balance *n* [Lat *bilanx* having two scale pans]
Maintenance of equilibrium.

balance organs *np* [Lat *bilanx* having two scale pans; Gk *organon* tool, sense organ]
The organs of the inner ear that provide information about head position and acceleration, comprising three semicircular canals (anterior, posterior, and horizontal) and the otolith organ (saccule and utricle) of each inner ear.

Baller-Gerold syndrome *np* Named after two German physicians, F. Baller (b 1883), who described an affected female in 1950, and M. Gerold, who described two affected individuals in 1959.
A syndrome characterized by craniosynostosis (premature fusion of skull bones) as well as abnormalities in the arms and hands. Signs and symptoms include steep forehead, high nasal bridge, misshapen ears, underdeveloped or missing thumbs, and dislocated hip.

band, frequency *np*
A range of frequencies between specified limits.

band-pass filter *np*
A filter that allows only frequencies within a certain range to pass.

band-reject filter *np*
Also: notch filter, band-stop filter, band elimination filter
A filter that stops the passage of a band of frequencies, but allows frequencies to pass in a band both above and below the range of frequencies that have been filtered out.

band spectrum *np* [Lat *spectrum* spectre, apparition]
Graphic representation of sound, displayed as sound-pressure levels in specified frequency bands.

band-stop filter *np*
A filter that stops the passage of a band of frequencies, but allows frequencies to pass in a band both above and below the range of frequencies that have been filtered out.

bandwidth (frequency) *n*
A range of frequencies within a specified band. The width, or the difference between the upper and lower frequency limits, of that band.

bar *n* [Gk *baros* weight]
A unit of pressure equal to 100,000 Newtons per square meter (N/m2). 1 N/m2 = 1 Pascal (Pa).

Bárány box *np* bă'răně Named after Robert Bárány (1876–1936), an Austrian-born physician, who introduced caloric irrigation. He was awarded a Nobel Prize in 1914 for his work on the physiology and pathology of the vestibular system. He was professor of otolaryngology at the University of Uppsala in Sweden from 1926–1936.
A mechanical source of masking noise.

Bárány caloric test *np* [Lat *calor* heat] Named after Robert Bárány (1876–1936). See "Bárány box."
Irrigation of the ear canal with warm and cool water to invoke nystagmus to test vestibular function.

Bárány chair *np* Named after Robert Bárány (1876–1936). See "Bárány box." A rotating chair used in vestibular testing.

Bárány sign *np* Named after Robert Bárány (1876–1936). See "Bárány box." A lack of nystagmus in response to caloric stimulation.

Bárány syndrome *np* Named after Robert Bárány (1876–1936). See "Bárány box."
Also: arachnoiditis pontocerebellaris
A central vestibular disorder caused by inflammation of the arachnoid, the middle of the three membranes covering the brain. Symptoms include rotary vertigo and one-sided headaches at the back of the head, tinnitus, and fluctuating hearing loss on the same side of the head as the headache, and an inability to point a finger accurately.

barbiturate *n*
A drug that depresses the central nervous system and is used as a sedative, anticonvulsant, and anesthetic.

barbula hirci *np* ˈbahbyūla ˈhersē [Lat *barbula hirci* little goat's beard]
Hairs growing at the entrance of the ear canal.

bar chart *np*
A graph consisting of rectangular bars with lengths proportionate to their value.

Bardet-Biedl syndrome (BBS) *np* Named after Georges Louis Bardet (1885–1970), a French physician, who established the syndrome in 1917, and Artur Biedl (1869–1933), a Hungarian pathologist and endocrinologist.
Also: Laurence-Moon-Bardet-Biedl syndrome
A genetic condition that affects many parts of the body. Characteristics include learning difficulty, retinitis pigmentosa, extra digits, obesity, and hearing loss.

Bark scale *n* Named after Heinrich Barkhausen (1881–1956), a German physicist and professor of electrical engineering at Dresden Technical University, who proposed the first scale of subjective loudness in 1916.
A psychoacoustical scale that corresponds to the first 24 critical bands of hearing, where each bark is of equal width and one bark represents the width of one critical band. (The bandwidth of human auditory filters increases and the accuracy of perception decreases with increasing frequency). The scale therefore provides a representation of frequency perception.

barotitis *n* [Gk *baros* weight, pressure + Gk *ous* ear]
Inflammation of the middle ear caused by a sudden pressure change.

barotrauma *n* [Gk *baros* weight, pressure + Gk *trauma* injury, wound]
Injury to the middle ear caused by a change in pressure, e.g., due to diving.

barrel effect *np*
Perception of one's own voice being too loud or echoing when the ear canal is blocked with an earplug, earmold, or custom hearing aid shell.

barylalia *n* [Gk *barus* deep + Gk *lalia* talk]
1. An unusually deep voice. 2. Heavy sounding, indistinct speech that can be a result of a lesion in the central nervous system.

basal *adj* [Gk *basis* base]
Forming the base or lowest level. In the cochlea, the basal end is the part where the high frequencies are coded.

basal cell carcinoma *np* [Gk *basis* base; Gk *karkinos* crab + Gk *-oma* denoting tumor, swelling]
Also: rodent ulcer
The most common type of skin cancer. It grows slowly and rarely spreads to other parts of the body. It is often caused by excessive exposure to sunlight and may occur on the pinna.

basal ganglia *np* [Gk *basis* base; Gk *ganglion* junction of nerves]
A mass of nerve tissues containing cell nuclei.

base form *np*
The original word when all affixes have been removed, usually applied to verbs. Words tend to be used in this form in speech or sign by a deaf person.

base level *np*
A parameter used in cochlear implant mapping that sets the lowest amplitude level for stimulation.

baseline *n*
1. Starting point. 2. The initial audiogram, taken prior to exposure to noise or ototoxic medications, during hearing monitoring procedures. 3. Preintervention measurement of an individual's performance.

basement membrane *np* [Lat *membrana* covering]
The part of the Reissner membrane that separates the mesothelial cells facing the perilymph of the scala vestibuli from the epithelial cells facing the endolymph of the scala media.

basic frequency *np*
The fundamental frequency.

basilar *adj* [Gk *basis* base]
Pertaining to the base.

basilar macula *np* [Gk *basis* base; Lat *macula* spot]
A group of embryonic cells that develop into the basilar membrane.

basilar membrane *np* [Gk *basis* base; Lat *membrana* covering]
The membrane that forms the floor of the scala media and that supports the organ of Corti along the length of the cochlea.

basilar papilla *np* [Gk *basis* base; Lat *papilla* nipple]
The organ of Corti in mammals, and the equivalent sensory structure in non-mammals.

bass *adj/n* bās
–*adj* Low in pitch. -*n* Tones of a low pitch.

bass increase at low levels (BILL) *np*
A type of sound processing that reduces low frequency amplification in response to high intensity input.

battery *n*
1. A collection of different tests. 2. A cell or cells that provide a source of electricity.

battery drain *np*
The amount of current drawn from the battery.

baud *n* bawd Named in 1926 after Jean Maurice Émile Baudot (1845–1903), a French telecommunications pioneer, who developed the first means of digital transmission in 1874.
A unit measure of transmission speed used in computing that corresponds to one information-carrying pulse per second. Originally used to mean one Morse code dot per second.

beam-forming *adj*
Pertaining to a signal processing technique that controls the directionality of the reception or transmission of a signal, thus allowing for a more narrow focus.

beam-forming microphone *np*
An array of directional microphones positioned so they focus on the sound sources at which they are pointed and thus pick up less ambient noise.

Beasley Report *np*
The report of the United States Public Health of 1935–6, which was directed by W.C. Beasley. This established an average normal hearing level that formed the basis of the ASA standards of 1951.

beat *n*
A periodic variation in sound intensity level resulting from the interaction that occurs when two adjacent frequencies are superimposed.

Beckwith-Wiedemann syndrome *np*
'běkwĭth-'vēdəmăn Named after John Bruce Beckwith (b 1933), an American pediatric pathologist, and Hans-Michael Weidemann (1915–2006), a German pediatrician, who both independently reported cases of the syndrome in the mid-1960s.
A congenital syndrome that can include macroglossia (large tongue), gigantism, hemihyperplasia (asymmetrical body overgrowth), umbilical hernia, neonatal hypoglycemia (low blood sugar), transverse linear creases on the ear lobes, and small pits at the back of the ear. Hearing loss is sometimes present. Complications of the syndrome include congestive (an abnormal accumulation of blood) heart failure and an increased risk of certain types of childhood cancer, notably Wilms tumor of the kidney and hepatoblastoma of the liver. The mortality rate is approximately 20%.

beclamide *n*

An anticonvulsant drug, the side effects of which may include dizziness.

Beethoven deafness *np* 'bāthōven
Named after Ludwig van Beethoven (1770–1827), a German composer who continued composing music despite increasing deafness.
Also: Paget disease; osteitis deformans
A skeletal condition in which excessive bone absorption is followed by poor abnormal bone formation, such that new bone is weak and bulky and prone to deformation and fracture. Bones affected can include those of the skull; the condition can lead to tinnitus, vertigo, and sensorineural hearing loss related to loss of bone mineral density in the cochlear capsule. Generally occurs in older Caucasian adults and is more common in males. Cause may be genetic and/or environmental.

behavior (behaviour) *n*

Anything that an organism does involving action and response to stimulation.

behavior (behaviour) modification *np*

The use of operant conditioning (and other behaviorist methods) to change people's behavior. Requires an active response.

behavioral (behavioural) observation audiometry *np*

Hearing tests requiring conditioning to elicit a specific response when an acoustic stimulus is heard.

behind-the-ear hearing aid *np*
Also: postural hearing aid; postauricular hearing aid
A hearing instrument that has all the electronic components housed within a case that sits behind the ear.

Békésy audiometer *np* bākāshē ('bā-kᴀshē) Named after Georg von Békésy (1899–1972), a Hungarian biophysicist, who carried out experimentation on the cochlea. He also developed a patient-operated audiometer in 1946. He was awarded the Nobel Prize in Physiology or Medicine in 1961 for his discoveries concerning the physical mechanism of stimulation within the cochlea.
An automated audiometer, used to assess hearing, which presents continuous and interrupted tones. The patient presses a signal button when tones are heard and releases the button when no tones are heard. The intensity of the tone decreases as long as the button is depressed and increases when it is released. The audiogram is usually displayed as a zigzag trace.

Békésy audiometry *np* Named after Georg von Békésy (1899–1972). See "Békésy audiometer."
Audiometric tests using a Békésy audiometer. The patient records his or her own thresholds on an audiogram using an automated audiometer. Continuous and interrupted tones are presented and the comparison between the two results can be useful in diagnosis as well as providing audiometric thresholds.

Békésy comfortable loudness test *np*
Named after Georg von Békésy (1899–1972). See "Békésy audiometer."
A variation of Békésy audiometry that utilizes tones presented at a comfortable level rather than at threshold.

Békésy tracing types *np* Named after Georg von Békésy (1899–1972). See "Békésy audiometer."
Classification of patterns of audiometric results produced in Békésy audiometry. The patterns are generally classified into five types, which may suggest certain hearing disorders.

Békésy traveling wave *np* Named after Georg von Békésy (1899–1972). See "Békésy audiometer."
A wave that progresses along the basilar membrane and changes amplitude as it moves through the cochlea. The point along the basilar membrane, where the amplitude is greatest, depends on the frequency of the stimulus sound wave.

bel *n* Named after Scottish-born Alexander Graham Bell (1847–1922), most famous for developing the telephone in Boston, Massachusetts, in 1876. There is some debate regarding whether Bell or Elisha Gray was the first to develop the telephone, but Bell was awarded the patent. Bell also invented the audiometer to detect minor hearing problems.

A logarithmic unit indicating the ratio of a physical quantity to some reference value; a unit for expressing ratios in base 10 logarithms. A tenth of a bel (a decibel) is more useful to describe real-world quantities

bell-shaped curve *np*
A graph showing the normal spread of statistical data, which is known as the normal distribution. The graph produced has a bell shape because most scores will fall near to the central point (95% of scores fall within 2 standard deviations of the mean).

Bell palsy *np* Named after Charles Bell (1774–1842), a Scottish surgeon and anatomist, who first described the condition in 1821.
Idiopathic facial nerve palsy, i.e., paralysis of the facial nerve.

belled *adj*
Term used to describe widening of the bore of an earmold at its tip.

belt region *np*
The area surrounding the auditory core of the cerebral cortex.

bending wave *np*
Also: flexural wave
The name for waves propagating in a bar or plate, which are a hybrid of transverse and longitudinal waves.

benign *adj* be'nīn
1. Having no significant effect, no threat to health or life. 2. Not malignant or cancerous and therefore not going to spread to different sites in the body.

benign paroxysmal positional vertigo (BPPV) *np* [Lat *benignus* benign; Gk *paroxunein* exasperate; Lat *vertigo* dizziness] Short episodes of rotary vertigo following a change in head position.

benorylate *n*
A drug derived from paracetamol, which may have tinnitus as a side effect.

benzodiazepine *n*
A psychoactive tranquilizer, used as a sedative, e.g., valium, ativan, diazepam. The side effects may include hearing loss, hyperacusis, and tinnitus.

Berger prescriptive formula *np* 'berjer Named after Kenneth W. Berger (1924–1994), Director of Audiology at Kent State University, Ohio. He is best known for the development of a hearing aid prescription method (1976) based on the premise that sounds should be amplified to average speech spectrum levels.
A hearing aid prescription method developed from the "half-gain rule" providing targets for gain and output at each frequency.

beta rhythm/waves *np* 'bīta [Gk *beta* (second letter of alphabet); Gk *rhuthmos* flow]
Electrical activity, with a frequency range 12–30 Hz, found within many parts of the nervous system including the cortex of the brain and associated with attention, perception, and cognition.

bethanidine *n*
A drug used to treat hypertension.

Bezold abscess *np* Named after Friedrich Bezold (1842–1908), a German otologist, who is best known for developing tuning fork tests and for providing an understanding of mastoiditis.
A collection of pus that occurs deep in the neck and which suppurates into the mastoid cells.

Bezold mastoiditis *np* bātsŏlt Named after Friedrich Bezold (1842–1908). See "Bezold abscess."
A form of mastoiditis in which pus has escaped into the neck, causing a deep neck abscess.

Bezold triad *np* Named after Friedrich Bezold (1842–1908). See "Bezold abscess." Three characteristics, i.e., low-frequency hearing loss, conductive hearing loss, and a negative Rinne test result, which may suggest otosclerosis.

bi- *prefix* bī- [Lat prefix *bi-* double]
Two or double.

biauricular *adj* bīawˈrĭkyūlah [Lat prefix *bi-* double + Lat *auris* ear]
Also: binaural; binotic
Pertaining to both ears.

bias *n*
A prejudice.

biased sampling *np*
The overrepresentation of a participant category in a study, such that the sample is not representative of the population.

bibliography *n* [Gk *biblion* book + Gk *graphe* writing]
A list of books used by the author when writing a book but are not specifically mentioned in the text.

bifid *adj* bīfĭd [Lat prefix *bi-* double + *findere* to split]
Divided into two parts.

bifurcate *adj/v* [Lat *bifurcare* to fork]
-adj Forked or split into two parts. *-v* To split into two parts.

bilabial *adj* [Lat prefix *bi-* double + Lat *labia* lips]
Formed with both lips placed together, as in the production of the speech sounds /p/, /b/, and /m/.

bilateral *adj* [Lat prefix *bi-* double + Lat *latera* sides]
Relating to both sides.

bilateral contralateral routing of signals (BiCROS) *np*
A hearing aid system for an asymmetric hearing loss, with a microphone at each ear feeding into one amplifier and receiver positioned on the better ear.

bilingual *adj* [Lat prefix *bi-* double + *lingua* language, tongue]

Using two languages fluently, e.g., spoken English and British sign language (BSL).

bilirubin *n* bĭlēˈrūbĭn [Lat *bilis* bile + Lat *ruber* red]
One of the products of the natural breakdown of red blood cells, with distinctive yellow color. Bilirubin is formed from the breakdown of red blood cells and is secreted in the bile and excreted in feces. Large amounts of bilirubin in the blood can cause jaundice.

bilirubinemia (bilirubinaemia) *n* bĭlēˈrū-bĭnēmēa [Lat *bilis* bile + Lat *ruber* red + Gk *haima* blood]
The presence of bilirubin in the blood. Bilirubin is normally removed from the blood by the liver. Jaundice occurs when there is too much bilirubin in the blood (hyperbilirubinemia). In a neonate the brain barrier is not fully developed and excessive bilirubin can cause neurological damage (kernicterus).

bimastoid *adj* [Lat prefix *bi-* double + Gk *mastos* breast + Gk *–oides* in the shape of]
Pertaining to both mastoids.

bimodal *adj* [Lat prefix *bi-* double + Lat *modus* type]
1. The use of a hearing aid on one ear and a cochlear implant on the other to provide binaural hearing. 2. In statistics, a type of frequency distribution where there are two most frequent values of a set of data.

binary *adj* [Lat *binarius* two together]
Composed of two elements, items, or terms, e.g., the two digits (conventionally zero or one) in a binary system such as used in computing.

binaural *adj* bĭˈnoral [Lat prefix *bi-* double + Lat *auris* ear]
Also: biauricular; binotic
Using both ears.

binaural advantage *np*
The advantage of using both ears rather than only one. Includes improved hearing thresholds (by about 3 dB), the ability to

localize sound, and improve listening in situations of background noise.

binaural beats *np* [Lat *binarius* two together]
Pulsations in perceived loudness when two tones of slightly different frequencies are played one into each ear.

binaural fusion *np*
Also: binaural integration; binaural re-synthesis
Integration of separate sounds introduced to left and right ears so they are heard as a single sound.

binaural hearing aids *np*
A system in which each ear is independently aided.

binaural separation *np*
Also: binaural integration; binaural re-synthesis
The ability to perceive sound in one ear while ignoring (different) sound in the other.

binaural squelch *np*
The improvement of hearing performance in noise when two ears are used rather than one. The effective improvement in the signal compared to the background noise is due to the differences in the sound reaching each ear, i.e., differences in the sound level and time of arrival.

binaural summation *np* [Lat prefix *bi-* double + Lat *auris* ear; Lat *summatio* an adding up]
The enhancement of hearing that occurs when listening with both ears, i.e., approximately 3 dB–6 dB increase in loudness in comparison with monaural listening.

Bing test *np* Named after Albert Bing (1844–1922), a German otologist, who was the first to report the use of this test in the diagnosis of hearing disorders in 1891.
Also: occlusion test
A monaural tuning fork test in which the individual is asked to compare the loudness of a tuning fork applied to the mastoid, when the canal on that side is first open and then occluded.

binotic *adj* bīn'ŏtĭk [Lat prefix *bi-* double + Gk *ota* ears]
Also: biauricular; binaural
Using both ears.

bio- *prefix* [Gk *bios* life]
Living.

bioacoustics *n* [Gk *bios* life + Gk *akousia* hearing]
Science of the effect of sound on living things.

biocompatible *adj* [Gk *bios* life]
Acceptable to the body; not rejected.

biofeedback *n* [Gk *bios* life]
A training technique for people to control alterations in certain body processes that normally happen involuntarily, such as heart rate, blood pressure, muscle tension, and skin temperature.

biofilm *n* [Gk *bios* life]
A colony of antibiotic resistant bacteria, formed when bacteria attach to surfaces and to each other to form a protective matrix. These may be found on the middle ear tissue of children who suffer from chronic ear infections and may also cause infection after cochlear implantation.

biologic *adj* [Gk *bios* life + Gk *-logia* study of]
Belonging to biology.

biologic calibration *np*
Audiometric threshold based on normal average hearing for a particular acoustic stimulus.

biologic check *np*
A listening check, e.g., of an audiometer.

biopsy *n* [Gk *bios* life + Gk *opsis* sight]
Removal of living body tissue for the purpose of diagnosis.

biphasic *adj* [Lat prefix *bi-* double + Gk *phasis* appearance]
Having two phases, as in a time-limited event with a negative and a positive part.

bipolar *adj* [Lat *bipolaris* with two poles]
Having two poles. 1. An electrode pair that measures action potentials at two

separate points. 2. A mood disorder with episodes of depression and elation.

bisensory *adj*
Combining two senses, e.g., visual and auditory.

bisyllabic *adj* [Lat prefix *bi-* double + Gk *sullabe* (from Gk *sun-* together + Gk *lamba-nein* to take)]
Having two syllables.

bit *n*
A unit of computer information reflecting the result of a choice between two alternative states, e.g., on or off.

bite block *np*
Also: colloq mouth prop
A solid structure, placed between the teeth, used to hold the jaw open.

bithermal *adj* [Lat prefix *bi-* double + Gk *thermos* hot]
Pertaining to heat and cold.

bithermal caloric stimulation *np* [Lat prefix *bi-* double + Gk *thermos* hot; Lat *cal-or* heat]
Irrigation of the ear canal with warm and cool water or air to test vestibular function.

Bixler syndrome *np* Named after David Bixler (b 1940), who first described the syndrome in 1975.
Also: Antley-Bixler syndrome; Harper dwarf; trapezoidocephaly
An autosomal recessive syndrome characterized by bone and cartilage malformations. Signs and symptoms include short stature, delayed psychomotor development, heart murmurs, microtia, cleft lip, hypoplastic pinnae, etc.

Björnstad-Crandall syndrome *np* Named after Roar T. Björnstad (1908–2002), who first reported the syndrome in 1965, and Barbara F. Crandall (b 1927), who reported a similar syndrome in three brothers in 1973.
Deafness due to irregular twisting of the hair cells. Two similar syndromes: Björnstad syndrome includes alopecia and hearing loss; Crandall syndrome includes hypogonadism (lack of sex development).

Blainville ears *np* Named after Henri Ducrotay de Blainville (1777–1850), a French zoologist and anthropologist.
Asymmetrical pinnae—of different size or shape.

blast- *prefix* [Gk *blastos* germ, sprout]
An immature primitive cell.

bleb *n*
1. A blister or small swelling. 2. A bubble of air.

blend *n*
1. A combination. 2. In speech, a consonant cluster.

blind experiment *np*
An experiment in which certain information is deliberately withheld from the subject to avoid bias.

Bliss symbols/blissymbols *np/n* Named after Charles K. Bliss (1897–1985), who was born Karl Kasiel Blitz, a Jewish Austro-Hungarian engineer who emigrated to Australia in 1946. He had intended it as a system of writing in pictures that could be universally understood and called it" Semantography." However, it was never used in this way.
A communication system that consists of more than 2000 graphic symbols that is used by physically and communicatively impaired persons.

block *v/n*
-v To obstruct, arrest, or interrupt, as in arresting the passage of a nerve impulse. *-n* A solid obstruction, e.g., an otoblock that is used to block the ear canal to stop the passage of impressions beyond the block.

blood–brain barrier *np*
The semipermeable barrier that prevents some substances from leaving the blood and crossing capillary walls into the brain.

blood pressure *np*
The pressure of blood against the walls of the main arteries. Measured in millimeters of mercury. Normal average blood pressure for a young adult is approximately 120/80, where 120 is the systolic pressure, when the ventricles contract, and 80 is the diastolic pressure, when the ventricles relax.

blooming effect *np*
An artifact that occurs when a compression hearing aid is tested using a pure tone signal rather than a broadband signal. Appears as an increased low-frequency response because frequency-dependent compression has not been activated by the pure tones.

blue eardrum *np*
A variant of otitis media with effusion in which the fluid is bluish in color due to bleeding.

bluetooth *n/adj* Bluetooth was developed in 1994 by the Swedish company Ericsson to unify wireless connectivity. The process was named after King Harald of Denmark (910–986) who was nicknamed "Bluetooth" (probably because of a filed and pigmented tooth decoration). King Harald united Denmark and part of Norway into one kingdom.
-n Short-range wireless connectivity. *-adj* With short-range wireless connectivity.

bobbing oscillopsia *np* ŏsĭlŏpsī̆a [Lat *oscallare* to swing + Gk *opsis* vision]
Also: Dandy syndrome
Involuntary eye movements that cause objects to appear to bounce about. May be caused by streptomycin or gentamycin toxicity. Characteristic of bilateral vestibular damage.

body baffle *np*
A marked increase in low-frequency amplification caused when the microphone of a hearing aid is positioned on the body rather than at or in the ear, or behind the pinna.

body language *np*
Nonverbal communication, e.g., gesture, facial expression, and body posture.

body-worn hearing aid *np*
Also: pocket aid
A hearing aid in which the microphone and amplifier are housed in a case, usually worn on the chest, connected by a cord to the receiver and earmold.

boilermaker's deafness *np obs*
Noise-induced hearing loss.

Bondy's procedure *np* Named after Gustav Bondy (1870–1954), a German otologist who developed the procedure.
A variation of the modified radical mastoidectomy procedure that used a perforation in the pars flaccida (the upper portion of the ear drum) to avoid entering the middle ear space to preserve hearing. It may also be carried out through an incision behind the pinna. The procedure may be used to remove large attic cholesteatomas where the middle ear is not diseased.

bone *n*
Strong hard connective tissue that forms the skeleton.

bone-air gap *np*
The difference between air conduction and bone conduction readings on an audiogram symptomatic of conductive hearing loss. More commonly referred to as air-bone gap.

bone-anchored hearing aid (BAHA) *np*
A hearing aid with a bone conduction transducer that is attached directly to the bone of the skull.

bone, compact *np*
Hard bone that forms the exterior of bones and that supports and protects the body.

bone conduction *np* [Lat *conducere* to lead]
Transmission of sound through bones, generally of the skull.

bone-conduction thresholds *np*
Hearing thresholds established during pure-tone audiometric assessment using signals transmitted through the bones of the skull to the cochlea. Comparison with air conduction thresholds can identify an air-bone gap, which indicates a conductive hearing loss.

bone conductor *np*
Also: bone vibrator
The transducer used during pure-tone audiometry to produce audible stimuli by vibration of the bones of the skull.

bone, flat *np*
Thin and broad bones, e.g., the cranial bones of the skull and the ribs.

bone, irregular *np*
Bone that does not fit into any other category, e.g., some bones of the skull.

bone, long *np*
Bones that are thick and longer than they are wide, e.g., the bones of the upper arms or forearms.

bone, petrous *np* ˈpĕtrʊs [Gk *petros* stone]
A dense stone-like part of the temporal bone, of pyramidal shape, that contributes to the base of the skull and contains the middle and inner ear.

bone, sesamoid *np* [Gk *sesame* + Gk suffix *-oid* in the shape of (i.e., in the shape of a sesame seed)]
Bone embedded within a tendon, e.g., the kneecap (patella).

bone, short *np*
Bones with no significant difference in length or width, but thicker than flat bones, e.g., the bones of the wrists.

bone, spongy *np*
Bone composed of a network of branching bony spicules that has the appearance of a sponge, with bone marrow contained in the spaces. Spongy bone is normally found in the ends of the long bones and in the vertebrae. In otosclerosis, spongy bone forms around the footplate of the stapes.

bone vibrator *np* [Lat *vibrare* to shake]
Also: bone conductor
The transducer used during pure-tone audiometry to produce audible stimuli by vibration of the bones of the skull.

bonelet *n*
A small bone.

bony labyrinth *np* [Gk *laburinthos* maze]
Also: osseous labyrinth
The cavity in the temporal bone that forms the cochlea and semicircular canals.

boom microphone *np* [Gk *mikros* small + Gk *phone* sound]
A microphone fixed to a pole to reach some distance away.

boot *n*
Also: shoe
A coupling device used with some behind the ear hearing aids, e.g., for direct audio input.

border cells *np*
Columnar supporting cells, i.e., cells that support the inner hair cells, on the medial portion of the basilar membrane.

bore *n*
The long, cylindrical hollow part of a tube or similar apparatus, e.g., earmold bore.

bore, earmold (earmould) *np*
The hole within an earmold through which the amplified signal is delivered to the ear canal.

Böttcher, cells of *np* ˈbertcher Named after Jakob Ernst Arthur Böttcher (1831–1889), a German pathologist, who is known for his study of the organ of Corti.
Supporting cells that lie on the high frequency area of the basilar membrane below the cells of Claudius.

bottom-up process *np*
A perceptual process driven by the raw data or sensory input in contrast to a top-down process which would be driven by knowledge, experience, etc.

bound morpheme *np* [Fr *morphème* (from Gk *morphe* form)]
A prefix or suffix that cannot stand on its own, e.g., "bi-."

brace *v*
To give firmness and support to improve safety, e.g., the procedure for taking an ear impression involves bracing against the face to protect the ear from injury if the individual should move unexpectedly.
Deriv: -adj bracing

brachium *n* ˈbrākēum *pl* brachia [Lat *brac(c)hium* arm]
1. A bundle of fibers. 2. The upper arm.

brachium of inferior colliculus *np* [Lat *brac(c)hium* arm; Lat *colliculus* little hill]
The bundle of fibers leading to the medial geniculate body.

brachy- *prefix* ˈbrăkē [Gk *brakhus* short]
Short.

bracketing *adj*
A method of finding a change point by alternately increasing and decreasing the value of a stimulus.

brady- *prefix* ˈbrădē [Gk *bradus* slow]
Slow.

bradyacusia *n* brădēakyūsĭs [Gk *bradus* slow + Gk *akousis* sense of hearing]
Dull hearing.

bradykinesia *n* brădēkĭnēsēa [Gk *bradus* slow + Gk *kinesis* movement]
A slowness in carrying out purposeful movements, e.g., as can occur in Parkinson disease.

bradylalia *n* brădēlālēa [Gk *bradus* slow + Gk *lalia* talk]
Abnormally slow speech.

brainstem *n*
The central portion of the brain that consists of the midbrain, pons, and medulla (oblongata). It connects the midbrain and cerebral hemispheres with the spinal cord.

brainstem evoked response audiometry (BSER, BERA) *np*
Hearing assessment to measure neural activity up to and including the level of the brainstem in response to clicks or tone bursts.

brainstem implant *np*
An auditory prosthesis in which electrodes are implanted in the cochlear nucleus of the brainstem.

branchial *adj* ˈbrăngkēul [Gk *brankhia* gills]
Related to gills.

branchial arches *np*
1. The curved bony or cartilaginous rings that support the gills of a fish. 2. Six (usually) embryonic arches that, in higher vertebrates, develop into specialized structures in the head and neck, including the outer and middle ear structures.

branchio-oto-renal (BOR) syndrome *np* [Gk *brankhia* gills + Gk *ous* ear + Lat *renes* kidneys]
An autosomal dominant syndrome that includes underdeveloped or absent kidneys and resultant renal failure. Ear abnormalities may include malformations of the outer and middle ear and deafness that may be conductive, sensorineural, or mixed.

branchio-oto-ureteral syndrome *np* [Gk *brankhia* gills + Gk *ous* ear + Gk *oureter* urinary duct]
A variable expression of the BOR syndrome that includes severe sensorineural hearing loss with the presence of preauricular tags or pits and duplication of ureters or bifid renal pelvis, i.e., the renal pelvis is divided into two.

breakthrough *n*
Also: 1. cross-talk
1. An unwanted signal appearing from another part of the circuit, e.g., breakthrough from the interrupter circuit in an audiometer can lead to audible background noise from the transducer. 2. A significant advance.

brevicollis n brĕvĭkŏlĭs [Lat *brevis* short + Lat *collis* neck]
Also: Klippel-Feil syndrome
A disorder characterized mainly by fusion of the upper cervical spine. Characteristics may include short neck, low hairline, decreased range of motion, and bilateral sensorineural hearing loss.

bridge n
1. An electrical instrument for measuring resistance, capacitance, inductance, or impedance. 2. The part of an earmold that extends from the canal to the helix.

bridge circuit np
An electrical circuit in which two circuit branches are bridged by a third branch.

brief tone np
Also: tone pip
A sinusoidal signal of less than 200 ms duration.

Bright syndrome np Named after Richard Bright (1789–1858), an English physician, sometimes known as the Father of Nephrology. He was the Physician Extraordinary to Queen Victoria and a pioneer of kidney disease research.
Also: nephritis
Inflammation of the kidneys sometimes accompanied by sensorineural hearing loss. Prevalent in males, mostly under 10 years of age.

broadband noise np
Noise that has equal distribution across the frequency range.

Broca area np Named after Pierre Paul Broca (1824–1880), a French neurologist, who demonstrated that the left frontal lobe of the brain controlled speech.
An area in the left cerebral hemisphere; Brodmann areas 44 and 45. Damage in this area can cause communication difficulties known as Broca aphasia.

Brodmann areas np Named after Korbinian Brodmann (1868–1918), who studied the cortex of mammals.

Regions of the cerebral hemispheres of the brain that are identified by numbering based on their function and anatomic place.

bronchus n pl bronchi [Gk *bronkhos* windpipe]
One of two tubes that branch off from the trachea and lead to the lungs.
Deriv: –adj bronchial

Brown-Vialetto-Van Laere syndrome (BVVL) np Named after Charles H. Brown, an American physician who first documented the syndrome in 1894. Further accounts have been made since, which have led to additions to the syndrome name.
Also: Brown syndrome; pontobulbar palsy
A rare genetic type of muscular dystrophy, in which there is progressive sensorineural deafness accompanied by or followed by paralysis of a number of cranial nerves. Occurs mostly in females. Characteristics include progressive deafness, clumsiness, weakness of the arms, shaking, slurred speech, and swallowing and respiratory difficulties.

bruit n brūt [Old Fr *bruit* noise (from *bruire* to roar)]
An abnormal swishing or blowing noise that can be heard with a stethoscope, often due to turbulent blood flow past an obstruction.

brux v bruks [Gk *brukhein* to grind the teeth]
To grind one's teeth.

buccal cavity np ˈbŭkʉl [Lat *bucca* cheek, mouth]
The mouth.

buclizine n byūklĭzēn
An antihistamine with antiemetic and sedative properties, which is sometimes used in the management of vertigo.

buffer n
An area of computer memory that temporarily holds a digital signal.

bulla *n* ˈbŭlɑ *pl* bullae [Lat *bulla* bubble, blister]
Blister. Containing serous fluid.
Deriv: –adj bullous

bulla ossea *np* ŏsēɑ [Lat *bulla* bubble, bliste; Lat *osseus* bony]
An enlarged part of the bony section of the external auditory meatus.

bumetanide *n* byūmĕtɑnīd
An ototoxic diuretic.

bundle *n*
A group of muscle or nerve fibers that run in the same direction.

bundle of Rasmussen *np* ˈrăsmŭsen
Named after Grant Litster Rasmussen (1904–1989), an American anatomist, who discovered the olivocochlear system in 1946.
Also: olivocochlear bundle
A group of efferent nerve fibers that exit the brainstem on the vestibular nerve and joins the cochlear nerve in the inner ear and terminates on outer hair cells.

bursa *n* [Lat *bursa* bag, purse]
A fluid-filled sac.

burst *n*
A sudden, more intense peak of energy. In acoustic phonetics this occurs when a plosive sound is released.

butacaine *n* ˈbyūtɑkān
A local anesthetic that is sometimes used in ear, nose, and throat surgery.

button *adj*
Small and round, e.g., a button battery cell.

byte *n*
A unit used to describe digital data; eight bits equal one byte.

C

C-weighting *n*
The flattest, broadest weighting scale scale (dBC, dB'C' or dB(C)). It has essentially equal sensitivity at all frequencies from 10Hz to 20,000 Hz. It has a standardized frequency response based on the 100 phon equal loudness curve. It is often used to measure peak noise and noise above 100 dB.

café au lait spots *n* kăfā-ō-'lā
Spots on the skin associated with neurofibromas.

caffeine *n*
An alkaloid drug found in coffee and tea that has a stimulant effect on the nervous system.

Cagot ear *np* ˈkăgō (ˈkăgō) Named after the Cagots, an outcast race found in the Pyrenees, one of whose genetic features was a lack of ear lobes.
Also: Aztec ear
An ear that has no lobe.

caisson syndrome *np* ˈkāson
Also: colloq the bends
Occurs in divers and workers in diving bells or caissons, when they are not slowly decompressed back to atmospheric pressure. Bubbles of nitrogen are released into the blood and migrate to different tissues. Symptoms include headache, nausea, vertigo, nystagmus, hearing loss, and tinnitus.

calcification *n* [Lat *calx* pebble, limestone + Lat *facere* to make]
Calcium salts deposited in the tissues.

calcium (Ca) *n* [Lat *calx* pebble, limestone]
A common white metallic mineral that is an important component of bones.

calcium carbonate (CaCO$_3$) *np*
A mineral compound that occurs naturally as chalk, limestone, and marble.

calibrate *v* [Ital *calibro* mold]
To adjust the performance of an instrument to established specifications.
Deriv: -n calibration

calibration, biologic *np*
Calibration based on average normal values for a particular signal.

calibration tone *np*
The 1 kHz tone used to ensure an accurate output level of speech stimuli on an audiometer.

caloric *adj* [Lat *calor* heat]
Pertaining to heat.

caloric inversion *np*
Caloric stimulation that has the opposite effect of normal.

caloric irrigation *np*
Also: caloric stimulation
The method of introducing warm and cool water into the ear canal to test vestibular function.

calvarial bone *np*
The top part of the skull or scalp.

canal *n* [Lat *canalis* pipe, groove, channel]
A channel or tubular cavity.

canal hearing aid *np*
Also: in-the-canal hearing aid (ITC)
A small hearing aid that fits mainly in the ear canal.

canal lock *np*
An earmold that includes a projection into the base of the concha to assist retention.

canal of Rosentahl *np* ˈrōsĕntahl Named after Isidor Rosentahl (1836–1915), a German physiologist and professor of physiology at the University of Erlangen.
The spiral canal of the modiolus of the cochlea that contains the spiral ganglion.

canales semicirculares ossei *np* kaˈnahlāz sĕmīserkyūˈlahrāz ˈōsēī (sĕmēserkyūˈlahrāz ˈōsāē) *sg* canalis [Lat *canales semicirculares ossei* bony semicircular canals]
The bony semicircular canals.

canaliculi perforantes *np* kănaʹlĭkyūlī (kănaʹlĭkyūlē) ʹperforăntēs
Small connecting channels in the tympanic shelf of the osseous spiral lamina.

canaliculus *n* kănaʹlĭkyūlus *pl* caniculi [Lat *canaliculus* small pipe, groove, channel]
A small canal.
Deriv: -adj canalicular

canaliculus cochleae *np* kănaʹlĭkyūlus ʹkŏklēī (ʹkŏklēī)
The small canal in the temporal bone that contains the endolymphatic duct.

canaliculus mastoideus *np* kănaʹlĭkyūlus măsʹtoidēus
The canal that carries the vagus nerve through the mastoid process.

canaliculus tympanicus *np* kănaʹlĭkyūlus tĭmʹpănĭkus
The canal that carries a branch of the glossopharyngeal nerve through the temporal bone to the tympanic cavity.

canalis *n* [Lat *canalis* pipe, groove, channel]
Canal or channel.

canalis spiralis cochlea *np* kaʹnălĭs spĭʹrălĭs ʹkŏklēa
The bony cochlear labyrinth.

canalis spiralis modiolus *np* kaʹnălĭs spĭʹrălĭs ʹmŏdīōlē (ʹmŏdēōlĭ)
The bony modiolus in which the cochlear nerve spiral ganglia are found.

canalith repositioning procedure *np* [Lat *canalis* pipe, groove, channel + Gk *lithos* stone]
Also: Epley maneuver
A maneuver of the head and body that aims to force any free otoconia to collect in the vestibule.

canalithiasis *n* kaʹnălĭthēahsĭs [Lat *canalis* pipe, groove, channel + Gk *lithos* stone]
Benign paroxysmal positional vertigo caused by free otoconia that collect near the cupula of the posterior semicircular canal.

cancellation *n*
The elimination of an acoustic stimulus when two identical stimuli occur 180° out of phase.

cancellous bone *np*
Also: trabecular bone; spongy bone
Bone composed of a network of branching bony spicules that has the appearance of a sponge, with bone marrow contained in the spaces.

cancer *n* [Lat *cancer* crab]
A malignant tumor.

canthus *n* [Gk *kanthos* corner]
The outer or inner angle where the two eyelids meet.

capacitance *n* [Lat *capax* that can contain]
A stored electric charge.

capacitor *n* [Lat *capax* that can contain]
Also: condenser
An electrical component used to store electricity. A capacitor allows high frequencies to pass and blocks low frequencies.

capillary *n* [Lat *capilaris* pertaining to hair]
A very narrow blood vessel with walls only one cell thick. Capillaries form a network in most tissues and facilitate the exchange of oxygen, nutrients, and carbon dioxide between the blood and the tissues.

capitulum *n* kaʹpĭchūlum [Lat *capitulum* small head]
A knob or protrusion at the head of a bone.

capitulum malleus *np* [Lat *capitulum* small head + Lat *malleus* hammer]
The head of the malleus.

capitulum stapes *np* [Lat *capitulum* small head + Lat *malleus* hammer]
The head of the stapes.

capreomycin *n* kăprēōʹmīsĭn
An ototoxic antibiotic used in treating tuberculosis.

capsule n [Lat *capsula* little box]
A receptacle.

capsule, otic np
The bone that surrounds the membranous labyrinth.

captioning n
Providing a heading or title.

captioning, closed np
The concealed text of the dialogue or narrative of programs on television or video that can be made visible when desired.

captioning, open np
The visible text of the dialogue or narrative of programs on television or video.

captioning, real-time np
Essentially instantaneous captioning.

Capute-Rimoin-Konigsmark syndrome
np Named after Arnold Capute (1923–2003), an American pediatrician; David Rimoin (b 1936), a Canadian-American geneticist and pediatrician; and Bruce Konigsmark (1928–1973), an American otolaryngologist; who first described the syndrome in 1969.
Also: leopard syndrome; multiple lentigines syndrome
Characteristics include lentigines (freckles) on the head and neck, dwarfism, and sensorineural deafness.

carbon microphone np
A microphone in which carbon granules are disturbed when sounds cause the diaphragm to move. This causes changes in resistance between the granules.

carboplatin n
An ototoxic antineoplastic drug.

carcinoma n kahrsĭnōma pl carcinomata
[Gk *karkinos* crab + Gk -*oma* denoting tumor, swelling]
Cancer derived from epithelial tissue.

carcinoma, basal cell np [Gk *karkinos* crab + Gk -*oma* denoting tumor, swelling; Gk *basis* base]
A type of skin cancer, commonly caused by excessive exposure to sunlight and usually found in sun-damaged areas, e.g., the top of the pinna. This type of skin cancer appears as a pearly nodule (usually brown, black, or blue) that grows slowly and rarely spreads to other parts of the body.

carcinoma, squamous cell np skwāmus
[Gk *karkinos* crab + Gk -*oma* denoting tumor, swelling; Lat *squamosus* scaley]
A type of skin cancer, commonly caused by excessive exposure to sunlight and usually found in sun-damaged areas, e.g., the top of the pinna. This type of skin cancer can vary widely in appearance. It tends to grow slowly, but occasionally spreads to nearby lymph nodes and other organs.

cardiac evoked response audiometry np
[Gk *kardiakos* pertaining to the heart]
An electrophysiologic technique that measures changes in heart rate in response to sound stimuli.

cardinal vowels np [Lat *cardinalis* pertaining to the points of the compass]
A system that gives reference points to describe the position of the vowels in the mouth.

cardioauditory syndrome np [Gk *kardia* heart + Lat *auditorius* pertaining to hearing]
Also: Jervell and Lange-Neilson syndrome
A type of long QT syndrome that causes congenital profound deafness and an irregular heart rhythm. An autosomal recessive genetic condition.

cardioid adj [Gk *kardia* heart + Gk -*oides* shaped like]
Heart shaped.

cardioid response np
A cardioid pattern of sensitivity in directional microphones.

cardiotachometry n [Gk *kardia* heart + *takhos* speed + *metron* measure]
Measurement of heart rate.

Carhart notch *np* Named after Raymond T. Carhart (1912–1975), an American audiologist, who reported the phenomenon in 1950. He also established the first academic program in audiology in the United States.

A reduction in bone conduction sensitivity at 2 kHz, which is associated with otosclerosis.

Carhart tone decay test *np* Named after Raymond T. Carhart (1912–1975), an American audiologist, who introduced the test. He also established the first academic program in audiology in the United States. The test was modified to a shorter version by Rosenberg in 1958.

A test in which a tone is presented just above threshold and the time for which it is audible is measured. Rapid decay indicates possible retrocochlear problems.

caroticotympanic artery *np* [Gk *karotis* drowsiness (compression of these arteries causes drowsiness) + Gk *tumpanon* drum; Gk *arteria* blood vessel, artery]

A branch of the petrous portion of the internal carotid artery that supplies the tympanic cavity.

carotid arteries *np* [Gk *karotis* drowsiness (compression of these arteries causes drowsiness) + Gk *tumpanon* drum; Gk *arteria* blood vessel, artery]

The two main arteries that supply the head and neck with oxygenated blood. At the thyroid cartilage (Adam's apple), they divide into two branches. One branch, the internal carotid artery supplies the middle ear, cerebrum, forehead, nose, and eyes.

Carpenter syndrome *np* Named after George Carpenter (1859–1910), an English physician, who reported the syndrome in two sisters in 1901.

Also: acrocephalopolysyndactyly
Symptoms include learning difficulty, craniofacial abnormalities, and webbed fingers. Additional symptoms may also include low-set ears, preauricular pits and conductive hearing loss.

carrier *adj/n*
Also: heterozygote
–*adj* Transporting or bearing.–*n* A person who bears the gene for an abnormal trait, but does not show signs of the disorder.

carrier frequency *np*
A frequency capable of being modulated by signals of other frequencies.

carrier phrase *np*
A phrase that is used in speech audiometry to precede the target word, used to ensure the client/patient is ready and listening, e.g., "Now say…"

cartilage *n* [Lat *cartilago* cartilage]
Dense network of connective tissue that is strong and resilient. Unlike other connective tissues, cartilage does not have blood vessels running through it to deliver nutrients to the cells.

cartilage, permanent *np*
Cartilage that retains its structure.

cartilage, temporary *np*
Connective tissue that is present early in life and subsequently changes to bone.

cartilago auriculae *np* kahti'lājō awr'ĭkyū-lĭ (kahti'lăgō ŏ'rĭkyūlĭ) [Lat *cartilago auriculae* cartilage of the ear]
Auricular cartilage.

carved shell *np*
A silicone shell earmold where the interior has been carved out to make it lightweight and flexible.

case history *np*
A record of a person's medical, communication, and social background.

cast *n*
A mass of dead cellular matter that forms within a canal or a cavity and takes its shape, e.g., a wax or keratin cast in the ear canal.

CAT scan *np*
Also: computed tomography (CT)
Computerized axial tomography. A scan that uses x-rays and computer technology to build up detailed images or tomograms.

catarrh *n* kɑtah [Gk *katarrhous* a flowing down]
Inflammation of mucous membrane causing excessive mucus.
Deriv: -adj catarrhal

categorical perception *np*
The ability to identify different objects or sounds as belonging to a particular category, e.g., cars, animals, vowels, etc. Perception becomes easier when an item can be categorized. Talkers are able to categorize the individual phonemes (/a/, /p/, /m/, etc.) that are present in running speech even though they are not discrete units.

catheter *n* [Gk *katheter* something let down]
A long tubular instrument for passing down a canal to draw off fluid, e.g., Eustachian tube catheter.

cathode *n* [Gk *kathodos* way down]
The point at or path by which an electric current passes to the negative pole.

cation *n* kăt′ĭon [Gk *kation* going down]
A postively charged ion.

caudal *adj* ′kordɑl [Lat *caudalis* from Lat *cauda* tail]
Situated toward the tail or posterior end.

caudate nucleus *np* [Lat *caudatus* having a tail]
A mass of nerve cells located within the basal ganglia of the brain. Partly responsible for movement and coordination.

cauliflower ear *np*
Thickening and malformation of the cartilage of the pinna due to traumatic injury to the pinna.

causal *adj* [Lat *causa* cause]
Acting as the cause.

cauterize (cauterise) *v* ′korterīz
To burn or sear.
Deriv: –n cautery

cavernous hemangioma (haemangioma) *np* ′hēmănjēōmɑ
A vascular tumor consisting of large dilated blood vessels.

cavity *n* [Lat *cavus* hollow]
A hollow space within a structure.

cavum *n* ′kāvum [Lat *cavus* hollow]
A hollow or space.

cavum, concha *np*
The main lower part of the concha of the pinna.

cavum tympani *np*
The tympanic cavity. A hollow chamber in the temporal bone located between the Eustachian tube and the mastoid. Contains the ossicles.

cecum (caecum) *n* ′sēkum [Lat *caecus* blind]
A blind pouch.

cecum cupulare *np* [Lat *caecus* blind + Lat *culparis* pertaining to a vault]
The blind end that is the tip of the cochlear duct.

cecum vestibulare *np* [Lat *caecus* blind; Lat *vestibularis* pertaining to the vestibule]
The blind pouch at the vestibular end of the cochlear duct.

ceiling effect *np*
The maximum performance available, or level possible, in an activity.

cell *n* [Lat *cella* small room, chamber]
The basic unit of all living organisms. Bounded by a cell membrane that encloses cytoplasm within which is suspended a nucleus.

cells of Böttcher *np* ′bertcher Named after Jakob Ernst Arthur Böttcher (1831–1889), a German pathologist, known for his study of the organ of Corti.
Supporting cells that lie on the high frequency area of the basilar membrane below the cells of Claudius.

cells of Claudius *np* Named after Friedrich Matthias Claudius (1822–1869), an Austrian anatomist and professor at the University of Marburg.
Large supporting columnar cells in the organ of Corti that extend from the cells of Hensen.

cells of Deiters *np* ˈdētⲉrz Named after Otto Freidrich Karl Deiters (1834–1863), a German neuroanatomist, who is known for giving a detailed description of the nerve cell.
Finger-like supporting cells that rest on the basilar membrane.

cells of Held *np* Named after Hans Held (1886–1942), a German anatomist and neurologist, who described the development and structure of mammal and bird cochlea and isolated single hair cells in bird cochlea in 1926.
Also: border cells of Held
A layer of specialized nonsensory epithelial (hyaline) cells along the upper surface of the basilar membrane that support the inner hair cells. The number and height of the cells vary along the length of the basilar membrane, showing a spatial (tonotopic) correspondence with the frequency of sound.

cells of Hensen *np* Named after Christian Andreas Viktor Hensen (1835–1924), a German zoologist and professor of physiology at the University of Kiel, who described the organ of Corti including the structures bearing his name.
Supporting cells in the organ of Corti, between the outer hair cells and the cells of Claudius.

cellulitis *n* [Lat *cella* small room, chamber + Gk *-ites* denoting disease of]
Subcutaneous inflammation of connective tissue, e.g., in the pinna, often due to bacterial infection.

center (centre) *n/adj* [Lat *centrum* center]
-n The midpoint. *-adj* at the midpoint

center (centre) frequency *np*
The frequency at the center of a bandwidth.

center (centre) of gravity *np*
The point around which a body is balanced.

central *adj*
1. Pertaining to the central nervous system, e.g., central hearing loss due to a lesion in the brain or CNS. 2. In the center or central portion, e.g., a central perforation of the tympanic membrane.

central auditory nervous system *np*
The part of the central nervous system that relates to hearing, i.e., from cranial nerve VIII to the auditory cortex.

central auditory processing *np*
The functions of the central auditory pathways.

central auditory processing disorder *np*
Difficulty in differentiating, recognizing, or understanding sounds despite normal hearing and intelligence. Caused by disease or disorder in the central auditory pathways.

central masking *np*
Masking noise introduced into one ear causing a threshold shift of 5-10 dB in the opposite test ear. Considered to be due to interaction of signals from both ears at the level of the cortex.

central nervous system *np*
The brain and spinal cord. Integrates sensory impulses from all parts of the body.

central perforation *np*
A hole in the tympanic membrane, in the pars tensa.

central presbyacusis *np* ˈprĕzbīakyūsĭs [Gk *presbus* old man + *akousis* sense of hearing]
Age-related hearing problems due to central processing.

central tendency *np*
A typical value of a set of scores, e.g., the mean, median, and mode.

centrifugal *adj* sĕntrĭˈfyūgⲁl [Lat *centrum* center + Lat *fugere* flee]
Away from the center.

centripetal *adj* sĕntrĭˈpētⲁl [Lat *centrum* center + Lat *-petus* seeking (from *petere* to seek)]
Toward the center.

cephalad *adj* [Gk *kephale* head]
Also: cranial; rostral
Toward the head.

cephalic *adj* sĭfălĭk [Gk *kephale* head]
Situated in, or pertaining to, the head.

ceramic microphone *np* [Gk *keramikos* made of pottery; Gk *mikros* small + Gk *phone* sound]
A microphone in which a thin ceramic plate is attached to the diaphragm for transducing acoustic to electrical signals.

cerebellar pontine (cerebellopontine) angle (CPA) *np* [Lat *cerebellum* small brain; Lat *pons* bridge]
The space between the cerebellum and the pons.

cerebellopontine angle tumor *np* sĕrē-bĕlō'pŏntīn [Lat *cerebellum* small brain + Lat *pons* bridge; Lat *tumor* swelling]
Also: vestibular schwannoma
A benign tumor that grows from the vestibular branch of cranial nerve VIII, caused by an overgrowth of the Schwann cells of the myelin sheath. Unilateral hearing loss is often the first sign of the condition. Bilateral tumors are very rare, but may be associated with neurofibromatosis.

cerebellum *n* sĕrē'bĕlum [Lat *cerebellum* small brain]
The largest part of the posterior brain, situated behind the pons and the medulla (oblongata). It consists of two highly folded hemispheres lying at the base of the brain. The function is motor coordination and maintenance of muscle tone and equilibrium.
Deriv: –*adj* cerebellar

cerebral *adj* sĕr'ē'brʌl [Lat *cerebrum* brain]
Relating to the brain.

cerebral cortex *np* [Lat *cerebrum* brain; Lat *cortex* bark of tree, outer layer]
The convoluted outer grey matter of the brain which is divided into two hemispheres, each of which is divided into a frontal, parietal, temporal, and occipital lobe. The processing of auditory informa-

tion takes place mainly in the primary auditory cortex in the temporal lobe.

cerebral dominance *np*
The tendency of one side of the brain to control particular functions, e.g., the left side is usually dominant for language functions.

cerebral hemispheres *np*
The halves of the cerebrum, each consisting of four lobes.

cerebral palsy *np* [Lat *cerebrum* brain; Old Fr *paralisie* (from Gk *paralysis* paralysis)]
Paralysis, weakness, and lack of coordination caused by a brain lesion. Characterized by uncontrollable muscle spasms. Mild to moderate high-frequency hearing loss sometimes present.

cerebral vascular (cerebrovascular) accident (CVA) *np* [Lat *cerebrum* brain; Lat *vas* vessel]
Also: stroke
Interruption of the blood flow to the brain. A cerebral vascular accident may cause hearing loss, visual difficulty, speech disturbance, etc.

cerebrospinal fluid (CSF) *np* [Lat *cerebrum* brain; Lat *spina* thorn, spine]
The clear liquid in the subarachnoid space and ventricles that surrounds and cushions the central nervous system.

cerebrovascular *adj* [Lat *cerebrum* brain + Lat *vas* vessel]
Pertaining to the brain and the blood vessels supplying it.

cerebrum *n* sĕ'rēbrum [Lat *cerebrum* brain]
The largest and most highly developed part of the brain. Consists of the two hemispheres of the forebrain. Responsible for integrative functioning and sensory and motor function.
Deriv: –*adj* cerebral

cerumen *n* [Lat *cera* wax]
Waxy substance secreted by the ceruminous glands in the ear canal.
Deriv: –*adj* ceruminal, ceruminous

ceruminectomy *n* [Lat *cera* wax + Gk *ektome* excision]
The removal of impacted cerumen from the ear canal.

ceruminolytic/cerumenolytic *n* [Lat *cera* wax + Gk *lusis* loosening]
A substance used to soften cerumen.

ceruminoma *n obs* [Lat *cera* wax + Gk –*oma* denoting tumor, swelling]
A tumor of the ceruminous glands. May be a benign adenoma or a malignant adenocarcinoma. Term no longer used by the World Health Organization because it does not describe the benign or malignant nature of the lesion.

ceruminosis *n* [Lat *cera* wax + Gk –*osis* denoting a diseased state]
Build up of excess cerumen.

cervical *adj* [Lat *cervix* neck]
Of the neck.

cervical-ocular reflex *np*
An ocular stabilization reflex elicited by rotating the neck.

cervical tinnitus *np* [Lat *cervix* neck + Lat *tinnitus* ringing]
Tinnitus associated with movement of the neck.

cervicooculoacoustic syndrome *np* [Lat *cervix* neck + Lat *oculus* eye + Gk *akousis* sense of hearing]
Also: Wildervanck syndrome; otofaciocervical dysmorphia
A syndrome where two or more cervical vertebrae are fused. Similar to Klippel-Feil syndrome. Characteristics include narrow elongated face, short webbed neck, poorly developed neck muscles, facial asymmetry, deafness that may be total, prominent ears, preauricular fistulas, eyeball retraction, and nystagmus.

channel *n*
1. A frequency region (band) that is processed independently in a compression hearing aid. 2. A narrow hollowed course or way.

characteristic *adj/n* [Gk *kharakter* character]
-*adj* Indicating an essential quality. –*n* An essential quality.

characteristic frequency *np*
The frequency to which a neuron is most sensitive. Shown as the sharp tip on a normal psychoacoustical tuning curve.

Charcot-Marie-Tooth disease *np* shahr-kō-măr'ē-tūth Named after three physicians. Jean-Martin Charcot (1825–1893), a French neurologist and professor of neurology, and Pierre Marie (1853–1940), a student of Charcot, published a classic description of the condition in 1886. Howard Henry Tooth (1856–1925), an English physician, described the condition in the same year in his doctoral dissertation titled, *The peroneal type of progressive muscular atrophy.*
Also: hereditary motor and sensory neuropathy
A genetic condition that affects peripheral nerves and causes progressive muscle wasting that first affects the muscles of the legs. The condition is often associated with bilateral sensorineural hearing loss.

CHARGE syndrome *np* The name of the syndrome is an acronym of the characteristics.
A congenital disorder characterized by features that may include coloboma of the eye (a malformation that leaves a cleft, often in the iris), heart anomaly, choanal atresia, retardation, and genital and ear anomalies, which may include sensorineural or mixed hearing loss.

chemo- *prefix* [Arabic *alkimia: al* the + Gk *khemia* the art of transmuting metals]
Chemical

chemoradiotherapy *n* [Arabic *alkimia: al* the + Gk *khemia* the art of transmuting metals + Gk *therapeia* treatment]
Simultaneous chemotherapy and radiation therapy, often used in cancer treatment.

chemoreceptor *n* [Arabic *alkimiya: al* the + Gk *khemia* the art of transmuting metals + Lat *receptor* receiver]
A sensory organ that is activated by chemical stimulation.

chemosensory *adj*
Pertaining to smell or taste.

chemotherapy *n* [Arabic *alkimiya: al* the + Gk *khemia* the art of transmuting metals + Gk *therapeia* treatment]
The treatment of disease by chemical substances, e.g., cisplatin, which is ototoxic.

Chiari syndrome/malformation *np* kē'ahrē Named after Hans Chiari (1851–1916), a professor of pathological anatomy at the German University of Prague, who described the malformations in 1891. He also credited Julius Arnold (1835–1915), a professor of anatomy at the University of Heidelberg, for an earlier description, but this was not the same condition.
Also: cerebellomedullary malformation/syndrome; *obs* Arnold-Chiari malformation/syndrome
A malformation, most commonly congenital, of the cerebellum and brainstem. May cause symptoms such as muscle weakness, balance problems, head and neck pain, dizziness, hearing loss, and tinnitus.

chickenpox *n*
Also: varicella; varicella zoster virus (VZV)
Common childhood infection by the contagious *varicella-zoster* virus, the same virus that causes herpes zoster (shingles) in adults. Chickenpox causes itchy fluid-filled blisters and may result in ear infections. Hearing loss is a very rare direct complication. The virus can remain latent in the body and become active again later in life as shingles. If the auditory nerve is affected, sensorineural hearing loss with pain will result.

chi-square test *np* kī'skwĕa
A statistical procedure of probability that tests whether there is a significant difference between two variables.

chloral hydrate *np*
A sedative drug. May be used to sedate young children prior to evoked response audiometry.

chloropromazine/chlorpromazine *n*
An antipsychotic drug, sometimes also used as a tranquilizer and to enhance the effect of analgesics.

chloroquine *n*
Synthetic drug to replace quinine. Used to prevent and treat malaria and in the treatment of rheumatoid arthritis, lupus erythematosus, etc. Can be ototoxic.

cholesteatoma *n* kolĕstēatōma cholesteatomas, cholesteatomata [Gk *khole* bile + Gk *stereos* stiff + Gk *–oma* denoting tumor, swelling]
Also: epidermoid cyst
A benign tumor-like mass in the middle ear consisting mainly of cellular debris. Usually occurs secondary to otitis media or marginal tympanic perforation. May cause destruction of surrounding tissues.

cholesteatosis *n* kolĕstēa'tōsĭs [Gk *khole* bile + Gk *stereos* stiff + Gk *-osis* denoting a diseased state]
Fatty degeneration due to deposits of cholesterol in tissue.

cholesterol *n* [Gk *khole* bile + Gk *stereos* stiff]
A fat-like substance that is present in the blood and tissues.

cholesterol granuloma *np*
A cyst that forms in response to excessive cholesterol in the tissues. If it occurs in the middle ear, mastoid, or petrous apex, it may result in damage to bones and nerves, with consequent conductive or retrocochlear hearing loss.

chondroblastoma *n* [Gk *khondros* cartilage + Gk *blastos* germ, sprout + Gk *–oma* denoting tumor, swelling]
A tumor with the appearance of a mass of well-differentiated cartilage.

chondrodermatitis nodularis chronica helicis *np* [Gk *khondros* cartilage + Gk *derma* skin + Gk *–ites* denoting disease of]
Also: Winkler disease
A benign painful nodule on the external ear, most commonly on the helix of the pinna.

chondrodysplasia/chondrodystrophy/ chondrodystrophia *n* [Gk *khondros* cartilage + Gk *dus-* bad + Gk *plasis* formation; Gk *trophe* nourishment]
Also: Nance-Sweeney syndrome
A genetic disorder affecting the development of cartilage mainly in the long bones, leading to arrested growth and associated with sensorineural hearing loss.

chondrodystrophia fetalis *np* [Gk *khondros* cartilage + Gk *dus-* bad + Gk *trophe* nourishment; Lat *fetalis* pertaining to the fetus]
Also: achondroplasia
A disorder of cartilage formation in the fetus resulting in a small body with normal sized skull, protruding forehead, a button nose, middle and inner ear abnormalities, and associated conductive and sensorineural hearing loss.

chondroma *n* [Gk *khondros* cartilage + Gk *–oma* denoting tumor, swelling]
A benign cartilaginous tumor. Most common in the small bones of the hands and feet, but may occur in the bony external auditory meatus or in the middle ear.

chondrosarcoma *n* kŏndrōsah'kōma [Gk *khondros* cartilage + Gk *sarx* flesh + Gk *–oma* denoting tumor, swelling]
Cancer of the cartilage.

chorda tympani *n* [Gk *khorda* gut, string; Gk *tumpanon* drum]
A branch of the facial nerve (cranial nerve VII) that passes through the middle ear and across the eardrum and is responsible for taste sensation.

chordoma *n* [Gk *khorde* gut, string + Gk *–oma* denoting tumor, swelling]
Bone cancer that occurs in the spine and base of the skull. If it occurs in the base of the skull it may cause hearing loss, vertigo, double vision, difficulty swallowing, headache, and facial pain.

chromosome *n* [Gk *khroma* color + Gk *soma* body]
The genetic material in a cell nucleus. Composed of a long double thread-like filament of DNA.
Deriv: –adj chromosomal

chromosome 21-trisomy syndrome *np*
Also: Down syndrome
A congenital genetic disorder. Characteristics include some physical and cognitive impairments, together with distinctive facial features (such as slanting eyes, square-shaped face, and macroglossia) and a high incidence of conductive and sensorineural hearing loss.

chromosome 18q- syndrome *np*
Also: long arm 18 deletion syndrome
A rare condition in which the long arm (q) of chromosome 18 is missing. Characteristics are variable, but may include short stature; learning difficulties; malformation of hands, feet, and skull; underdeveloped midface; prominent ears; and hearing loss.

chronic *adj* [Gk *khronos* time]
1. Persistent, of long duration or frequent recurrence. 2. Referring to a specific long duration, depending on the condition, e.g., over 3 months in otitis media.

chronological age *np* [Gk *khronos* time + Gk *logos* reason]
The actual age or number of years lived.

ciliotoxic *adj* [Gk *cillium* eyelash + Gk *toxikon* poison]
Poisonous to the cilia.

cilium *n* *pl* cilia [Lat *cillium* eyelash]
A hair-like process extending from a cell surface, e.g., the cilia of the hair cells in the cochlea.
Deriv: –adj ciliated

cinchonism *n* 'sĭngkonĭzem
Temporary hearing loss due to ingesting quinine, a derivative of cinchona bark.

ciproflaxin *n*
A quinolone antibiotic (a group of synthetic antibiotics that inhibit an enzyme needed for replication of bacterial DNA) used to treat severe bacterial infections. May be ototoxic.

circuit *n* [Lat *circuitus* a going round]
The complete path of an electric current.

circuit, integrated *np*
An electronic circuit formed on a single body of semiconductor material.

circuitry *n*
The components of an electrical circuit.

circumambient *adj* [Lat *circum* around + Lat *ambire* go round]
Surrounding, especially of the air or environment.

circumaural *adj* [Lat *circum* around + Lat *auris* ear]
Surrounding the ear.

circumaural ear protection *np*
Earmuffs.

circumscribed *adj* [Lat *circum* around + Lat *scribere* to write]
Confined or restricted to a limited area, e.g., circumscribed labyrinthitis.

cisplatin *n*
An ototoxic drug used in cancer treatment.

class *n*
A classification or division.

class A amplifier *np*
A single-ended circuit design that results in constant current drain independent of the amplitude of the input signal. It is used in low-power applications.

class B amplifier *np*
A push–pull (double-ended) circuit design where two output stages alternate in sending current to a load (receiver), which prolongs battery life. It is used in high-power applications.

class C amplifier *np*
An amplifier used in radio transmission.

class D amplifier *np*
A pulse width modulated amplifier that operates with the output rapidly switching between on and off, which conserves current.

classroom *n*
A teaching space.

classroom accommodation *np*
1. A room to hold a certain number of students. 2. Adjustment of the classroom environment to improve accessibility for persons with hearing loss or other disabilities.

classroom acoustics *np*
The sound characteristics of a classroom.

classroom amplification *np*
An amplification system designed to improve the signal-to-noise ratio in a classroom.

Claudius cells *np* Named after Friedrich Matthias Claudius (1822–1869), an Austrian anatomist and professor of anatomy at the University of Marburg, Germany, who described these cells in 1856.
Large supporting columnar cells in the organ of Corti that extend from the cells of Hensen.

cleft *n*
A fissure or opening.

cleft palate *np* [cleft and Lat *palatum* palate]
Also: uranoschisis
A congenital fissure in the median line of the palate.

cleidocranial dysostosis *np* ˈklīdō ˈkrānēal dīsŏstˈōsĭs [Gk *kleido-* pertaining to the clavicle + Gk *kranion* skull; Gk *dus-* bad + Gk *osteon* bone + Gk *-osis* denoting a diseased state]
A disorder of bone development in the skull and clavicle with associated conductive and sensorineural hearing loss and a susceptibility to sinus and ear infections.

click *n*
A brief, transient broadband signal.

clicking tinnitus *np*
A sound heard in the ears or head caused by the rhythmical contraction of the middle ear muscles that have gone into spasm.

clinical *adj* [Gk *klinike* bedside]
Medical or pertaining to diagnosis and treatment.

clinical audiologist *np*
A professional who holds a master's degree in audiology and works in a clinical setting or in research.

clinician *n*
A healthcare professional.

clipping *n*
The action of cutting.

clipping, peak *np*
A method used in hearing aid circuits to prevent the output signal from exceeding a predetermined level.

clival chordoma *np* klēval kor'dōma [Lat *clivus* hill; Gk *khorde* string, cord + Gk – oma denoting tumor, swelling]
An intracranial tumor that occurs in the cliva, a sloping bony surface in the skull base. It may result in double vision, tongue and facial weakness, headache, hearing loss, vertigo, tinnitus, and intracranial pressure.

clonus *n* 'klōnus [Gk *klonos* spasm]
Muscular spasm.

closed *adj*
Confined.

closed captioning *np*
The concealed text of the dialogue or narrative of programs on television or video, etc., which can be made visible when desired.

closed head injury *np*
Brain injury due to a trauma with a blunt instrument.

closed-loop irrigation *np*
The process of injecting warm or cool water into an expandable balloon in the ear canal during caloric testing.

closed platform *np*
A digital circuit that cannot be modified or altered.

closed set *np*
A limited number of alternatives from which to choose.

closure *n*
1. The condition of being closed. 2. The process by which incomplete forms are perceived as whole.

closure, auditory *np*
The process whereby a word can be recognized despite missing one or more phonemes.

cluster *n*
Also: consonant blend
Two or more spoken consecutive consonants without an intervening vowel.

coarticulation *n* [Lat *co-* together + Lat *articulare* divide into parts]
1. Jointing of two bones. 2. The influence of a phoneme on the preceding or following phonemes in a word or phrase.

coblation *n*
Removal of soft tissue, e.g., tonsils and adenoids, using bipolar high-frequency electrical energy.

cochlea *n* [Lat *cochlea* snail shell, spiral]
The fluid-filled spiral cavity of the inner ear, containing the end organ for hearing.
Deriv: -*adj* cochlear

cochlear amplifier *np*
Enhancement of sound vibration in the inner ear due to action of the outer hair cells. Responsible for increased sensitivity and frequency resolution.

cochlear aqueduct *np* [Lat *cochlea* snail shell, spiral; Lat *aqueductus* an aqueduct]
A small channel in the temporal bone that connects the scala tympani to the subarachnoid space.

cochlear artery *np* [Lat *cochlea* snail shell, spiral; Gk *arteria* blood vessel, artery]
A branch of the labyrinthine artery.

cochlear conductive presbyacusis *np* [Lat *cochlea* snail shell, spiral; Gk *presbus* an old man + Gk *akousis* hearing]
Hearing loss caused by mechanical changes in the basilar membrane, spiral ligament, and other cochlear structures.

cochlear duct *np* [Lat *cochlea* snail shell, spiral; Lat *ductus* a channel]
Also: scala media; endolymphatic space
The cochlear portion of the membranous labyrinth.

cochlear echo *np* [Lat *cochlea* snail shell or spiral; Gk *ekho* an echo]
Sound emitted by the outer hair cells of the cochlea in response to an auditory stimulus.

cochlear fenestra *np* [Lat *cochlea* snail shell, spiral; Lat *fenestra* window]
The round window of the cochlea.

cochlear hearing loss *np*
Sensorineural deafness due to cochlear damage.

cochlear implant *np*
A device for persons with profound hearing loss, in which an electrode array is implanted in the cochlea to deliver impulses to the nerve; an external sound processor activates the electrodes.

cochlear labyrinth *np* [Lat *cochlea* snail shell, spiral; Gk *laburinthos* a labyrinth]
Also: canalis spiralis cochleae
The cochlear pathways in the petrous part of the temporal bone.

cochlear microphonic *np* [Lat *cochlea* snail shell, spiral; Gk *mikros* small + Gk *phone* a sound]
A tiny electrical potential from the outer hair cells of the cochlea that resembles the waveform of the input signal.

cochlear nerve *np*
One branch of cranial nerve VIII (the vestibulocochlear nerve) that carries impulses from the inner ear to the brain. The second branch is the vestibular nerve, concerned with balance information.

cochlear nucleus *np* [Lat *cochlea* snail shell, spiral; Lat *nucleus* nut kernal]
A cluster of neurons, in the medulla portion of the brainstem, that receive input from the cochlear nerve.

cochlear otosclerosis *np* [Lat *cochlea* snail shell, spiral; Gk *ous* ear + Gk *sklerosis* hardening]
Spongy bone formation at the stapes that invades the cochlea causing sensorineural hearing loss.

cochlear ramus *np* ˈrāmus [Lat *cochlea* snail shell, spiral; Lat *ramus* tree branch]
A branch of the vestibulocochlear artery that supplies the basal, high-frequency region of the cochlea.

cochlear recess *np*
A small depression on the inner wall of the labyrinthine vestibule in which the round window is situated.

cochlear reflex *np*
Also: cochleostapedial reflex; acoustic reflex
An involuntary activation of one or both of the middle ear muscles (tensor tympani and/or stapedius muscle) to high-intensity acoustic stimulation.

cochlear reserve *np*
The difference between the actual hearing level and the potential hearing level without any conductive element; equivalent to the air-bone gap.

cochlear window *np*
Also: fenestra cochlea; round window; fenestra rotunda
A membrane-covered opening in the bone, leading into the cochlea, i.e., the round window.

cochleariform process *np*
Also: trochleariform process; processus cochleariformus
A thin bony plate in the mesotympanum above the oval window and medial to the neck of the malleus. The tensor tympani muscle makes a right angle at this process before it runs laterally to attach at the neck of the malleus.

cochleogram *n* [Lat *cochlea* snail shell, spiral + Gk *gramma* something written]
An audiogram based on the detection of cochlear microphonic responses.

cochleoorbicular reflex *np* [Lat *cochlea* snail shell, spiral + Lat *orbis* ring]
Also: acousticopalpebral reflex; acoustopalpebral reflex; auropalpebral reflex; cochleopalpebral reflex
A rapid eye blink caused by a sudden loud sound.

cochleopalpebral *adj* ˈkŏklēōpălˈpebral [Lat *cochlea* snail shell, spiral + Lat *palpebra* eyelid]
Pertaining to the cochlea and the eyelid.

cochleopalpebral reflex *np*
Also: acousticopalpebral reflex; acoustopalpebral reflex; auropalpebral reflex; cochleoorbicular reflex
A rapid eye blink caused by a sudden loud sound.

cochleosaccular *adj* [Lat *cochlea* snail shell, spiral + Lat *sacculus* a little sac]
Pertaining to the membranous portion of the cochlea and saccule.

cochleosaccular degeneration, infantile *np*
Degeneration of the cochlea during infancy resulting in unilateral or bilateral profound sensorineural hearing loss.

cochleosaccular dysplasia *np* [Lat *cochlea* snail shell, spiral + Lat *sacculus* a little sack; Gk *dus-* bad + Gk *plasis* formation]
Also: Scheibe dysplasia
Gross malformation of the cochlea and saccule. The organ of Corti may be fully or partially missing and the cochlear duct collapsed or distended, resulting in congenital profound deafness.

cochleosacculotomy *n* [Lat *cochlea* snail shell, spiral + Lat *sacculus* a little sack + Gk *-tomia* a cutting]
A surgical procedure to insert a needle through the oval window to puncture a dilated saccule.

cochleostapedial reflex *np* [Lat *cochlea* snail shell, spiral + Lat *stapes* stirrup]
Also: acoustic reflex; cochlear reflex
An involuntary activation of one or both of the middle ear muscles (tensor tympani and/or stapedius muscle) to high-intensity acoustic stimulation.

cochleostomy *n* [Lat *cochlea* snail shell, spiral + Gk *-tomia* a cutting]
Opening the cochlea (e.g., for cochlear implant surgery) or destruction or removal of the cochlea.

cochleotoxic *adj* [Lat *cochlea* snail shell, spiral + Gk *toxikon* poison]
Poisonous to the ear and may produce temporary or permanent hearing loss, tinnitus, and/or balance problems.

cochleovestibular *adj* [Lat *cochlea* snail shell, spiral + Lat *vestibulum* vestibule, anteroom]
Pertaining to the cochlea and vestibule.

Cockayne syndrome *np* Named after Edward Alfred Cockayne (1880–1956), an English pediatrician at the Great Ormond Street Hospital for Sick Children in London, who reported the disorder in 1946.
Also: progeroid nanism
A progressive disorder characterized by dwarfism, an abnormally small head, sensitivity to sunlight, learning difficulty, and impaired development of the nervous system. Progressive later-onset sensorineural hearing loss, eye abnormalities, and bone abnormalities.

code of practice *np*
A set of rules regarding conduct, ethics, and professional practice, to which professionals are expected to conform.

coding strategy *np*
An algorithm used in cochlear implants for presenting the processed sound to the electrode array.

Cogan syndrome *np* ˈkōgan Named after David Glendenning Cogan (1908–1993), an American ophthalmologist, who described the disorder in 1945.

An autoimmune disorder that mainly affects children and young adults. It causes inflammation of the eyes, vertigo, and hearing loss.

cognition *n* [Lat *cognitio* the act of knowing]
The act of knowing.
Deriv: –adj cognitive

cognitive behavioral therapy (CBT) *np*
[Lat *cognitio* the act of knowing; Gk *therapeia* healing]
An approach to the treatment of psychological problems to help the individual to manage them by changing thoughts and behaviors.

cogwheeling *n*
1. Jerkiness of motion. 2. Inability of the eyes to keep pace with an oscillating target resulting in the abnormal presence of saccades during smooth pursuit.

coherence *n*
The extent to which two conditions are similar.

coherence, evoked potential *np*
The extent to which successive averages are similar.

coherence, hearing aid *np*
The extent to which the output is similar to the input.

cold-opposite warm-same (COWS) *np*
A mnemonic term, used when teaching caloric irrigation, to describe the direction of nystagmus toward the same or opposite ear in response to stimulation with warm or cold water or air.

collagen *n* ˈkŏlajen [Gk *kolla* glue + Fr suffix *–gène* produced, producing]
A protein that is a main constituent of bone, tendons, and other connective tissues, e.g., the cartilage of the pinna.

collapsed ear canal *np*
A condition in which pressure of a headphone placed on the pinna results in temporary occlusion of the canal. It most commonly occurs when the cartilage of

the external ear has lost elasticity, e.g., in old age.

colliculus *n* koˈlĭkyulus [Lat *colliculus* a little hill]
A small elevation.

colliculus, inferior *np*
The central auditory nucleus of the midbrain.

coloboma *n* kŏloˈbōma *pl* colobumata, colobomas [Gk *koloboma* a part taken away]
A congenital eye defect. A gap or cleft is left in the ocular tissue during development that often occurs in the iris but may be in other parts of the eye, e.g., in retina, eyelid, or optic nerve. It may be inherited and occurs in a number of inherited syndromes, e.g., Treacher-Collins and Charge syndromes.

coloboma lobuli *np* [Gk *koloboma* a part taken away; Gk *lobos* the lobe of the ear]
A congenital split in the earlobe.

color (colour) hearing *np*
A type of synesthesia (synaesthesia) in which there is a subjective experience of colors in response to sounds.

columella *n* [Lat *columella* small column]
1. The bony central axis of the cochlea. 2. The small column of bone in a bird's middle ear that is the equivalent of the ossicles in a human.

combination tone *np*
A harmonic that occurs when two pure tones are presented at the same time.

comfort level (C-level) *np*
Also: maximum level (M-level)
In hearing aids, the input level of an auditory stimulus that is judged to be comfortable by the patient; in cochlear implants, the current level that does not cause discomfort to the patient.

commissure *n* [Lat *comissura* junction]
A bundle of nerve fibers that join together two parts of the brain.

common *adj*
1. Shared, where parts meet. 2. Usual, normal. 3. Identical.

common cavity *np*
A bony labyrinth without the normal turns.

common crus *np* [Lat *crus* leg]
The place where the superior and posterior semicircular canals meet.

common electrode *np*
Also: reference electrode
The ground electrode (earth) used in electrophysiologic measurement, e.g., in auditory brainstem response audiometry, the common electrode often placed on the contralateral mastoid.

common mode rejection *np*
The subtraction, by a differential amplifier, of noise that is common or identical at two electrodes.

communication *n*
The exchange of information using a common system of symbols.

communication disorder *np*
A speech and/or language disorder.

communication, manual *np*
A visual communication system utilizing sign language, finger spelling, and gesture.

communication, oral-aural *np*
A verbally based communication system that utilizes speech and hearing.

communication science *np*
The study of human communication.

communication, total *np*
A communication philosophy that uses both signed and spoken language together.

communicologist *n obs*
A speech and language therapist.

communicology *n*
The science of communication.

comodulation masking release (CMR) *np*
An improvement of a listener's ability to use temporal and spectral information to detect signals embedded in noise by the addition of modulated masking energy in frequency regions remote from the signal frequency.

comorbidity *n* [Lat prefix *co-* together with + Lat *morbus* disease]
The presence of a coexisting, but unrelated disease or disorder.

compact bone *np*
Hard bone that forms the exterior of bones and that supports and protects the body.

comparative *adj*
Characterized by systematic comparison of similarities and differences.

compensated *adj*
Adjusted; having provided a means for counteracting a variation.

compensated tympanometry *np*
Immittance measurements that are adjusted by the removal of the contribution of the ear canal.

competence *n*
The ethical requirement for audiologists and other professionals to practice within the limits of their capacity to deal adequately with a situation or individual.

competing *adj*
In a state of rivalry.

competing message *np*
A speech signal that interferes with the target message.

complementary *adj*
Something that completes or perfects.

complementary distribution *np*
Phonetic variants that have a distinctive position in words, e.g., in the initial position.

complementary metal oxide semiconductor (CMOS) *np*
Also: real-time clock
A technology for designing and constructing integrated circuits. CMOS memory is used in computers to store details such as time, date, and hardware settings.

completely in the canal (CIC) *np*
A small hearing aid that fits in the ear canal.

complex *adj*
Consisting of various connected parts.

complex tone *np*
A sound consisting of more than one frequency.

compliance *n*
The degree of yielding (suppleness) or ease of transfer.
Deriv: -adj compliant

compliance, acoustic *np*
A measure of the ease of transfer of energy through the outer and middle ears.

compliance, electrical *np*
A term used with cochlear implants indicating that the signal level required has been presented.

composite *adj* [Lat *componere* to put together]
Made up of various parts.

composite noise *np*
The noise from all sources present.

composite noise rating *np*
A noise measurement system used to evaluate noise levels and predict annoyance levels.

composite signal *np*
A complex flat spectrum noise.

compound *adj*
Made up of several elements.

compound action potential *np*
1. A synchronous change in the electrical potential of a nerve. 2. The whole nerve potential of cranial nerve VIII which is the main component in wave 1 of the auditory brainstem response.

compound threshold shift *np*
The combined hearing loss due to both temporary and permanent threshold shift.

comprehension *n* [Lat *comprehendere* to understand]
Understanding.

compression *n* [Lat *comprimere* to compress]
1. A decrease in size or density. 2. Nonlinear amplifier that controls the dynamic range of an amplified signal, resulting in a reduction of variations in the speech signal at the output. 3. Method used to control gain in a hearing aid by adjusting the relationship between high and low input levels in accordance with a specified rationale, so as to control the level of the amplified output. 4. The positive phase of a sound wave in which there is an increase in local pressure.
Deriv: –adj compressional

compression, adaptive *np*
Also: variable compression
A compression circuit that automatically varies release time depending upon the (temporal) lengths of input signal segments.

compression, curvilinear *np*
A compression circuit in which the compression ratio increases as the input level increases.

compression, dynamic range *np*
A compression circuit that compresses a wide range of acoustic signals to within the listener's residual dynamic range.

compression, frequency dependent *np*
A compression circuit that applies compression at specific frequency ranges: (1) bass increase at low levels (BILL), (2) treble increase at low levels (TILL), (3) programmable increase at low levels (PILL), and (4) multiband compression.

compression, input *np*
A type of compression in a hearing aid where, as the volume control changes, the gain and output levels are locked together and are shifted up and down simultaneously depending on volume control setting, while the compression threshold remains constant. The volume control setting of the hearing aid does not affect the compression threshold be-

cause the level detector is positioned before the gain control.

compression, knee point *np*
The input level required to activate a change in gain.

compression, multiband *np*
A compression system in which each frequency band can be independently adjusted.

compression, output *np*
A type of compression circuit where gain is increased as the volume control is reduced, and vice versa. Although the compression threshold varies according to volume control setting, the output signal remains at a fixed level.

compression ratio *np*
The ratio of the input signal relative to the output signal in a compression system.

compression, syllabic *np*
Compression with a low threshold of activation, low compression ratio, and a short/fast attack and release time (shorter than a typical speech syllable). Intended to reduce the differences between vowels and consonants to make soft sounds louder without causing vowels to be too loud or consonants to be lost.

compression, wide dynamic range (WDRC) *np*
A type of compression that attempts to squeeze the extremes of normal environmental sound into the individual's reduced range of residual hearing. Soft sounds receive proportionately more gain than that given to louder sounds. In summary, the purpose is to make soft sounds louder, moderate sounds audible, and loud sounds comfortable.

compressional wave *np*
A pressure wave in an elastic medium traveling away from the source that causes an element of the medium to change its volume, but not its direction.

computed tomography (CT) *np* [Lat *computare* to prune, to calculate; Gk *tomos* slice + Gk *graphia* writing]
Also: computerized axial tomography (CAT)
A scan that uses x-rays and computer technology to build up detailed images or tomograms. The scans are recorded at various focal lengths to give sliced images of the target.

computer averaging *np*
Also: signal averaging
The averaging of successive samples to reduce unrelated signals and improve the measurement of the desired response.

computerized dynamic posturography *np*
A vestibular assessment focusing on the ability to maintain postural stability in a variety of simulated conditions.

concha *n pl* conchae [Lat *concha* shell]
The depression (bowl) on the outer surface of the pinna that leads to the ear canal.

concha cavum *np* [Lat *concha* shell; Lat *cavum* a cave]
The main lower part of the concha of the pinna.

concha cymba *np* [Lat *concha* shell; Gk *kumbe* a cup]
The upper part of the concha of the pinna, above the crus of helix.

concordance rate *np*
1. The probability that both of a pair of individuals, especially identical twins, will have (or lack) a characteristic or trait of interest. 2. The proportion of pairs of identical twins with a specified trait, especially in disease, e.g., for comparison with fraternal twins to establish whether a disease may have a genetic cause.

concurrent *adj* [Lat *concurrere* to run side by side]
Occurring together.

concurrent equalization (equalisation) *np*
Also: real-time equalization or leveling; online equalization or leveling
Correction (equalization) that is performed at the same time as the measurement. Used in probe microphone (real ear) measurements so that the level and spectrum of the test sound field remain the same from one test to the next.

concurrent validity *np*
The assessment of the ability to distinguish between groups as intended. Often measured by correlating with previously validated measures.

condensation *n*
The state of being condensed. In acoustics, an increased concentration of air particles (density) due to the displacement of a vibratory force.

condensation reaction silicone *np*
An impression material that cures by condensation polymerization. Alcohol is given off as a by-product of this reaction and consequently the material shrinks a little.

condenser *n*
Also: capacitor
1. That which makes dense. 2. An electrical component used to store electricity. A capacitor allows high frequencies to pass and blocks low frequencies.

condenser microphone *np*
Also: capacitor microphone, electrostatic microphone
A microphone that uses a capacitor to convert acoustical energy into electrical energy.

condition *n/v*
–*n* 1. A state of being. 2. The state of something with regard to its appearance, quality, or working order. A broad medical term that includes injuries, medical disorders, and normal health situations, e.g., pregnancy. –*v* To modify behavior by training a person to associate a desired

behavior with a specific stimulus.
Deriv: -n conditioning

conditioned orientation reflex (COR) *np*
Also: visual response audiometry (VRA)
A type of pediatric audiometry in which a correct response to presentations of sound is reinforced by a visual reward, e.g., a lighted toy or a pleasing digital image.

conductance *n* [Lat *conducere* to lead]
The ease of energy flow, the reciprocal of resistance.

conduction *n*
The transmission of energy flow through a medium.
Deriv: -adj conductive

conductive hearing loss *n*
Reduction in hearing due to a loss of sound transmission through the external and/or middle ear.

condyle *np* [Gk *kondulos* knuckle]
A rounded process at the end of a bone that articulates with another bone.

cone of light *n*
Also: light reflex
The triangular reflection on the eardrum of the light from an otoscope.

confidentiality *n*
The ethical requirement for audiologists and other health professionals to refrain from making public any personal or health information.

configuration *n*
A shape.

configuration, audiometric *np*
The unique arrangement (shape) of hearing thresholds across the test frequencies on an audiogram, e.g., sloping, flat, etc.

configuration of a map *np*
Manipulation of the threshold and comfort-level data for programming a cochlear implant.

confusion matrix *np*
A table of items used in pattern recognition as a means of depicting errors.

congenital *adj* [Lat *cum* together + Lat *genetalis* pertaining to birth]
Present at birth.

conjugate *adj* [Lat *coniugare* join together]
Paired or joined together.

conjugate eye movement *np*
Paired movement of the eyes in the same direction.

connected discourse *np*
Also: continuous discourse
Running speech, e.g., reading a story.

connected discourse tracking *np*
A measurement of the ability to follow connected speech, where the listener has to repeat back the words spoken by someone who reads from a text.

connective tissue *np*
The most abundant tissue of the body, e.g., blood, bone, cartilage. Its functions include supporting, binding together, separating, strengthening, protecting, and insulating. Connective tissue is made up of three basic components—cells, ground substance and fibers. The ground substance and fibers make up a nonliving extracellular matrix, which may be fluid, semifluid, gelatinous, fibrous, or calcified (containing mineral deposits, e.g., bone).

conotruncal abnormalities *np* ˈkōnō'-trŭnkəl [Gk *konos* a cone + Lat *truncus* a trunk]
Congenital defects of the outflow tract of the heart, e.g., interrupted aortic arch, double-outlet right or left ventricle, artery transposition, etc.

conotruncal anomaly face syndrome *np*
Also: velocardiofacial syndrome; DiGeorge syndrome; 22q 11.2 deletion syndrome
A rare (1 in 4000 live births) syndrome that is genetic in only about 10% of cases. The signs and symptoms are very variable and may include congenital heart defects, cleft palate, an asymmetric crying face, poor growth, autism, skeletal abnormalities such as spinal problems and extra fingers and toes, and external ear abnormalities. The syndrome is due to the deletion of a small amount of genetic material in on the short or q arm of chromosome 22.

consanguine *adj* [Lat *consanguineus* of the same blood]
Related by blood.
Deriv: -n consanguinity

consensual *adj*
1. Occurring by mutual consent. 2. Occurring independent of conscious intent. A reflex.

conservation *n*
Protection from damage.

conservation, hearing *np*
Protection against noise damage.

conservation, speech *np*
Therapy to maintain speech production following acquired hearing loss.

consonance *n* [Lat *consonare* sound together]
The blending of tones that are presented at the same time.

consonant *n* [Lat *consonare* sound together]
A class of voiced or unvoiced speech sounds produced by either constricting, shaping or closing one or more of the structures in the vocal tract during breath flow.

consonant, voiced *np*
A consonant speech sound made with voicing.

consonant, unvoiced *np*
A consonant speech sound made without voicing.

constricted ear *np*
Also: lop ear; cup ear
A pinna that has an abnormally tight helix.

constriction *n* [Lat *constringere* constrain]
A narrowing, e.g., of the vocal tract when making a consonant sound.

construct validity *np*
A term used in statistics to mean the extent to which a test measures what it is supposed to measure.

contextual cues *np*
Linguistic or situational clues that can improve speech understanding.

contingent *adj* [Lat *contingere* touch, happen, befall]
Coming into contact with.

contingent negative variation (CNV) *np*
An electrical event that is indicative of a state of readiness or expectancy.

continuant *n*
A speech sound in which the speech organs are held in position for a period of production, e.g., /s/.

continuous flow adapter/adaptation *np*
Also: Hillyard effect; auditory "N1" effect; readiness potential (RP)
A hard plastic connector that is inserted in the earmold and to which the tubing is attached. This maintains the tubing diameter in the earmold and facilitates quick and easy tubing changes.

continuous interleaved sampling process (CIS) *np*
A cochlear implant processing strategy in which brief pulses are presented at a high rate of stimulation to multiple electrodes in a nonoverlapping sequence.

contra- *prefix* [Lat *contra* opposite]
Against.

contraindications *n*
Conditions under which a given procedure should not be carried out.

contralateral *adj* [Lat *contra* opposite + Lat *latus* side]
Pertaining to the opposite side.

contralateral routing of signals (CROS) hearing aid *np*
A hearing aid for unilateral hearing loss, in which the microphone is placed at the hearing impaired ear and the signal is routed to the opposite ear that has mild or no hearing loss.

control group *np*
In an experiment, a carefully matched group of subjects who do not receive the independent variable. The control group is used as a standard for comparison. The researcher can attribute the difference between the control and the experimental group as being due to the effect of the independent variable.

conversion deafness *np*
A condition in which the patient presents with hearing loss without an organic cause. Psychological factors are judged to be associated with the hearing loss because a stressor has preceded the symptoms.

cookie-bite *adj colloq*
A trough-shaped audiogram configuration.

Cornelia de Lange (CDL) syndrome *np*
kor'nēlēa de 'lahnge Named after Cornelia de Lange (1871–1951), a Dutch pediatrician, who reported the syndrome in two unrelated children in 1933. She presented a third case in 1941. In fact, the syndrome had been described earlier (1916) by Winfred Robert Brachman (1888–1969), a German doctor. It was probably first described by Willem Vrolik (1801–1863), a Dutch anatomist and professor of anatomy and physiology at the Athenaeum Illustre in Amsterdam.
Also: de Lange syndrome; bushy syndrome; Brachman de Lange syndrome
A developmental disorder characterized by distinctive facial appearance, slow growth, small stature, psychomotor delay, severe learning difficulties, skeletal abnormalities involving the upper extremities, and distinctive facial features (e.g., bushy eyebrows that meet in the middle [synophrys] and low set ears). There may be conductive and/or sensorineural hearing loss ranging from mild to severe.

corner audiogram *np*
Also: left/bottom corner audiogram
An audiogram configuration of profound

deafness, i.e., graph showing hearing thresholds that are only measurable in the low frequencies and that may be vibrotactile rather than true hearing.

cornu *n* ˈkorn(y)ū *pl* cornua [Lat *cornu* a horn]
A horn-like projection.

corpora quadrigemina *np* ˈkorpora kwŏ-drĭgĕmĭna [Lat *corpora quadrigemina* four-fold bodies]
A generic name for the two pairs of protuberances, the inferior colliculi and superior colliculi, which extend from the dorsal surface of the midbrain. The superior colliculi are the visual reflex centers. The inferior colliculi are important auditory centers that receive crossed and uncrossed nerve fibers before they pass to the primary auditory cortex and that may participate in the integration of auditory reflexes.

correlation *n*
The degree to which two sets of measurements are related. A correlation of 0 indicates there is no relationship between two measures. A correlation of +1 indicates a perfect positive correlation, i.e., a high value of one measure relates perfectly to a high value of another. A correlation of -1 indicates a perfect negative correlation, i.e., a high value of one measure relates perfectly to a low value of another.

cortex *n* [Lat *cortex* tree bark, outer layer]
A thin layer of tissue that covers the outer portion of the cerebrum and cerebellum.
Deriv: -adj cortical

cortex, cerebral *np* [Lat *cortex* tree bark, outer layer; Lat *cerebrum* the brain]
The convoluted outer gray matter of the brain, which is divided into two hemispheres, each of which is divided into a frontal, parietal, temporal, and occipital lobe. The processing of auditory information takes place mainly in the primary auditory cortex in the temporal lobe.

Corti, organ of *n* Named after Alfonso Giacomo Gaspare Corti (1822–1876), an Italian anatomist, who described the structure of the organ situated on the basilar membrane in 1851.
The spiral ribbon-like sense organ of hearing that is situated along the entire length of the basilar membrane in the scala media of the cochlea. It contains the inner and outer hair cells that convert sound pressure waves into the electrical impulses that are transmitted via cranial nerve VIII to the brain. The frequency of the sound activates a particular area along the organ of Corti, e.g., high frequencies near the base and low frequencies near the apex.

cortical evoked response audiometry *np*
Also: slow vertex response (SVR)
A form of evoked response audiometry that records potentials from the auditory cortex.

corticosteroid/corticoid *n*
A steroid hormone used to treat inflammatory conditions.

cortilymph *n* [Gk *lumpha* water]
The fluid found in the tunnel of Corti.

coryza *n* kerˈīza [Gk *koruza* nasal mucous]
Acute inflammation of the upper respiratory tract; the common cold.

cosmetic *adj*
Affecting a person's appearance.

Costen syndrome *np* Named after James Bray Costen (1895–1962), an American otorhinolaryngologist, who described the syndrome in 1934.
Also: temperomandibular joint syndrome (TMJ)
Mandibular malocclusion that may be accompanied by tinnitus, hearing loss, and earache.

cough reflex *np*
An involuntary cough caused by stimulation of the vagus nerve when something is placed in the ear canal, e.g., during earmold impression taking.

Coulomb (C) *n* 'kūlŏm Named in honor of Charles-Augustin de Coulomb (1736–1806), a French physicist, who developed the inverse square law.
A unit of electricity transferred by a current of one ampere in one second.

Coulomb's law *np* Named in honor of Charles-Augustin de Coulomb (1736–1806), a French physicist, who developed the inverse square law.
Also: inverse square law
A law that states that the intensity of a sound decreases in proportion to the square of the distance from the source. In practical terms, the amplitude of the wave decreases by about half or reduces by 6dB every time the distance from the sound source doubles.

counseling (counselling) *n*
1. Professional guidance of an individual using various psychological methods. 2. Guiding an individual to explore personal, social, or psychological issues.

coupler *n*
A device to join two parts of a system.

coupler, acoustic *np*
A device to join two parts of an acoustic system.

coupler, 2 cc *np*
Also: reference coupler; standard coupler
A device that joins the receiver of a hearing aid to the microphone of a sound level meter. Designed with a standard volume of 2 cc. Used for measuring the acoustic output of hearing aids.

coupler, 6 cc *np*
Also: occluded ear simulator; Zwislocki coupler
An artificial ear used for the calibration of audiometer headphones.

cranial *adj* [Gk *kranion* skull]
Relating to the skull.
Deriv: -n cranium

cranial nerve *np*
One of twelve pairs of nerves that emerge from the brainstem. Cranial nerves (CN) that are important in audiology include the trigeminal nerve (CNV), facial nerve (CNVII), and the acoustic or vestibulocochlear nerve (CNVIII).

craniofacial *adj*
Involving both the skull and the face.

craniofacial dysostosis *np* [Gk *kranion* skull + Lat *facies* face; Gk *dus-* bad + Gk *osteon* a bone + Gk *-osis* denoting a diseased state]
Also: Crouzon syndrome
An autosomal dominant genetic disorder characterized by an abnormally shaped skull with a frontal prominence and a beak-like nose. May have low-set ears, middle ear abnormalities, and conductive or mixed hearing loss.

craniometaphysical/craniometaphyseal dysplasia *np* [Gk *kranion* skull + Gk *metaphusis* a change of nature; Gk *dus-* bad + Gk *plasis* formation]
Also: Pyle disease
A condition in which tubular bones widen and there is overgrowth of the facial and skull bones. Characteristics may include a large broad head and frontal bossing (swelling). Cranial nerves may be affected due to stenosis and narrowing of the foramina (openings in the skull through which the nerves pass), resulting in facial nerve paralysis, atrophy of the optic nerve, and sensorineural deafness.

craniopharyngioma *n* [Gk *kranion* skull + Gk *pharunx* the throat + Gk *–oma* denoting tumor, swelling]
A benign slow-growing brain tumor that may behave like a malignant tumor. It tends to occur in children and is thought to arise from cells left over from early fetal development.

cribriform plate *np* [Lat *cribrum* sieve + Lat *forma* form]
1. A thin layer of bone. 2. The floor of the nasal cavity. It contains many holes that allow the passage of small olfactory nerve fibers.

cricoid *adj* ˈkrīkoid [Lat *cricoides* ring-shaped]
Ring-shaped.

cricoid cartilage *np*
The complete ring of cartilage around the trachea.

criss-CROS *adj*
Where both left to right and right to left contralateral routing of signals (CROS) systems are utilized simultaneously on an individual.

crista *n pl* cristae [Lat *crista* crest, plume]
The sense organ within the ampulla of the vestibular system, which reacts to changes in the rate of head movement.

critical band *np*
1. The minimal band of frequencies around a pure tone which mask that tone. 2. A measure of the effective bandwidth of an auditory filter.

cross hearing *np*
The perception of sound in an ear that is transmitted by either air conduction or bone conduction across or through the head from the contralateral ear under test.

cross links *n*
The connecting filaments between the stereocilia of the cochlear hair cells.

cross masking *np*
Overmasking, where masking sound delivered to the nontest ear is audible in the test ear.

crossover frequency *np*
The cut-off frequencies of filters that divide a frequency range into different bands.

crossover study *np*
A commonly used design method in which the participants are randomly as-signed to a sequence of treatments or trials, e.g., for hearing aid trials half the wearers would wear hearing aid A followed by hearing aid B, while the other half would wear hearing aid B followed by hearing aid A.

cross-talk *np*
A situation where unwanted signals from one electrical or acoustic system leak into another.

Crouzon syndrome *np* Named after Louis Edouard Olive Crouzon (1874–1938), a French neurologist, who described the syndrome in 1912.
Also: craniofacial dysostosis
An autosomal dominant genetic disorder characterized by an abnormally shaped skull with a frontal prominence and a beak-like nose. There may also be low-set ears, middle ear abnormalities, and conductive or mixed hearing loss.

crown *n*
The top of a structure, e.g., the top of the head.

crus *n pl* crura [Lat *crus* leg]
Any anatomical part that resembles a leg or pair of legs, e.g., the antihelix divides into the two crura that mark out the triangular fossa of the pinna.

crust *n*
A hard outer surface.

cryptophthalmos *n* krīptofˈthălmus [Gk *kruptos* hidden + Gk *ophthalmos* eye]
Also: Fraser syndrome
A syndrome that is characterized by eyelid malformation, i.e., eyelids that hide the eyes. The syndrome is often accompanied by underlying visual problems and malformation of the external and middle ear, including atresia and mixed hearing loss.

crystal microphone *np* [Gk *krystalos* ice, crystal]
A microphone that uses crystals that produce voltages when deformed. A thin strip of piezoelectric material attached to a diaphragm is used in a crystal micro-

phone. When the crystal is deflected by the diaphragm, the two sides of the crystal acquire opposite charges.

CT (computed tomography) scan *np* [Gk *tomos* slice + Gk *graphia* writing]
Also: computerized axial tomography (CAT)
A scan that uses x-rays and computer technology to build up detailed images or tomograms.

cubic centimeter (cc) *np*
A unit of measurement for volume where 1 cc = 1 ml.

cue *n*
A signal or clue to the articulation, perception or meaning of a word. An aspect that enables discrimination between two similar words, e.g., an acoustic cue is a signal that provides identifying speech information.

cued speech *np*
A system of hand signals combined with speech reading to discriminate between sounds that are visually similar and cannot be differentiated by lipreading alone.

cuniculum internum *np* [Lat *cuniculum* tunnel; Lat *internus* internal]
Also: tunnel of Corti; inner tunnel; canal of Corti
The triangular channel formed by the inner and outer pillars of the organ of Corti.

cupula/cupola *n* ˝kūpyulə/ˈkŭpolə *pl* cupulae [Lat *cupula* a dome]
1. A domed process or organ. 2. A gelatinous structure, concerned with rotational acceleration, within each of the semicircular canals.

cure *v/n*
-*v* 1. Altering a substance by chemical or other means for keeping or other use. 2. To recover; to make better.-*n* A substance that cures.

curette *n*
A medical instrument that includes a loop or scoop, used to remove ear wax or abnormal tissues.

current *n/adj*
-*n* 1. A flow marked by force or strength. 2. The flow of electricity through a conductor. -*adj* In progress.

curve walking *np*
The retrospective charting of the probable time course of noise induced hearing loss from a knowledge of the exposure pattern. The daily noise exposure and the time periods must be known.

curvilinear compression *np*
A compression circuit in which the compression ratio increases as the input level increases.

custom/customized *adj*
Made to individual specification.

cuticular plate *np* [Lat *cuticularis* pertaining to the skin]
A dense network of actin filaments that form a rigid platform in the organ of Corti, to which the apical ends of the cochlear hair cells are attached and through which their stereocilia project.

cycle *n* [Gk *kuklos* a cycle]
A period in which a recurring succession of an event is completed.

cycle per second (cps) *np obs*
Also: Hertz (Hz)
The completion of one cycle in one second.

cyclizine *n*
An antihistamine drug, used as a labyrinthine sedative to treat nausea and vomiting.

cycloserine *n*
An antibiotic, e.g., used in the treatment of tuberculosis (TB), which can be toxic to the central nervous system and may cause hearing loss.

cymba concha *np* ˈsĭmbə ˈkŏnchə [Gk *kumbe* cup; Lat *concha* shell]
The upper part of the concha of the pinna, above the crus of helix.

cyst *n* sĭst [Gk *kustos* vessel]
An abnormal sac containing air, liquid, or semisolid matter, which most often

forms on an organ or in the spaces between skin and muscle tissues.

cytocochleogram *n* ˈsītō ˈkŏklēōgrăm [Gk
kutos vessel + Lat *cochlea* shell + Gk *gramma* something written]
A graph showing the number of intact
and missing hair cells along the cochlea.

cytomegalovirus (CMV) *n* [Gk *kutos* vessel + Gk *megalos* big + Lat *virus* slime, poi-
son]
Also: cytomegalic inclusion disease
A herpes infection that causes symptoms
similar to a mild cold in an adult but
which, when passed to an unborn child,
may result in serious central nervous system damage, including brain damage,
seizures, vision loss, and hearing loss.

D

D-weighting (dBD) *n*
A standardized weighting network in a sound level meter used to measure aircraft noise based on annoyance rather than loudness. The scale has been removed from international standards and is rarely used.

dactyl *adj* ˈdăktᵻl [Gk *daktulos* finger]
Relating to a finger or a toe.

dactyl speech *np*
Also: finger spelling
A manual alphabet, for use by deaf people.

daily noise exposure (LEP,d) *np*
Equivalent continuous noise exposure, measured in dBA over an 8-hour period.

damp *v*
To diminish an activity or intensity.

damper *n*
A filter in an earhook, tubing, or earmold that reduces amplitude and smooths peaks in the frequency response of a hearing aid.

Dandy syndrome *np* Named after Walter Edward Dandy (1886–1946), an American neurosurgeon, who described the syndrome and who was also known for his pioneering intracranial vascular surgery.
Also: bobbing oscillopsia
Involuntary eye movements that cause objects to appear to bounce about and which may be caused by streptomycin or gentamycin toxicity or other cause. Characteristic of bilateral vestibular damage.

Darwin's ear *np* Named after Charles Darwin (1809–1882), an English naturalist, who first published a description of this condition. Darwin is best known for establishing the theory of evolution.
Also: tuberculum auriculae
A congenital condition in which the upper edge of the pinna does not roll over to form the helix.

Darwin's tubercle *np* Named after Charles Darwin (1809–1882), an English naturalist, who first published a description of this condition. Darwin is best known for establishing the theory of evolution.
A congenital condition where there is a small projection from the upper part of the helix.

data *n, pl* *sg* datum [Lat *datum* something given]
A fact, usually numerical, collected for research or reference.

data logging *np*
Information stored in a hearing aid regarding the wearing habits of the user, e.g., the number of hours worn and the volume control setting changes made by the user.

de- *prefix*
Remove, reverse, or reduce.

de Lange syndrome *np* *de* ˈlahrng*a*
Named after Cornelia de Lange(1871–1951), a Dutch pediatrician, who reported the syndrome in two unrelated children in 1933. She presented a third case in 1941. In fact, the syndrome had been described earlier (1916) by Winfred Robert Brachman (1888–1969), a German doctor. It was probably first described by Willem Vrolik (1801–1863), a Dutch anatomist and professor of anatomy and physiology at the Athenaeum Illustre in Amsterdam.
Also: bushy syndrome; Brachman de Lange syndrome
A developmental disorder characterized by distinctive facial appearance, slow growth, small stature, psychomotor delay, severe learning difficulties, skeletal abnormalities involving the upper extremities, and distinctive facial features (e.g., bushy eyebrows that meet in the middle [synophrys] and low set ears). There may be conductive and/or sensorineural hearing loss ranging from mild to severe.

dead *adj*
1. Having a short reverberation time. 2. Having no apparent life or function.

deaf *adj*
Unable to hear.

Deaf *adj*
Also: colloq big D Deaf
A cultural label referring to the community of those unable to hear who use sign language as their preferred mode of communication.

deaf-blind *adj*
Having both impaired hearing and impaired sight.

Deaf culture *np*
The beliefs, values, and traditions of communities of deaf people using sign languages as their main means of communication.

deafened *adj*
Becoming deaf after the acquisition of language due to accident, illness, etc.

deca- *prefix* [Gk *deka* ten]
Ten.

decade *n*
1. A logarithmic unit of frequency corresponding to a ratio of 10 to 1. 2. A period of 10 years.

decaPascal (daPa) *n*
A unit of pressure; 1 daPa equals 10 Pascals.

decay *n*
1. Gradual decrease in function or perception. 2. Fatigue or decrease in response to amplitude with continued stimulation. 3. Decrease in sound pressure level over time.

deci- *prefix* [Lat *decimus* tenth]
One tenth.

decibel (dB) *n* Named after Alexander Graham Bell (1847–1922), born in Scotland to a deaf mother and a father who taught speech to deaf people, who became a teacher of the deaf in Boston, Massachusetts, and later professor of the mechanism of speech at the University of Boston. In February 1876, both Alexander Graham Bell and Elisha Gray (1835–1901) had separately invented a telephone, but Alexander Graham Bell patented his first (by a few hours) and is therefore credited with the invention of the first telephone.
A unit of relative magnitude measured on a logarithmic scale, thus compressing large sound pressure differences into a manageable range of numbers. One decibel is equal to 1/10 Bel.

decibels hearing level (dBHL) *np*
A decibel scale referenced to accepted standards for average normal hearing.

decibels normalized hearing level (dBnHL) *np*
The decibel level referenced to the average behavioral threshold of a group of normal-hearing subjects.

decibels per decade *np*
The gradient on a graph of decibels versus frequency in decades.

decibels per octave *np*
The gradient on a graph of decibels versus frequency in octaves.

decibels sensation level (dBSL) *np*
A sound level value that is above and referenced to a subject's audiometric threshold.

decibels sound pressure level (dBSPL) *np*
A sound level that has 0.00002 Pa or 20 µPa as its reference pressure level.

decimation *n* [Lat *decimare* take a tenth]
In digital signal processing, a reduction of the original sampling rate. A technique used in noise shaping, where internal noise from an analog to digital converter is moved to frequencies above the audible frequency range.

decompression *n*
1. Reduction in atmospheric pressure. 2. The surgical reduction of pressure on a body part.

decongestant *n*
A drug that reduces nasal congestion.

decussate *adj/v* [Lat *decussare* to divide crosswise (from Lat *decussis* figure X, denoting 10)]
Crossing over/to cross over, particularly of the crossing over of the nerve fibers in the central nervous system.

dedicated *adj*
Used only for one thing.

deep *adj*
Far down.

deep brain stimulation (DBS) *np*
Electrical stimulation intended to alter brain function, delivered through an implanted probe.

deep canal fitting *np*
A hearing aid worn deep within the ear canal.

defender *n*
Also: ear muff; ear defender
Hearing protection that encloses the pinna.

degeneration *n*
Progressive deterioration and loss of function.

degree of hearing loss *np*
Hearing loss may be classified by its severity, i.e., mild, moderate, severe, or profound.

degrees of freedom (df) *np*
In statistics, independent values that are free to be varied.

dehiscence *n* dĭˈhĭsᴇns [Lat *dehiscere* gape open]
A gaping open, e.g., superior canal dehiscence, where bone is missing over the superior (top) semicircular canal.

Deiters cells *np* Named after Otto Freidrich Karl Deiters (1834–1863), a German neuroanatomist, who is known for giving a detailed description of a nerve cell. His great work, which included descriptions of the cells of Deiters, was published posthumously in 1865.
Also: phalangeal cells

Finger-like supporting cells that rest on the basilar membrane.

delay *n*
Stopped, hindered, or slowed for a time, e.g., speech or language delay.

delayed auditory feedback test *np*
A speech listening test, sometimes used in cases of nonorganic hearing loss, in which the individual's voice is fed back to him/her with a time delay of about 100 ms. If the feedback is above the individual's threshold of hearing, it will cause stuttering.

dementia *n* [Lat *demens* out of one's mind]
A progressive decline of cognitive function in a previously unaffected person.

demyelinating *adj* [Lat *de-* decrease + Gk *muelos* bone marrow]
Destruction of the myelin sheath surrounding nerve fibers. If affecting the auditory nerve, it results in retrocochlear hearing loss.

dendrite *n* [Gk *dendrites* tree-like]
A filament of a neuron that conducts impulses to a cell body.

density *n*
The ratio of mass to unit volume.

dental *adj* [Lat *dens* tooth]
Formed with the tip of the tongue toward the back of the teeth, as in the production of the speech sounds "t" and "d."

deoxyribonucleic acid (DNA) *np*
Various nucleic acids, located in the cell nucleus, that form the molecular basis of heredity.

dependent variable *np*
An aspect in an experiment or study that is affected by the action of another (independent) variable.

depolarization (depolarisation) *n*
A sudden decrease in the electrical potential from a large negative value to a lesser negative value in a cell.

depression *n*
A persistent low mood that interferes with normal functioning.

deprivation *n*
A lack of or being deprived from.

deprivation, auditory *np*
A lack of sound stimuli over time. 1. Auditory deprivation in early childhood may cause permanent changes in the auditory pathways, making the child less able to process auditory information. 2. Auditory deprivation in adults is a decrease in ability to hear in an ear that has been unaided. Full or partial recovery may occur when binaurally aided.

deprivation effect *np*
Reduced auditory performance associated with deprivation.

derecruitment *n*
A condition, in which increasing intensity results in a slower than normal loudness growth.

derm- *prefix* [Gk *derma* skin]
Skin.

dermal *adj*
Pertaining to the skin.

dermatitis *n*
Inflammation of the skin.

descending method *np*
A method of finding hearing threshold by reducing the signal intensity until the signal is no longer heard.

desired sensation level (DSL) method *np* Developed by Richard Seewald (b 1946), a pediatric audiologist and distinguished professor emeritus at the University of Western Ontario. The method was first published in 1985.
A method designed for prescribing the amount of amplification required when fitting hearing aids to infants and children. It calculates the level above the threshold of hearing needed to amplify speech to an audible level across the frequency range.

desquamation *n* dĕskwaʹmāshon [Lat *desquamare* remove scales from]
The process of shedding the outer layer of skin.

destructive surgery *np*
Medical intervention to destroy an organ or body part, e.g., vestibular nerve section may be used to stop the flow of balance information to the brain in some cases of severe vertigo.

desynchronize (desynchronise) *np* [Lat *de-* decrease + Gk *sunkhronos* occurring at the same time]
To cause to occur at unrelated times.

detection *n*
The determination of the presence of a signal.

detection differential *np*
The amount by which the signal exceeds the noise level for any specific listener and condition.

detection threshold *np*
The signal level that is just audible.

developmental *adj*
Associated with a stage or process in the maturation of the body.

developmental age *np*
The age at which children normally acquire certain skills.

deviated septum *np* [Lat *deviare* to deviate; Lat *septum* a fence]
The condition in which the cartilage in the nose, which should be central and divide the nostrils evenly, leans to one side.

dextr- *prefix* [Lat *dexter* right]
To the right.

di- *prefix* [Gk *dis* twice]
Two or twice.

dia- *prefix* [Gk *dia* through]
Through or across.

diabetes *n* [Gk *diabetes* siphon (from Gk *diabainein* go through)]
Usually used to refer to diabetes mellitus, a metabolic disorder of carbohydrate metabolism in which sugars are not oxy-

dized due to lack of insulin, and appear in the blood and urine.

diabetes insipidus *np* [Gk *diabetes* siphon; Lat *insipidus* without taste]
A condition in which the kidneys cannot conserve water because of damage to the thalamus or the pituitary gland.

diabetes mellitus *np* [Gk *diabetes* siphon; Lat *mellitus* honeyed, sweet]
A condition caused by insulin deficiency. Type 1 is due to the production of insufficient insulin by the body. Type 2 is due to the body's inability to use insulin effectively.

diabetes mellitus optic atrophy and deafness (DIDMOAD) *np* [Gk *diabetes* siphon; Lat *mellitus* honeyed, sweet; Gk *optikos* pertaining to the eyes; Gk *-a* without + Gk *trophe* nourishment]
Also: Wolfram syndrome
A progressive neurodegenerative syndrome that includes sensorineural hearing loss and visual impairment with diabetes mellitus and diabetes insipidus. There may also be other features, e.g., limited joint mobility and heart malformations. Onset is usually in late childhood or early adulthood.

diacritic *adj* [Gk *diakritikos* distinguishing (mark)]
A mark near or through a character used to distinguish different sounds, e.g., indicating which syllable to stress.

diagnostic *adj* [Gk *diagignoskein* discern, discover]
Serving to discover or identify the site or cause of a problem.
Deriv: –n diagnosis

dialect *n* [Gk *dialektos* way of speaking]
A form of spoken language used in a specific geographical area.

diaphragm *n* [Gk *dia* through + Gk *phragma* fence]
1. A thin circular sheet in a microphone or earphone that is the sound reception or production element. 2. A thin partition that separates two areas. 3. A muscular membranous partition separating the abdominal and thoracic cavities.

diastrophic dwarfism *np* [Gk *dia* through + Gk *strophe* turn]
A recessive craniofacial disorder, characterized by short stature, deformed hands, and club feet. The pinnae develop multiple cystic swellings that may become calcified. Hearing loss may be associated and is typically congenital and sensorineural.

diathesis *n* dĭ'ăthĭsĭs [Gk *diathesis* disposition]
A tendency, often familial, to develop a specific disease or disorder.

dichlorphenamide *n*
A diuretic used to treat glaucoma.

dichotic *adj* dĭ'kŏtĭk [Gk *dikho* apart + Gk *ous* ear]
1. Divided into two parts. 2. Where a different signal is presented to each ear simultaneously.

Dickinson syndrome *np* Named after William Howship Dickinson (1832–1913), an English physician and medical writer, who reported familial albuminurea (a sign of kidney damage in Dickinson syndrome) in 1875.
Also: Alport syndrome; deafness nephropathy
A syndrome that is characterized by progressive kidney disease, sensorineural hearing loss, and visual difficulties. It mostly affects males.

dicyclomine *n*
A drug that reduces muscle spasms. Side effects may include dizziness and vomiting.

dielectric *adj* [Gk *dia* through + Gk *elektron* amber (which causes electrostatic effects when rubbed)]
An insulating medium through which electricity may pass by induction, but not by conduction.

diencephalon *n* dĭĕn'sĕ'fălŏn [Gk *dia* through + Gk *en* in + Gk *enkephalos* brain]

The posterior part of the forebrain consisting of the epithalamus, thalamus, hypothalamus, and ventral thalamus. It serves as a relay and integration center for sensory input to the cortex.

difference limen (DL) *np* 'līmen [Lat *limen* threshold]
Also: just noticeable difference (JND); difference threshold; differential threshold
The minimum detectable change in a stimulus (50% of the time), e.g., the smallest detectable change in intensity of a pure tone.

difference tone *np*
A combination tone created when two primary tones are sounded simultaneously. Its frequency will be the difference between the two primary tones, e.g., for primary tones of 1 kHz and 1.1 kHz, the difference tone is 100 Hz.

differential *adj*
1. Showing or depending on a distinctive difference. 2. Producing an effect because of quantitative differences, e.g., in voltage or pressure.

differential amplifier *np*
An amplifier with two inputs that subtracts the voltage of one from the other, and then increases the amplitude of the voltage difference.

differential diagnosis *np*
The process of distinguishing one condition from other conditions with similar signs and symptoms.

differential threshold *np*
Also: difference limen; just noticeable difference; difference threshold
The minimum detectable change in a stimulus (50% of the time), e.g., the smallest detectable change in intensity of a pure tone.

diffraction *n* [Lat *diffringere* break in pieces]
A change in direction of a sound wave after meeting an object in its path.

diffuse field *np* [Lat *diffusus* scattered]
A sound field with uniform energy density and random direction of propagation.

DiGeorge syndrome *np* Named after Angelo M. DiGeorge (1921–2009), a professor of pediatrics at Temple University in Philadelphia, Pennyslvania, who first described the syndrome in 1968.
Also: velocardiofacial syndrome; conotruncal anomaly face syndrome; 22q 11.2 deletion syndrome
A rare (1 in 4000 live births) syndrome that is genetic in only about 10% of cases. The signs and symptoms are very variable and may include congenital heart defects, cleft palate, an asymmetric crying face, poor growth, autism, skeletal abnormalities, e.g., spinal problems and extra fingers and toes, and external ear abnormalities. The syndrome is due to the deletion of a small amount of genetic material in on the short or q arm of chromosome 22.

digital *adj* [Lat *digitus* finger]
Operating on numeric data.

digital signal processing (DSP) *np*
Conversion of an analog input to a binary stream of ones and zeroes representing signal amplitude and subsequent manipulation of the signal using mathematical algorithms.

digitally programmed hearing aid *np*
A hearing aid that is programmed via a computer.

dihydrostreptomycin *n*
An ototoxic antibiotic (a hydrogenated form of streptomycin) that can cause permanent sensorineural deafness and which used to be used to treat tuberculosis.

dilation *n* [Lat *dilatare* spread out]
Enlargement.

diltiazem *n* dĭl'tī*az*ĕm
A calcium antagonist (i.e., a substance that reduces the intake of calcium into the cells, especially of the heart and arteries) used in the treatment of angina and high blood pressure.

dimeric tympanic membrane *adj* [Gk *dis* twice + Gk *meros* part]
A thin area on the eardrum, having an abnormal appearance, where the elastic layer has not regrown following perforation.

dimethisterone *n*
A synthetic sex hormone used to treat disorders of the womb lining.

dimorphic *adj* [Gk *dis* twice + Gk *morphe* form]
Having two forms.

dioctyl sodium sulphosuccinate *np*
A softening agent sometimes used in solutions to soften ear wax.

diode *n* [Gk *dis* twice + Gk *odos* way]
A two terminal electronic component that allows current flow in one direction only.

diotic *adj* [Gk *dis* twice + Gk *ous* ear]
Where an identical signal is presented to both ears simultaneously.

diphasic *adj* [Gk *dis* twice + Gk *phasis* appearance]
In or having two phases, e.g., electrical variation consisting of one positive and one negative stage, or a disorder that fluctuates between two distinct phases, e.g., diphasic nystagmus, also called biphasic nystagmus.

diphenhydramine *n*
A sedating antihistamine used to treat motion sickness.

diphenyl hydantoin *np*
An anticonvulsant drug

diphthong *n* [Gk *dis* twice + Gk *phthongos* sound]
A gliding vowel consisting of two sounds, e.g., as in "eye."

diplacusis *n* dĭplaˈkyūsĭs [Gk *diplos* double + Gk *akousis* sense of hearing]
Also: diplacusia
A condition in which the same tone presented to both ears appears to be a different pitch in each ear.

diplacusis, monaural *np* [Gk *monos* single + Lat *auris* ear]
A condition in which a tone applied to one ear is perceived as two sounds.

diplegia *n* dĭˈplēja (dĭˈplējēa) [Gk *dis* twice + Gk *plege* stroke]
Paralysis of corresponding parts of both sides of the body, most commonly the legs.

direct *adj*
1. Open, without the effect of any boundaries. 2. In one direction.

direct audio input *np*
A direct connection between a hearing aid and an external sound source, e.g., the television.

direct current (DC) *np*
An electric current that flows continuously in one direction.

direct field *np*
The part of the sound field where the sound pressure level of the free field is greater than that of the diffuse field.

directional *adj*
Having sensitivity or tendency greatest in one direction.

directivity factor *np*
The ratio of sounds incident at 0° to random sounds incident from around an imaginary sphere.

directivity index *np*
The directivity factor converted to decibels.

dis- *prefix* [Lat *dis-* expressing separation or negation]
Deprive of, exclude or expel from, opposite or absence of.

disability *n*
Restriction of ability to perform an activity; a disqualification, restriction, or disadvantage.

disablement *n*
A measure of disability, usually for the purpose of compensation.

disarticulation *n*
A separation of two bones at a joint, e.g., of the ossicular chain.

discharge rate *np*
The rate at which a neuron is able to fire.

discomfort level *np*
Also: uncomfortable loudness level (ULL/UCL)
The sound level at which the listener begins to experience discomfort. The preferred term is uncomfortable loudness level (ULL).

discordance *n* [Lat *discors* discordant (from Lat *dis-* expressing negation + *cor* heart)]
1. A mix of sounds not in harmony. 2. The presence of a given genetic trait in only one sibling of a twin set.

discourse *n* [Lat *discursus* argument (from Lat *discurrere* run to and fro)]
A written or oral communication.

discourse, connected *np*
Continuous speech, used in speech audiometry where a talker reads a passage.

discrete *adj*
Individually distinct. Not part of a continuous spectrum, e.g., discrete frequencies are represented by separate lines in a line spectrum.

discrimination *n* [Lat *discriminare* to discriminate]
1. Ability to differentiate one sound from another. 2. Unfair behavior toward members of a group, in comparison with other groups.

discrimination loss *np*
The difference between an individual's word recognition score and 100%.

disease *n*
An illness; a condition of the body that disturbs normal function.

disequilibrium *n*
A disturbance in balance function.

disorder *n*
A disturbance or abnormality of bodily or mental function, e.g., a speech disorder is any difficulty with the production and/or reception of linguistic units.

dispense *v* [Lat *dispendere* to dispense, weigh out]
To prescribe and distribute.

dispersion *n* [Lat *dispergere* to scatter]
1. A change in the speed of sound with frequency. 2. A measure of the scatter or variability in a set of scores, e.g., range and standard deviation.

dissipate *v* [Lat *dissipare* to scatter]
1. To disperse; to lose intensity as sound energy travels over time and distance. 2. To convert sound energy to heat.

dissonance *n* [Lat *dis-* expressing negation + Lat *sonare* to sound]
The quality of being harsh and inharmonious, lack of agreement.

distal *adj*
Situated away from the origin or center.

distance index *np*
An index that compares a directional microphone to an omnidirectional microphone and indicates the increase in distance away from the sound source possible while maintaining the same signal-to-noise ratio.

distinctive *adj*
Differentiating.

distinctive feature *np*
The element of a phoneme that differentiates it from another phoneme, e.g., the place of articulation.

distortion *n*
Also: noise
Unwanted changes in waveform.

distortion, amplitude *np*
Undesired changes in a sound wave pattern occuring when an output signal is not proportionate to the input signal in an amplifying system.

distortion, frequency *np*
When different frequency components of an input signal undergo unequal degrees of amplification in a system or device.

distortion, harmonic *np*
The occurrence of additional whole number multiples (harmonic components) in a sound wave's frequencies.

distortion, intermodulation *np*
Distortion that occurs when two or more signals are passed through a nonlinear system. Additional frequencies are present in the output that are equal to the sums and differences of those frequencies already present.

distortion product *np*
Acoustic energy that occurs when two pure tones are presented to the cochlea at the same time.

distortion product, otoacoustic emission (DPOAE) *np*
Also: colloq cochlear echoes; Kemp echoes
Tiny sounds produced by the outer hair cells. These can be recorded in the ear canals of most normal ears.

distraction *n*
Prevention from concentrating.

distraction testing *np*
Manipulating a child's attention while test sounds are presented and observing if they turn toward the test sounds.

distribution *n*
Grouping of data into categories.

distribution, normal *np*
A frequency graph in which most scores are clustered in the mid range, with a tail at each end of the highest and lowest scores. This produces a bell-shaped curve.

diuretic *n* dīyer'rĕtĭk [Gk *diouretikos* pertaining to urination]
Also: colloq water tablets
A drug that increases the production of urine, generally by inhibiting the reabsorption of sodium in the kidney. Some diuretics are ototoxic.

Dix-Hallpike maneuver (manoeuvre) *np*
A diagnostic maneuver used to identify benign paroxysmal positional vertigo (BPPV).

dizygotic *adj* [Gk *dis* twice + Gk *zygotos* yoked]
Formed by twinned but separately fertilised eggs, i.e., fraternal twins.

DNA *np abbr*
Also: deoxyribonucleic acid

Doerfler-Stewart test *np* dūfle-styūwert
Named after Leo G. Doerfler (1919–2004), an American audiologist, and K.C. Stewart, who published the test in 1946.
A test that may be used in cases of suspected nonorganic hearing loss (malingering). The test involves presenting speech with masking. The malingerer may incorrectly assume the level of masking used would interfere with hearing speech and therefore stop repeating the test words.

domiciliary *adj* [Lat *domus* house]
Relating to, or occurring at, the home, e. g., domiciliary visits are those made to a home or residence.

Doppler effect *np* Named after Christian J. Doppler (1803–1853), an Austrian-American mathematician and physicist, who showed how frequency appears to shift when the source is in motion relative to the listener (and vice versa).
The apparent change in the pitch of a sound when the source passes a listener at speed. Pitch increases when the sound approaches and decreases as the sound moves away.

dorsal *adj* [Lat *dorsum* back]
Posterior; toward the backbone.

dosemeter/dosimeter *n* dō'sĭmĭter [Gk *dosis* giving, gift + Gk *metron* measure]
A personal sound level meter worn by the individual to provide a measure of the noise exposure over a period of time.

double-blind *adj*
Where two test conditions are administered and neither the subjects nor the examiner know under which test condition the subject is operating.

double hearing protection *np*
The use of earplugs under ear muffs used for very high noise exposure. This provides an additional 3 dB of protection.

down sampling *np*
Also: subsampling
The process of reducing the sampling rate of a signal. This is usually done to reduce the data rate or the size of the data.

Down syndrome *np* Named after John Langdon Down (1828–1896), a London surgeon, who described this syndrome and termed it "mongolism." The World Health Organization officially dropped the term "monogolism" in 1965.
Also: trisomy 21; *obs* mongolism
A congenital genetic disorder characterized by learning difficulty, certain physical features including distinctive facial features (such as slanting eyes, square-shaped face, and macroglossia [large tongue]), and a high incidence of conductive and sensorineural hearing loss.

downward spread of masking *np*
The masking of low-frequency sound by intense high-frequency sound.

drain *n*
1. In a hearing aid, the amount of current drawn from the battery. 2. A surgical tube and/or valve to allow fluid to flow out of the body, e.g., sometimes used in cases of Ménière disorder to drain excess endolymph and reduce pressure.

drainage *n*
The drawing off of fluid, e.g., fluid from the middle ear.

drift *n*
A slow continuous change.

drop attack *np*
Sudden loss of balance without loss of consciousness, usually seen in elderly women.

Duane syndrome/Duane retraction syndrome *np* dwān (dūw'ān) Named after Alexander Duane (1858–1926), an American ophthalmologist, who contributed to the study of the eye and vision and analyzed the movement of the eye muscles. He discussed this syndrome in detail in 1905.
A congenital genetic disorder that limits the movement of the eye due to paralysis of cranial nerve VI. The eye disorder may be the only disorder, but it may also be accompanied by fusion of the neck vertebrae and malformations of the external and middle ears. A congenital nonprogressive conductive or sensorineural hearing loss may be present.

duct *n* [Lat *ductus* duct, passage]
A passage.

duct of Hensen/ductus reuniens *np* [Lat *ductus* duct, passage; Lat *reuniens* joining together] Named after Christian Andreas Viktor Hensen (1835–1924), a German zoologist and professor of physiology at the University of Kiel, who studied the organs of hearing and described the ductus reuniens and the supporting cells in the organ of Corti.
Also: Reichert canal
A short membranous tube in the inner ear that connects the scala media in the cochlea with the saccule of the vestibular system.

dura mater *np* 'dyur*a* 'māt*a* ('dur*a* 'māt*a*) [Lat *dura mater* hard material]
The fibrous membrane surrounding the brain and spinal cord.

duty cycle *np*
The time a signal is on compared with the total time on and off, usually given as a percentage.

dyacusis *n* [Gk *dus-* bad + Gk *akousis* sense of hearing]
Also: dysacusia/dysacusis
1. A disturbance in the perception of sound quality, pitch, or loudness (but not primarily a loss of hearing level), resulting in a distortion of hearing. 2. A condition in which ordinary sounds cause discomfort or pain.

dynamic *adj* [Gk *dunamis* power]
Not steady state.

dynamic microphone *np* [Gk *dunamis* power; Gk *mikros* small + Gk *phone* sound]
A microphone that uses electromagnetic induction.

dynamic range *np*
1. The full range of operation, maximum to minimum, usually expressed in dB. 2. The difference between threshold and the uncomfortable loudness level, usually expressed in dBHL. 3. An electrical measure of the difference between the threshold level and the comfort level, obtained via a cochlear implant.

dyne *n obs* [Gk *dunamis* power]
A unit of force. The force needed to accelerate 1 gm to a velocity of 1 cm per second.

dys- *prefix* [Gk *dus-* bad, difficult]
Poor.

dysacusia/dysacusis *n* [Gk *dus-* bad + Gk *akousis* sense of hearing]
Also: dyacusis
1. A disturbance in the perception of sound quality, pitch, or loudness (but not primarily a loss of hearing level), resulting in a distortion of hearing. 2. A condition in which ordinary sounds cause discomfort or pain.

dysarthria *n* [Gk *dus-* bad + Gk *arthron* joint, articulation]
A neurologic condition affecting the motor functioning of speech production.

dyschondrosteosis *n* dĭs̆'k̆ŏndr̆ŏst̄ēōs̄ĭs [Gk *dus-* bad + Gk *khondros* cartilege + Gk *-osis* denoting a diseased state]

Also: Madelung disease; Leri-Weill syndrome; multiple symmetric lipomatosis (MSL)
A bone dysplasia, characterized by an uncommon congenital wrist deformity (known as Madelung deformity), fat deposits at the neck, and short stature. Conductive hearing loss may also be present.

dyscrasia *n* [Gk *dus-* bad + Gk *krasis* mixture (of the humors, which would cause a diseased state)]
A diseased state.

dysfunction *n* [Gk *dus-* bad + Lat *fungere* to function]
An inability to function normally.
Deriv: –adj dysfunctional

dysgenesis *n* [Gk *dus-* bad + Gk *genesis* generation, creation]
1. Lack of or partial fertility. 2. Abnormal development of an organ.

dysgeusia *n* dĭ's̆juz̄ēa [Gk *dus-* bad + Gk *geusis* taste]
Impairment of the sense of taste.

dysgraphia *n* [Gk *dus-* bad + Gk *graphia* writing]
An inability to write, with poor handwriting and often an inability to express thoughts in the written form.

dyslexia *n* [Gk *dus-* bad + Gk *lexis* speech; by confusion with Lat *legere* to read]
A neurologic disorder causing difficulty in reading, writing, and spelling.

dyslexia, phonological *np*
A reading disorder in which a person can read by the whole word method, but is unable to identify the individual sounds within words.

dyslexia, surface *np*
A reading disorder in which a person can read phonetically, but has difficulty reading irregularly spelled words by whole word recognition.

dysmorphic *adj* [Gk *dus-* bad + Gk *morphos* shape]
Malformed.

dysphagia *n* [Gk *dus-* bad + Gk *phagia* swallowing]
Difficulty swallowing.

dysosmia *n* [Gk *dus-* bad + Gk *osme* sense of smell]
Also: parosamia
A disorder of smell or olfaction.

dysostosis *n* [Gk *dus-* bad + Gk *osteon* bone + Gk *-osis* denoting a diseased state]
Defective or incomplete bone ossification, especially of fetal cartilage.

dysphasia *n* [Gk *dusphatos* difficult to utter]
A neurologic condition impairing communication, including difficulty in speech production.

dysphemia *n* dĭsfīmīa [Gk *dus-* bad + Gk *phemi* I speak]
A speech disorder of psychological origin characterized by stammering or stuttering.

dysphonia *n* [Gk *dus-* bad + Gk *phone* sound]
A disorder of vocal cord function or respiration that impairs speech production.

dysplastic *adj* [Gk *dus-* bad + Gk *plasis* formation]
Misshapen, characterized by abnormal growth of tissues or organs.
Deriv: –n dysplasia

dysprosody *n* [Gk *dus-* bad + Gk *prosoidia* tone of a syllable (from Gk *pros* toward + Gk *oide* song)]
An impairment of suprasegmental features of speech, e.g., stress, intonation, etc.

dyssynchrony *n* [Gk *dus-* bad + Gk *sunchronos* happening at the same time]
Also: auditory neuropathy (AN)
A disorder in which responses to non-speech sounds are normal, but the ability to decode speech and language is impaired.

dystonia *n* [Gk *dus-* bad + Gk *tonos* tone]
Impaired muscle tone of one or more muscles.

dystrophy *n* [Gk *dus-* bad + Gk *trophe* nourishment]
A wasting disorder due to defective nutrition, e.g., muscular dystrophy.

ear *n*
The organ of hearing.

earache *n*
Also: otalgia
Pain in the ear.

ear advantage *np*
Dominance of one ear over the other.

ear canal *np*
Also: external auditory/acoustic meatus
The passage between the pinna and the eardrum.

ear canal resonance *np*
The constructive enhancement of sound, by about 10 dB at frequencies between 2.5 and 3.5 KHz. that occurs in the ear canal.

ear candle *np*
Hollow candle used as a home remedy for wax removal. The method is ineffective for wax removal and can be dangerous.

ear defender *np*
Also: earmuff; defender
Ear protection that encloses the pinna.

eardrum *n colloq*
The common term for the tympanic membrane, which is a thin, semitransparent membrane separating the external ear from the middle ear.

ear, external *np*
The part of the ear that is normally visible, i.e., the pinna and ear canal.

ear hook *np*
Also: elbow
The part of a behind-the-ear hearing aid that hooks over the pinna and connects to earmold tubing.

ear impression *np*
A cast of the concha used to make an earmold or hearing aid shell.

ear insert *np*
A device to direct sound from an earphone into the ear canal.

ear light *np*
Also: otolight; otoprobe
A handheld probe with a battery-powered light, used for the insertion of an otoblock into the ear canal.

ear lobe *np*
The small lobule at the bottom of the pinna that contains fat but no cartilage.

earmold (earmould) *np*
A device fitted within the outer ear and connected to a behind-the-ear hearing aid by means of tubing that channels amplified sound into the ear.

earmold (earmould) acoustics *np*
The influence of an earmold on a hearing aid's frequency response.
Deriv: colloq earmold plumbing

earmold (earmould), custom *np*
An earmold made from an individual's ear impression.

earmold (earmould) plumbing *np colloq*
Also: earmold acoustics
The influence of an earmold on a hearing aid's frequency response.

earmold (earmould), skeleton *np*
Also: ear defender
An earmold in which the central concha portion has been cut away.

earmuff *n*
Also: ear defender
Ear protection that encloses the pinna.

ear, nose, and throat (ENT) *np*
Also: otolaryngology; otology; otorhinolaryngology
The medical specialty that deals with the diagnosis and treatment of diseases of the ear, nose, and throat.

earphone *n*
An electroacoustic transducer fitting into or over the ear, which converts electrical signals from equipment such as media players and telephones into audible sound.

earpiece *n*
An earmold for a hearing aid or an earphone.

ear pip *np*
1. A small ready-made ear insert. 2. A short duration tone burst.

ear plug *np*
A device made from pliable material designed to fit into the ear canal to block the entry of sound, water, or foreign objects.

ear plug, musician's *np*
An ear plug that attenuates sounds equally across the frequency range to ensure sound clarity is maintained at a reduced, safer volume.

ear protector *np*
Generic term for devices designed to shield the ear from loud sounds or water, including earmuffs and helmets.

ear simulator *np*
A device used to calibrate air conduction audiometry earphones, designed to simulate the acoustic impedance of the average human ear.

ear trumpet *np*
A nonelectric trumpet-shaped device designed to amplify sound by collecting it and directing it to the ear canal.

ear wax *np*
A protective waxy secretion produced by the glands (ceruminous, sebaceous, and apocrine) in the outer part of the ear canal.

early *adj*
Occurring relatively near the beginning.

early childhood intervention *np*
A support system for families who have a child with a developmental disability or delay, to ensure they receive the required resources to maximize their child's development.

early intervention *np*
Assessment and habilitation provided as soon as possible after diagnosis or intervention, especially for children under 2 years of age, to facilitate normal speech and language development and prevent further developmental delays.

early latency response *np*
The classification of auditory evoked potentials that occur within a few milliseconds following the auditory signal generated by the cochlea, e.g., an electrocochleogram or cochlear microphonic.

ec- *prefix* [Gk *ek* out of]
Out of.

echo *n* *pl* echoes [Gk *ekho* echo]
A delayed return of sound, perceived as a repetition of the original sound produced by reflected waves.

echoacousia *n* [Gk *ekho* echo + Gk *akousis* sense of hearing]
The subjective perception of echoes when sound has ceased.

echogram *n* [Gk *ekho* echo + Gk *gramma* a written thing]
A record of the very early reverberatory decay of sound in a room.

echolalia *n* ĕkō'lālēa [Gk *ekho* echo + Gk *lalia* speech]
1. The meaningless involuntary repetition of someone else's words or phrases. 2. Imitation of speech patterns by a child that is learning to speak.

ecto- *prefix* [Gk *ektos* outside]
On the outer side.

ectodermal *adj* [Gk *ektos* outside + Gk *derma* skin]
The outer layer of the embryo at the earliest stage that divides into layers of cells that will form the various parts of the body.

ectodermal abnormalities *np*
Disorders, including many syndromes with hearing loss, that occur due to abnormalities in the outer layer of the embryo during development.

ectodermal dysplasia *np* [Gk *ektos* outside + Gk *derma* skin; Gk *dus-* bad + Gk *plasis* formation]
Also: Marshall syndrome; lobster-claw syndrome; saddle nose and myopia
A rare genetic pigmentary disorder characterized by distinctive facial features

that include a flattened nasal bridge, up-turned nose and widely spaced eyes, also lobster-claw deformity of hands and feet, nearsightedness, cataracts, and congenital progressive moderate-to-severe sensorineural, conductive, or mixed hearing loss and poor vestibular function.

-ectomy *suffix* [Gk *ektome* excision]
Surgical removal.

ectopic *adj* [Gk *ek* outside + Gk *topos* place]
Located away from the normal position, e.g., ectopic carotid artery in the middle ear.

eczema *n* [Gk *ekzema* a boiling over]
A noninfectious inflammatory skin condition characterized by itching, reddening, and vesicle formation. Can occur on the pinna or in the ear canal.

edema (oedema) *n* ĕ̄'dēmᴀ [Gk *oedema* swelling]
The presence of excessive fluid in, around, or discharging from body cells or tissue.

educational audiologist *np*
A specialized audiologist working in an educational setting.

Edwards syndrome *np* Named after John Hilton Edwards (1928–2007), a British geneticist and professor of human genetics at the University of Birmingham, who is credited with the first description of this syndrome in 1960.
Also: trisomy 18
A genetic disorder caused by the presence of three copies of chromosome 18. Characteristics include microcephaly (abnormally small head) with triangular shape due to prominent chin, undernourished appearance, heart disease, renal abnormalities, cleft lip, malformed ears, and learning difficulty.

effective *adj*
1. Having a desired result or outcome. 2. Real world, e.g., an effective compression ratio utilizes real world stimuli.

effective masking *np*
The minimum level of masking noise that will just mask a given signal.

effective masking level *np*
The masking noise level that is equal to the hearing level of a pure tone at the same frequency.

efferent *adj* [Lat *efferre* to carry out]
Pertaining to the neural pathway from higher to lower level, i.e., carrying nerve impulses away from the central nervous system to muscles or glands.

efficacy *n* [Lat *efficere* to achieve, accomplish]
The capacity to produce a desired effect.

effusion *n* [Lat *effundere* to pour out]
1. Escape of fluid 2. Fluid that has escaped.

egocentric speech *np* [Lat *ego* I + Lat *centrum* center]
The speech that young children use to themselves during their play. It is not intended as a form of communication and dies out as the child develops social communication.

eighth cranial nerve *np*
Also: CN VIII
The auditory and vestibular nerves (vestibulocochlear nerve), responsible for transmitting vestibular and auditory information from the ear to the brain.

elastic *adj* [Gk *elastikos* stretchable]
Being able to return to the original shape.

elbow, hearing aid *np*
Also: ear hook
The part of a behind-the-ear hearing aid that hooks over the pinna and connects to earmold tubing.

electret microphone *np*
A type of condenser microphone that utilizes permanently polarized dielectric material. Widely used in hearing aids.

electric and acoustic stimulation (EAS) *np*
The use of natural hearing (usually low

frequency) and a cochlear implant in the same ear.

electric response audiometry (ERA) *np*
Measurement of auditory function using acoustic signals to evoke electrical potentials that are measured to give information about hearing function and the site of lesion.

electrical potential *np*
A difference in electrical charge measured between two electrodes.

electro- *prefix* [Gk *elektron* amber (which causes electrostatic effects when rubbed)] Pertaining to electricity.

electroacoustic *adj*
Pertaining to an electrical or electronic method used to amplify, generate, or measure acoustic signals.

electrocochleogram *n* elĕctrōˈkŏklēō-grăm (elĕctrōˈkŏklēōgrăm) [Gk *elektron* amber (which causes electrostatic effects when rubbed) + Lat *cochlea* snail shell, spiral + Gk *gramma* written thing]
A graph that shows the magnitude of the summating potential, cochlear microphonic and action potential on the vertical axis, and time on the horizontal axis.

electrocochleography (ECoG/ECochG) *np* [Gk *elektron* amber (which causes electrostatic effects when rubbed) + Lat *cochlea* snail shell, spiral + Gk *graphos* writing]
Evoked response audiometry where an electrode is placed on the cochlear promontory or in the ear canal to enable auditory evoked potentials to be recorded from the cochlea and eighth cranial nerve.

electrode *n* [Gk *elektron* amber (which causes electrostatic effects when rubbed) + Gk *hodos* way]
A conductor through which electrical energy is applied to or measured from the body. Electrodes are arranged in pairs for recording electric potential changes. One pair of electrodes, consisting of an active and reference electrode, makes up a channel.

electrode, active *np*
The positive or noninverting electrode that is placed nearest to the site of activity being recorded and which determines the potential at that position, e.g., in auditory brainstem response audiometry the active electrode may be attached to the ipsilateral mastoid, behind the ear receiving the signal.

electrode anomalies *np*
Problems with the electrodes of a cochlear implant.

electrode array *np*
An arrangement of electrodes, e.g., a cochlear implant uses a multiple electrode array.

electrode, bipolar *np*
A system of electrodes in which the contacts are adjacent. When current is passed through, it passes between the pair of contacts. Electrodes are symmetrical.

electrode, common *np*
The ground electrode (earth) used in electrophysiologic measurement, e.g., in auditory brainstem response audiometry, the common electrode may be placed on the contralateral mastoid.

electrode, extratympanic *np*
An electrode resting against the ear canal, skin, or tympanic membrane surface. Used in electrocochleography.

electrode, hybrid *np*
A small thin electrode that may be used in cochlear implantation in an attempt to retain the residual hearing. Hybrid refers to the aim of using electrical and auditory stimulation to the same ear.

electrode impedance *np*
Opposition to the flow of current at the interface between the scalp and the electrode. Electrode impedance refers to AC current and is numerically equal to electrode resistance, which refers to DC current.

electrode, recording configuration *np*
The placement pattern of electrodes used, e.g., during electrophysiologic measurements.

electrode, reference *np*
The inverting, indifferent, or dispersive electrode. An electrode placed away from the source of recorded activity so that its potential is assumed to be negligible, e.g., in auditory brainstem response audiometry, the reference electrode may be placed on the vertex (forehead).

electrode, surface *np*
An electrode that is placed on the surface of the skin, e.g., electrodes used in auditory brainstem response audiometry.

electrode, transtympanic *np*
An electrode inserted through the eardrum and placed in the middle ear, on the cochlear promontory. Used in electrocochleography.

electrodermal *adj* [Gk *elektron* amber (which causes electrostatic effects when rubbed) + Gk *derma* skin]
Pertaining to the measurement of electrical properties of the skin, with reference to changes in resistance.

electrodermal audiometry *np*
Pertaining to the measurement of electrodermal responses to sound following conditioning.

electrodynamic *adj* [Gk *elektron* amber (which causes electrostatic effects when rubbed) + Gk *dunamis* power]
Pertaining to the force excited by one magnetic current on another.

electroencephalography (EEG) *n* elĕk'trōĕnsĕfălŏgrafē [Gk *elektron* amber (which causes electrostatic effects when rubbed) + Gk *en* in + Gk *kephalos* head + Gk *graphos* writing]
The recording of background electrical activity from the brain.

electrolyte *n* [Gk *elektron* amber (which causes electrostatic effects when rubbed) + Gk *lutos* released]

A solution that is capable of conducting an electric current.

electromagnet *n*
A piece of iron surrounded by a coil of wire through which an electric current is passed that renders the iron temporarily magnetic.
Deriv: -adj electromagnetic

electromagnetic field *np*
An area in which electrically induced magnetic changes occur. These changes can be picked up by the induction coil in a hearing aid.

electromechanical *adj*
1. Pertaining to the application of electricity to a mechanical process. 2. Pertaining to the conversion of electrical energy to mechanical energy.

electromotility *n* [Gk *elektron* amber (which causes electrostatic effects when rubbed) + Lat *motus* motion]
The movement that occurs in the outer hair cells, located in the cochlea of the inner ear, in response to electrical stimulation.

electronystagmography (ENG) *n* elĕk'trōnĭstagmŏgrafē [Gk *elektron* amber (which causes electrostatic effects when rubbed) + Gk *nustagmos* nodding, blinking, drowsiness + Gk *graphos* writing]
A battery of tests used to assess the vestibular system. Small electrodes are placed on the skin to facilitate recording and analyzing eye movements while following a moving target.

electrooculography (EOG) *n* elĕk'trōŏkyūlŏgrafē [Gk *elektron* amber (which causes electrostatic effects when rubbed) + Lat *oculus* eye + Gk *graphos* writing]
The recording of changes in electrical activity caused by eye movements. Used as the basis for electronystagmography (ENG).

electrophonic *n* [Gk *elektron* amber (which causes electrostatic effects when rubbed) + Gk *phone* sound]

Pertaining to electronically produced sound.

electrophonic effect *adj*
The sensation of hearing due to the effect of electromagnetic radiation on the head.

electrophysiology *n* [Gk *elektron* amber (which causes electrostatic effects when rubbed) + Gk *phusis* nature + Gk *-logia* study of]
The study of electrical activity in the body.

electrostatic *adj* [Gk *elektron* amber (which causes electrostatic effects when rubbed) + Gk *statikos* causing to stand]
Pertaining to static electricity, an electrical effect in a body that cannot conduct a current.

electrostatic noise *np*
Interference due to static electricity, e.g., from fluorescent lights. Can cause interference with acoustic signals during audiometric testing.

electrostatic pressure *np*
The overall result of ionic attraction (where positively and negatively charged ions are attracted to each other) and repulsion (where ions of the same charge repel each other).

electrotactile effect *np* [Gk *elektron* amber (which causes electrostatic effects when rubbed) + Lat *tactilis* touchable (from *tangere* to touch)]
Touch sensation, produced by electrical stimulation of the skin to transmit some speech information via tactile sensation.

elevated *adj*
Raised.

elevated threshold *np*
A threshold that is poorer than normal and therefore occurs at a raised decibel level.

ellipse *n*
A regular oval shape in which the sum of the distances of any point from the foci (two fixed points) remains the same. An ellipse can be formed by taking a section across a cone that is not parallel or perpendicular to its base.
Deriv: -adj elliptical

embolism *n* [Gk *embolismos* blockage (from *emballein* to insert)]
A blockage of a blood vessel due to a clot.

embryo *n* [Gk *embruon* fetus]
1. An unborn baby. 2. A fetus early in pregnancy (usually before the third month)
Deriv: -adj embryonic, embryonal

embryonal rhabdomyosarcoma *np* ĕm-brēōnạl răbdōmīōsahkōma [Gk *rhabdos* rod + Gk *mus* muscle + Gk *sarkoun* to become fleshy]
A malignant neoplasm that may arise in various parts of the body, e.g., the middle ear, and occurs in young children.

-eme *suffix*
A distinct unit of speech, e.g., phoneme.

eminence *n*
A prominence or protuberance.

emission *n* [Lat *emittere* to send out]
A discharge.

emission, otoacoustic (OAE) *np* [Lat *emittere* to send out; Gk *ous* ear + Gk *akousis* sense of hearing]
Also: cochlear echoes; Kemp echoes
Tiny sounds produced by the outer hair cells. Can be recorded in the ear canals of most normal ears.

empathy *n* [Gk *empatheia* (from Gk *en* in + Gk *pathos* feeling)]
The ability to share in the emotional state of another person.

empiric *adj* [Gk *empereia* experience]
Relying on observation and experience, rather than theory.

empyema *n* ĕmpīēma (ĕmpĭēma) [Gk *empuema* collection of pus]
A collection of pus.

empyema of the mastoid *np*
A type of acute mastoiditis in which pus collects in the mastoid cavity.

encephalic *adj* ĕnsĕ'fălĭk [Gk *enkephalos* brain]
Pertaining to the brain.

encephalitis *n* ĕnsĕfăl'ītĭs [Gk *enkephalos* brain + Gk *-ites* denoting disease of]
Inflammation of the brain.

encephalopathy *n* ĕnsĕfă'lŏpăthē [Gk *enkephalos* brain + Gk *pathos* illness]
Brain disease.

endemic *adj* [Gk *endemios* native]
Prevalent among a group of people or in a country.

endo- *prefix* [Gk *endo-* inside]
Within.

endocochlear potential *np* [Gk *endo-* inside + Lat *cochlea* snail shell, spiral]
The resting electrical potential of the endolymph in the scala media, relative to the perilymph in the scala vestibuli and scala tympani. The endocochlear potential is generated by the scala media and is approximately +80mV.

endocrine system *np* [Gk *endo-* inside + Gk *krinein* to sift]
Made up of glands that produce and secrete hormones to regulate the body's growth, metabolism, and sexual development and function.

endoderm *n* [Gk *endo-* inside + Gk *derma* skin]
1. The inner layer. 2. The innermost layer of the three primary embryonic layers.

endogenous *adj* 'ĕndōjenu̯s [Gk *endo-* inside + Gk *genes* born, type]
1. Growing from within. 2. Evoked potentials in response to an external event, e.g., due to perception or cognition. 3. Genetically caused.

endogenous hearing loss *np*
Deafness of genetic origin.

endolymph *n* 'ĕndōlĭmf [Gk *endo-* inside + Lat *lympha* liquid]
The clear fluid in the scala media of the cochlea, which is high in potassium and low in sodium.
Deriv: -*adj* endolymphatic

endolymphatic duct *np*
The passage carrying endolymph from the endolymphatic sac to the utricle and saccule.

endolymphatic hydrops *np*
Also: Ménière syndrome/disease/disorder
A disorder in which there is excessive endolymph within the inner ear, characterized by recurrent episodes of spontaneous vertigo, aural fullness, tinnitus, and progressive low-frequency sensorineural hearing loss.

endolymphatic potential *np*
The direct current (DC) standing electrical potential within the endolymphatic space. The electrical potential is approximately +70-90 mV relative to perilymph.

endolymphatic sac *np*
A membranous bag containing endolymph that is connected to the main membranous labyrinth by the endolymphatic duct.

endolymphatic space *np*
Also: scala media; cochlear duct
The middle chamber of the cochlear duct that is filled with endolymph and contains the organ of Corti.

endomastoiditis *n* [Gk *endo-* inside + Gk *mastoeides* breast-shaped + Gk *-itis* denoting illness of]
Inflammation of the mastoid cavity and cells.

endoplasmic reticulum *np* [Gk *endo-* inside + Gk *plasma* shape, mould; Lat *reticulum* small net]
Parallel layers of membrane found in the cytoplasm of cells.

endoplasmic reticulum, rough *np*
An organelle of cells that synthesizes proteins.

endoplasmic reticulum, smooth *np*
An organelle of cells that synthesizes lipids.

end organ *np*
The terminal structure of a sensory or motor nerve fiber.

endorphin *n*
Any of the opioid polypeptide neurotransmitters in the brain.

endosalpingitis *n* [Gk *endo-* inside + Gk *salpinx* trumpet]
Inflammation of the mucous membrane lining of the Eustachian tube.

endoscope *n* [Gk *endo-* inside + Gk *skopein* to look at]
An illuminated tubal instrument that can be inserted into organs and cavities in the body, e.g., the sinuses can be viewed using an endoscope via the nose.

endosteal hyperostosis *n* ĕndŏst'ēal [Gk *endo-* inside + Gk *osteon* bone; Gk *hyper* beyond + Gk *osteon* bone + Gk *-osis* denoting a diseased state]
Also: Van Buchem syndrome; hyperostosis corticalis generalisata; generalized cortical hyperostosis; gout
A genetic bone disorder characterized by overgrowth of the mandible and thickening of the long bones and the forehead and brow area. The bone growth may trap cranial nerves, causing facial palsy and hearing loss.

endosteum *n*
The internal periosteum (dense vascular connective tissue that lines the cavities of bones).

endothelium *n* [Gk *endo-* inside + Gk *thele* nipple]
The layer of cells that lines internal cavities in the body.

Engelmann syndrome/disease *np*
Named after Guido Engelmann (1876–1959), a German surgeon, who reported the syndrome in 1929 in a boy aged 8. It was first described by Cockayne in 1920, and in 1922 Camurati suggested it was a genetic disorder.
Also: progressive diaphyseal dysplasia (PDD); Camurati-Engelmann syndrome

A skeletal disorder, characterized by muscle weakness, bone pain, and difficulty in walking due to progressively thickening bones. It may be accompanied by progressive sensorineural hearing loss as the skull bones may thicken and constrict the passages carrying nerves and blood vessels.

enkephalin *n*
A pentapeptide neurotransmitter that occurs in the brain, spinal cord, cochlea, and gastrointestinal tract and has an opiate-like pain killing effect.

envelope *n*
1. That which wraps around. 2. A curve formed by joining the peaks of a wave.

envelope analysis *np*
Frequency analysis of the shape of the original time signal.

envelope following response *np*
Also: auditory steady state reponse; amplitude modulation following response
A steady-state evoked response, i.e., one that is phase-locked to the modulation envelope.

environmental *adj*
Surrounding.

environmental microphone *np*
An additional microphone that provides environmental sounds to the listener in addition to the direct signal, e.g., an environmental microphone on a radio hearing aid facilitates hearing other pupils in class in addition to the voice of the teacher.

enzymatic *adj*
Pertaining to the termination of the postsynaptic potential through the destruction of the neurotransmitter by an enzyme. It is thought that postsynaptic potentials are terminated in this way for only one neurotransmitter, acetylcholine.

enzyme *n*
A molecule that acts as a catalyst, speeding up the rate of chemical reactions without itself being used up.

ephedrine *n*
A stimulant that speeds up the heart and central nervous system. Used to increase energy, enhance fitness training, for slimming, and in some cold remedies. Uncommonly may be related to hearing loss due to cochlear ischemia (restriction of blood supply).

epi- *prefix* [Gk *epi* above]
Above.

epicanthal fold *np* [Gk *epi* above + Gk *kanthos* corner (of the eye)]
A layer of skin at the inner angle of the eyes. A feature of Waardenburg syndrome.

epidemic *n* [Gk *epidemia* prevalence of disease]
A disease prevalent in a community at a particular time, e.g., the rubella epidemic in 1963–1965, which caused many cases of permanent sensorineural deafness.

epidemiology *n* [Gk *epidemia* prevalence of disease]
1. The study of disease in a population. 2. The branch of medicine that treats epidemics.

epidermis *n* [Gk *epi* above + Gk *derma* skin]
The outer layer of the skin.

epidermoid *adj*
Pertaining to the epidermis.

epidermoid carcinoma *np* [Gk *epi* above + Gk *derma* skin + Gk *-oides* in the shape of; Gk *karkinos* crab + Gk *–oma* denoting tumor, swelling]
A cancerous tumor derived from epithelial tissue. May be found in the external or middle ear or mastoid. Most epidermoid carcinomas are of the squamous cell type.

epidermoid cyst *np obs* [Gk *epi* above + Gk *derma* skin + Gk *-oides* in the shape of; Gk *kustos* a box]
Also: cholesteatoma
A benign tumor-like mass in the middle ear consisting mainly of cellular debris.

Usually occurs secondary to otitis media or marginal tympanic perforation. May cause destruction of surrounding tissues.

epiglottis *n* [Gk *epi-* above + Gk *glotta* the tongue]
A thin triangular structure of elastic cartilage that projects from the base of the tongue in front of the glottis. The epiglottis folds back to cover the larynx during swallowing to prevent food and liquids from entering the larynx and the lungs.

epiotic *adj* [Gk *epi* above + Gk *ous* ear]
Above or near the ear.

epiphenomenon *n* [Gk *epi* above + Gk *phainomenon* thing appearing to view]
A secondary symptom.

episodic *adj* [Gk *epeisodion* thing coming in besides]
Occurring in repeated incidents or episodes.

epithelium *n* [Gk *epi* above, on top of + Gk *thele* nipple]
A nonvascular tissue forming the outer layer of the skin and mucous membranes. A term generalized from the nipples to the rest of the body.

epitympanic *adj* [Gk *epi* above + Gk *tumpanon* drum]
Above the eardrum.

epitympanic recess *np*
Also: epitympanum; attic
The attic or upper part of the middle ear cavity above the eardrum, which contains the head of the malleus and the body of the incus.

Epley maneuver *np* Named after John M. Epley (b 1930), an American neurotologist (neurootologist), who introduced the procedure in 1980.
Also: canalith repositioning procedure (CRP)
Head and upper body exercises to move detached calcium carbonate crystals from the posterior or anterior semicircular canals into the utricle. The crystals are destroyed in the utricle preventing

false information regarding spatial movements being sent to the brain. The main treatment for benign paroxysmal positional vertigo (BPPV).

Epstein syndrome *np* Named after Charles Joseph Epstein (1933–2011), an American geneticist and professor of medical genetics at the University of California–San Francisco, who first reported the syndrome in two families in 1972.
A rare autosomal dominant disease associated with progressive sensorineural hearing loss of childhood onset. Characterized by progressive renal failure, a reduction in normal blood platelets (required for clotting) and the presence of giant platelets.

equalization (equalisation) *n*
Adjusting the frequency response and/or level of a device or system to achieve a flat response.

equalizer (equaliser) *n*
A filtering network to modify the frequency response.

equal loudness contour *np*
Also: phon curve
The loudness level curve that maps the sound pressure levels required to produce a specified phon level for normal hearing across the frequency range. Equal loudness contours plot the intensity that is heard (on average) as being of the same loudness at each frequency as a 1 kHz tone.

equally tempered scale *np*
A musical scale in which the octave is divided into 12 equal intervals.

equilibration *n*
The maintenance or restoration of a balanced state, e.g., the steady state following the initial burst in neural activity when a neuron fires.
Deriv: –v. equilibrate

equilibrium *n*
The condition of being evenly balanced.

equivalent *adj*
Equal in value.

equivalent continuous A-weighted sound level *np*
The sound level that conveys the same sound energy as the actual time-varying A-weighted sound level.

equivalent continuous sound level (Leq) *np*
A time-weighted energy average that represents the total sound energy experienced, averaged over a given period of time, usually 8 hours. Used where sound levels vary over time.

equivalent ear canal volume *np*
An estimate of the volume between the probe tip and the eardrum. It is the volume of an air-filled cavity with the same acoustic admittance as that of the system it represents.

equivalent input noise level *np*
A measure of the level of internal noise generated.

equivalent rectangular bandwidth (ERB) *np*
A psychoacoustic scale that weights the perceptual importance of differences in the frequency of human auditory filters by modeling them as rectangular bandpass filters, i.e., the filters represent auditory frequency resolution.

equivalent volume *np*
Changes from probe tone sound pressure level (SPL) to volume, such that a decrease in SPL appears as an increase in volume and vice versa.

erysipelas *n* ĕrĭ'sĭpelas [Gk *eruthros* red + Gk *pella* skin]
A skin inflammation that can affect the external ear.

erythema *n* ĕrĭ'thēma [Gk *eruthainein* to be red]
Temporary reddening (due to capillary dilation) of skin that is inflamed.

erythroblastosis fetalis *np* [Gk *eruthros* red + Gk *blastos* germ, sprout]
Also: hyperbilirubinemia (hyperbilirubinaemia)
An abnormally large amount of bilirubin present at birth which results in jaundice. A risk factor for sensorineural hearing loss.

erythromycin *n* [Gk *eruthros* red + Gk *mukes* fungus]
A macrolide antibiotic used to treat respiratory and other bacterial infections, (as an alternative to penicillin). Can be ototoxic causing high-frequency sensorineural hearing loss especially in elderly individuals with liver or kidney disease.

esophagus (oesophagus) *n* ē'sŏfagus [Gk *oesophagus* esophagus]
The passage between the pharynx and the stomach.

ethacrynic acid *np*
A loop diuretic used to treat water retention, e.g., in renal disease. Can be ototoxic.

ethics *n* [Gk *ethikos* pertaining to morals]
A set of principles of acceptable conduct.

ethmoid bone *np* [Gk *ethmos* sieve + Gk *eidos* shape]
A bone located anterior to the sphenoid bone and inferior to the medial portion of the frontal bone. Forms part of both orbits, part of the nasal cavity, and part of the floor of the skull.

ethmoid sinuses *np* [Gk *ethmos* sieve + Gk *eidos* shape; Lat *sinus* recess, bend]
A collection of many small spaces situated beside the bridge of the nose.

etiology (aetiology) *n* [Gk *aetia* a cause + Gk *-logia* study of]
1. The study of the causes of disease. 2. The cause of a specific disease.

etymotic gain *np* [Gk *etumos* true]
Also: insertion gain; real ear gain; transmission gain
The difference between the sound pressure level in the ear canal without and with a hearing aid. Measured in dB. Often used for comparison with a prescription target.

Eustachian tube *np* yū'stāshan Named after Bartolomeo Eustachius (1500–1574), an Italian anatomist, who described many anatomic structures including the Eustachian tube.
Also: auditory tube
The tube joining the middle ear tympanic cavity to the nasopharynx. Opened during swallowing. Functions to maintain middle ear pressure equal to external atmospheric pressure and to drain the middle ear. If the Eustachian tube is blocked so that middle ear pressure becomes negative in relation to atmospheric pressure, a conductive hearing loss can occur.

evaluation *n*
1. Appraisal. 2. To assess the value.

evoked *adj*
Activated in response to a stimulus.

evoked otoacoustic emissions *np*
Also: colloq cochlear echoes; Kemp echoes
Tiny sounds produced by the outer hair cells in response to acoustic stimulation. Can be recorded in the ear canals of most normal ears.

evoked potential *np*
Electrical activity of the brain in response to an external stimulus or sensory stimulation, e.g., sound.

evoked response audiometry (ERA) *np*
Measurement of auditory function using acoustic signals to evoke electrical potentials that are measured to give information about hearing function and the site of lesion.

excitation *n*
Arousal of a response, e.g., the triggering of neural activity.

executive functioning *np*
High-level cognitive processes that control and regulate thoughts and behavior.

exo- *prefix* [Gk *exo* outside]
Outside.

exocytosis *n* [Gk *exo* outside + GK *kutos* a box + GK *-osis* denoting a diseased state]
The cellular process in which vesicles in the cytoplasm fuse with the plasma membrane and secrete their contents, e. g., the process by which neurotransmitters are secreted into the synapse.

exogenous *adj* [Gk *exo* outside + Gk *genes* born, type]
From an external source.

exogenous hearing loss *np*
Deafness due to environmental factors, e. g., noise, ototoxins, infections.

exostosis *n* ĕksŏ'stōsĭs [Lat *ex* out + Gk *osteon* bone + Gk *-osis* denoting a diseased state]
Also: colloq surfer's ear
The growth of bone on another bone or cartilage. Commonly occurs from the bony portion of the ear canal in people participating in water-related sports like swimming or surfing because of prolonged exposure to cold water.

expansion *n*
Also: squelch; noise-gating
Adaptive processing, designed to reduce the amount of amplification of low-level inputs. Increases gain with increasing input, i.e., the opposite of compression. Frequently recommended for hearing aid users with near-normal hearing thresholds to reduce complaints of audible internal noise in hearing aids that use wide dynamic range compression. Due to the nature of wide dynamic range compression (WDRC) amplifying low-level inputs, it is able to help reduce overamplification of low-level environmental noise such as air conditioning. Expansion can provide improved sound quality, but may also reduce the recognition of low-level high-frequency speech sounds.

explantation *n*
The removal of an implanted part, e.g., cells, tissues, cochlear implant, etc.

exponent *n*
A symbol that denotes the number of times that a base is to be taken to produce the power indicated.

exponential *adj*
Occurs when the growth rate of a mathematical function is proportional to the function's current value. Exponential growth starts slowly and increases rapidly as time increases.

expression *n*
1. The extent to which a genetic trait appears. 2. To convey feeling or meaning.

external *adj*
Outside.

external acoustic/auditory meatus *np*
The passage between the pinna and the eardrum.

external ear *np*
The pinna and ear canal ending at the eardrum.

external validity *np*
The extent to which results of a study or experiment can be generalized beyond the sample used for the study.

external vent *np*
A vent where there is insufficient room for the entire vent to be within the earmold due to a small ear canal.

extirpation *n* [Lat *exstirpare* uproot]
Surgical removal.

extra- *prefix* [Lat *extra* outside]
Outside.

extraaxial *adj*
Outside the brainstem.

extracochlear *adj*
Outside the cochlea.

extrapolate *v* [Lat *extra* outside + Lat *polare* to polish]
To estimate the values or to continue a curve on the assumption that the trend or pattern, demonstrated inside the range or graph, will continue outside.

extrinsic *adj*
From the outside.

extrinsic redundancy *np*
The abundance of superfluous information present in a speech or other message that improves understanding.

extrude *v*
To force out.
Deriv: –n extrusion

exudate *n* [Lat *exsudare* to sweat out]
Fluid or semisolid matter that contains protein and cellular debris, e.g., enzymes and dead tissue. Exudate oozes from blood vessels when their permeability is increased due to injury or inflammation and is deposited in tissues or on tissue surfaces.

exudate, purulent *np*
Pus that secretes from tissues.

eye-blink reflex *np*
Also: auropalpebral reflex; acoustopalpebral reflex; cochleo-orbicular reflex; cochleopalpebral reflex; startle reflex
A rapid eye-blink caused by sudden loud sound.

Fabry syndrome *np* ˈfĕbrē Named after Johannes Fabry (1860–1930), a German dermatologist, who described the syndrome in 1898. It was also discovered independently in the same year by William Anderson, an English surgeon, and is therefore sometimes referred to as Fabry-Anderson syndrome.
An X-linked metabolic disorder that gives rise to vascular malfunction. Characteristics include clusters of dark nodules on the skin, renal failure, headaches, seizures, high-frequency sensorineural hearing loss, and vestibular dysfunction.

faceplate *n*
The front part of a custom hearing aid, which usually contains the battery door, microphone, and any user controls, e.g., volume control.

face validity *np*
The degree to which test items represent what they claim to test.

facial canal *np*
Also: Fallopian aqueduct
The small canal, in the petrous part of the temporal bone, that runs from the internal auditory canal to the stylomastoid foramen and contains the facial nerve.

facial nerve *np*
Also: seventh cranial nerve
Cranial nerve VII, which provides innervation to the facial muscles and conveys sensation from the tongue and soft palate.

facies *n* ˈfāshēz [Lat *facies* face]
The facial appearance or expression, characteristic of a particular disease, disorder, or physical irregularity.

facies, adenoidal *np*
The facial appearance of someone with adenoidal problems.

factitious *adj*
A psychiatric disorder in which a person intentionally exaggerates or falsifies symptoms not for external gain, but to assume a sick role.

falling *n*
1. The result of an attempt to correct movement that does not exist due to vertigo, causing a fall in the opposite direction to the sense of rotation caused by the vertigo. 2. A description of an audiogram that slopes, usually from low to high frequencies.

fall-off rate *np*
The rate at which a signal's amplitude diminishes.

Fallopian aqueduct *np* faˈlōpēan Named after Gabriel Fallopius (1523–1562), an Italian anatomist and professor of anatomy at Padua, who discovered the various anatomic structures now bearing his name.
Also: facial canal
The small canal, in the petrous part of the temporal bone, that runs from the internal auditory canal to the stylomastoid foramen and through which the facial nerve passes.

fall time *np*
The time taken for a signal to decay by 60 dB from its steady state.

false fundus *np* [Lat *fundus* a base, bottom]
An accumulation of epithelial-covered granulation tissue that closes the ear canal at the bony cartilaginous junction. This blind end can be seen instead of the normal view during otoscopic examination of the eardrum. May result following severe injury to the canal lining. Usually causes a moderate to severe conductive hearing loss.

false-negative/positive *np*
1. False-negative or false-positive responses. A false-positive response occurs when a patient responds in the absence of a signal. False-positives may occur with tinnitus where the patient mistakes the tinnitus for the signal. A false-negative response occurs when a patient fails

to respond to a signal that is audible to them. False-negatives may occur if the patient is malingering, but may also occur, for example, if the patient is tired. 2. False-negative or positive test results or findings. A false-negative test result incorrectly suggests the absence of a condition that turns out to be present. A false-positive test result incorrectly suggests the presence of a condition that turns out not to be present.

familial *adj* [Lat *familia* family]
Occurring in a family at a rate greater than chance. Usually due to heredity.

familiarization *n*
The act of making a patient accustomed to the test surroundings or requirements before the proper test begins.

Fanconi pancytopenia syndrome/Fanconi anemia (anaemia) syndrome *np*
Named after Guido Fanconi (1892–1979), a professor of pediatrics at the University of Zurich and regarded as a pioneer of pediatrics. Fanconi made some important contributions to pediatrics, but he is not considered to have been the identifier of this syndrome.
Also: renal tubular acidosis
A rare condition that may be genetic or acquired, characterized clinically by progressive bone marrow failure, skeletal deformities, and a predisposition to neoplasia. Signs include patchy brown pigmentation, short stature, microcephaly, kidney problems, delayed puberty, learning difficulty, extra or fewer digits. The external ear may be malformed and there may be conductive and sensorineural hearing loss.

farad *n* Named after Michael Faraday (1791–1867), an English bookbinder, who became interested in electricity. He was a self-taught physicist who made his discoveries, which included electromagnetic induction, through experimentation.
The standard international unit of electric capacitance. A farad (F) is the capacitance of a capacitor between the plates of which a potential of 1 volt is created by a charge of 1 coulomb (the electricity conveyed in 1 second by a current of 1 amp).

far (sound) field *np*
A region in the sound field, further away from the sound source than the near field, where acoustic changes are small as the sound pressure level decreases according to the inverse square law, i.e., decreases by 6 dB with every doubling of distance from the sound source. In this region the sound particle velocity is in phase with the sound pressure. The far field is divided into the direct field, dominated by direct radiated sound and the reverberant field, dominated by reflected sound.

farmers' ear *np*
Occupational hearing loss associated with farming, e.g., due to noise or infection occurring as a result of farming.

fascia *n* [Lat *fascis* bundle]
A layer of fibrous connective tissue covering body structures, such as muscles, blood vessels, and nerves.

fascia lata *np* [Lat *fascis* bundle; Lat *lata* wide]
A layer of dense connective tissue surrounding the thigh muscle. May be used during surgery as a graft material.

fasciculus *n* [Lat *fasciculus* small bundle]
A small bundle of nerve or muscle fibers.

fast Fourier transform (FFT) *np* Named in honor of John Baptiste Joseph Fourier (1768–1830), a French mathematician and physicist, for his investigation of Fourier series, i.e., transforming a function into its composite frequencies.
The mathematical procedure for Fourier analysis, used to calculate the spectrum of a signal, by converting the signal from the time domain into the frequency domain.

fast phase nystagmus *np*
The rapid recovery eye movement following a slow drift of the eyes in the other direction, during jerk nystagmus.

fatigue, auditory *np*
A brief temporary reduction in hearing threshold after exposure to sound.

feature *n*
A notable or prominent characteristic.

febrile *adj* [Lat *febris* fever]
Pertaining to fever.

Fechner's law *np* Named after Gustav Theodor Fechner (1801–1887,) a professor of philosophy at the University of Leipzig, who is credited with developing this law.
Fechner's law states that sensation is linearly related to the logarithm of the stimulus.

feedback *n*
1. A signal derived from the output signal returned to the input. 2. Hearing one's own voice. 3. Evaluative information in response to a particular process or activity.

feedback, acoustic *np*
In acoustical equipment, the unwanted interaction between the output and the input of the system; e.g., in hearing aids, this is a high-pitched squeal created when sound leaks from the receiver of the hearing aid and is picked up by the microphone and reamplified.

feedback, auditory *np*
The hearing of one's own voice (which is important for monitoring vocalizations).

feedback, internal *np*
1. Feedback that is due to electrical or mechanical causes within a hearing aid. 2. The information received from the body, e.g., heart rate, used to monitor one's own physical state.

feedback, negative *np*
1. Feedback that reduces the output of a system. 2. In an amplifier, feedback that is out of phase with the input signal and results in a decrease in amplification of the signal. 3. *colloq* Criticism.

feedback, positive *np*
1. A self-accelerating disturbance or change. 2. In an amplifier, feedback that is in phase added to an input stage resulting in increased amplification of the signal, which may possibly lead to acoustic feedback. 3. *colloq* Praise.

Fehr's corneal dystrophy *np* Named after Oskar Fehr (1871–1959), a German Jewish ophthalmologist, who moved to Great Britain in 1939 after he was forced by the Nazis to resign. He became a British citizen in 1947 and continued operating until the age of 80.
Congenital corneal dystrophy usually detected during the first decade of life, leading to blindness by about age 40, together with progressive sensorineural hearing loss of late onset.

fence *np*
A limit, barrier, or enclosure.

fence, low *np*
The accepted lower limit of hearing impairment, i.e., the slight hearing loss in comparison to average normal hearing, which is still considered to be within the normal range. This is lower for children than for adults because children are still developing language and learning. The low fence is approximately 15 dB for children and approximately 20 dB for adults.

fenestra *n* [Lat *fenestra* window]
Also: window
A small anatomical window-like opening.

fenestra ovalis *np* [Lat *fenestra* window; Lat *ovalis* oval]
Also: fenestra vestibule
The oval window of the cochlea.

fenestra rotunda *n* [Lat *fenestra* window; Lat *rotundus* round]
Also: fenestra cochlea; fenestra rotunda
The round window of the cochlea.

fenestration *np*
1. An opening in a structure such as a membrane. 2. The surgical creation of an artificial opening in the bony labyrinth of

the cochlea. Previously used in the treatment of otosclerosis. 3. The placement of an external groove in an earmold.

fetal (foetal) alcohol syndrome (FAS) *np*
A lifelong condition caused by consumption of excessive alcohol by the mother during pregnancy, which leads to central nervous system damage in the unborn fetus. Characteristics include low birth weight, small head, cognitive impairment, short nose, heart and joint abnormalities, conductive hearing loss due to chronic otitis media, and occasionally cleft palate.

fetus (foetus) *n* *pl* fetuses (foetuses) [Lat *fetus* offspring]
A developing baby, beginning from the ninth week after fertilization. The fetus is considered full-term from 37 weeks' gestational age.
Deriv: -adj fetal/foetal

fiber (fiber) *n* [Lat *fibra* fiber]
A long threadlike anatomical structure, e. g., a nerve fiber.

fibril *n* [Lat *fibra* fiber]
A thread-like component of a fiber.

fibroblast *n* [Lat *fibra* fiber + Gk *blastos* sprout, germ]
Spindle-shaped cells in connective tissue that secrete protein substances, e.g., collagen, elastic and reticular fibers, to provide a structural framework for many tissues and for wound healing.

fibrocartilage *n*
Cartilage that contains compact thick parallel bundles of collagen fibers.

fibroid/fibroma *n* [Lat *fibra* a fiber + Gk *eidos* shape; Gk *–oma* denoting tumor, swelling]
A benign tumor of fibrous or connective tissue.

fibrosis *n* [Lat *fibra* a fiber + Gk *-osis* denoting a diseased state]
The formation of excess fibrous or scar tissue as a reparative or reactive process or as the result of inflammation, irrita-

tion, or healing.
Deriv: -adj fibrotic

fibrosis, medial canal *np*
The formation of solid fibrous tissue in the ear canal.

fidelity, high *np* [Lat *fides* faith]
The reproduction of sound with minimal distortion.

field *n*
1. An area over which a sound wave dissipates. 2. An area of specialization or interest.

field effect transistor (FET) *np*
A type of transistor, usually made of semiconductors, used for amplifying or switching very low power signals, e.g., in digital memory circuits.

field, free *np*
A sound field with minimal boundary effects.

field, sound *np*
1. Any environment that contains sound. 2. A region through which sound waves, standing or progressive, propagate from a sound source. 3. An enclosed space in which the diffused sound waves are random in magnitude, phase, and direction, constituting reverberant sound.

filter *n*
A frequency selective device that modifies the spectrum of a signal by blocking the passage of some frequency energy, while allowing that selected to pass.

filter, acoustic *np*
Filters that smooth the hearing aid response and help to avoid peaks of gain, mainly in the mid-frequencies between 1 kHz and 3 kHz.

filter, active *np*
A filter that uses reactive elements to produce the required characteristics. Active filters can use operational amplifiers, as well as resistors and capacitors and provide precise filtering. 1. Active filters used in hearing aids. 2. The nonlinear response of the basilar membrane, which is

partially determined by the mechanical action of the outer hair cells.

filter, adaptive *np*
A filter that has a frequency response that self-adjusts according to the input.

filter, band-pass *np*
A filter allowing only frequencies within a certain range to pass.

filter, band-reject/band-stop *np*
A filter allowing most frequencies to pass, but rejecting a specific frequency range.

filter, high pass/low-cut *np*
A filter allowing only high-frequency sounds to pass.

filter, low pass/high-cut *np*
A filter allowing only low-frequency sounds to pass.

filter, narrow-band *np*
A filter with a narrow bandwidth, usually of no more than 0.5 octave.

filter, notch *np*
A filter that attenuates a narrow frequency range, but allows sounds of higher and lower frequency to pass.

filter, octave *np*
A filter with a bandwidth of one octave.

filter, passive *np*
An electronic filter that uses no amplifying elements and does not require an external power source.

filter, sintered *np*
A filter made of fused metal ordinarily placed in the earhook or tubing of a hearing aid for reduction of the amplified signal.

filter skirt *np*
The range of frequencies either side of the center frequency.

finger spelling *np*
Also: dactyl speech
A manual alphabet used by deaf people.

first arch syndrome *np* Named after Edward Treacher-Collins (1862–1932), an English ophthalmologist, who first reported the condition.
Also: Treacher-Collins syndrome; mandibular dysostosis
A syndrome characterized by craniofacial deformities including downward sloping eyelid fissures, depressed cheek bones, receding chin, large fish-like mouth, and abnormalities of the external and middle ear, e.g., pinna abnormalities, atresia, and middle ear deformities. Hearing loss is usually severe conductive, but may be mixed if there is also inner ear deformity.

first-order neurons *np*
First-order neurons carry signals from the peripheral nerves (end organs) to the spinal cord.

fissure *n* [Lat *fissio* a crack]
A cleft or groove.

fistula *n* [Lat *fistula* pipe]
An opening, e.g., an endolymphatic fistula is an unhealed rupture of the cochlear duct.

fistula test *np*
The air pressure in the middle ear is altered while eye movements are recorded. If a fistula is present, pressure changes will affect the inner ear and may produce a type of eye movement known as nystagmus.

fixation *n*
An inability to move.

fixation, index *np*
1. A method of summarizing genetic differences within and between populations. 2. A method for analyzing a patient's ability to suppress vestibular nystagmus during a caloric test, by comparing the nystagmus intensity before and after visual fixation.

fixation, stapes *np*
Restriction of the movement of the stapes due to otosclerosis.

fixation suppression *np*
The ability to suppress vestibular nystagmus. In normal individuals, nystagmus

intensity is strongly reduced by visual fixation.

fixed frequency response *np*
A frequency response that does not change with input level changes.

flaccid *adj* [Lat *flaccus* flaccid]
Without elasticity; floppy.

flap *n*
1. A sound produced by rapid vibration of an articulator. 2. Tissue that has been surgically separated and used in grafting to fill a defect, e.g., a tympanic membrane perforation.

flat *adj*
Equal across the range.

flat audiogram *np*
Hearing threshold levels that do not vary by more than 5-10 dB per octave on an audiogram.

flat response *np*
Amplification that is approximately equal across the frequency range.

floating footplate *np*
Fragments of the stapes footplate dislodged during stapedectomy surgery.

floor effect *np*
When test results or statistical data cannot have a value lower than a particular number. Having a floor effect may lead to the inability to discriminate between the participant's test scores in a study or experiment due to the use of an inappropriately difficult measuring device. Clinical decline will therefore not indicate a change in score despite worsening of function.

fluctuating *adj* [Lat *fluctuare* to fluctuate]
Varying.

flutter *n*
1. The first feeling of sound pressure, which is too low in frequency to be heard as a tone. 2. A beating or drumming sensation in the ear, sometimes due to twitching ear muscles or pulsations from blood vessels in the ear.

follicle *n* [Lat *folliculus* little bag]
A depression in the skin from which a hair grows.

footplate *n*
The flat part of the stapes bone that rests in the oval window of the cochlea.

footplate, floating *np*
Fragments of the stapes footplate dislodged during stapedectomy surgery.

foramen *np* *pl* foramina [Lat *foramen* opening, passage]
An opening in a bone.

foramen, stylomastoid *np* [Lat *foramen* hole, opening; Gk *stulos* a pillar + Gk *mastos* breast + Gk *eidos* shape]
A passage into the bone between the styloid and mastoid processes; where the facial nerve canal ends.

force *n*
1. A change of motion. 2. A product of mass and acceleration applied.

forced choice *np*
A situation in which the listener must choose between two or more presented signals or items.

forebrain *n*
The most anterior of the three major divisions of the brain. It includes the telencephalon and the diencephalon.

forensic audiology *np* [Lat *forum* market place (where the court cases were held); Lat *audire* to hear + Gk *-logia* study of]
Investigative audiology related to resolving medicolegal cases, e.g., serving as an expert witness in hearing loss compensation claim cases and other forms of litigation.

formant *n* [Lat *formare* to form]
A peak in the frequency spectrum of a vowel sound caused by vocal tract resonance.

forward masking *np*
The brief inability to hear a sound immediately after a masking noise has been removed.

fossa *n pl* fossae [Lat *fossa* ditch]
A depression or dip, e.g., the triangular fossa of the pinna.

Fountain syndrome *np* Named after R.B. Fountain, a British physician, who reported the syndrome in 1974.
A rare syndrome characterized by learning difficulty, sensorineural hearing loss, skeletal abnormalities, and a coarse face with full lips.

Fourier analysis *np* ˈfūrīā Named after Joseph Fourier (1768–1830), a French mathematician, for his contributions to mathematics and physics.
A mathematical subdivision of a signal waveform into its sinusoidal components.

fracture *n/v* [Lat *frangere* to break]
-n A break. *-v* To break.

fracture, longitudinal *np*
A fracture that follows the long axis or length of a bone.

fracture, transverse *np*
A fracture across the bone, at right angles to the long axis.

Frank sign up *np* Named after Sandes T. Frank (b 1938), an American chest physician.
An acquired crease in the ear lobe that is associated with diabetes, coronary disease, and hypertension (high blood pressure).

Fraser syndrome *np* Named after George R. Fraser (b 1932), a British geneticist, who described the syndrome in 1962. *Also:* cryptophthalmos
A syndrome that is characterized by eyelid malformation, i.e., eyelids that hide the eyes. The syndrome is often accompanied by underlying visual problems and malformation of the external and middle ear, including atresia and mixed hearing loss.

free *adj*
Without boundary effects.

free field *np*
A sound field with minimal boundary effects where sound radiates uniformly in all directions without reflections.

free progressive wave *np*
A sound wave propagated within a free field.

frenulum *n* [Lat *frenulum* a little bridle]
A fold of membrane that restrains or supports, e.g., the lingual frenulum restrains the tongue.

Frenzel glasses/goggles/lenses *np* Named after Hermann Frenzel (1895–1967), a German otologist, who developed the glasses to measure vertigo.
Illuminated magnifying glasses used for observing eye movements during vestibular testing and removing fixation from the person under testing.

frequency *n*
The number of compression and rarefaction cycles per second in a vibrating system, reported in hertz (Hz).

frequency advantage *np*
An improved pattern of sound where the two ears hear differently across the frequency range in each ear, but the brain is able to combine the signals.

frequency analysis *np*
The procedure to determine the frequency spectrum of a signal.

frequency band *np*
A frequency interval between two limits.

frequency, carrier *np*
A frequency capable of being modulated by signals of other frequencies; generally the center frequency of a frequency modulated signal.

frequency, characteristic *np*
The frequency to which a neuron is most sensitive. Shown as the sharp tip on a normal psychoacoustical tuning curve.

frequency component *np*
One of the components of a signal waveform.

frequency , crossover *np*
The cut-off frequencies of filters that divide the frequency range into different bands.

frequency discrimination *np*
The ability to differentiate two sequential frequencies.

frequency distribution *np*
A table showing a distribution of data in different classes or categories.

frequency, fundamental *np*
Also: basic frequency
1. The frequency corresponding to the repetition rate. 2. The lowest frequency component or first harmonic in the acoustic spectrum of a complex sound; f0, e.g., speech where f0 is the fundamental frequency or first harmonic, f2 is the second formant or third harmonic, etc.

frequency modulation (FM) *np*
Variation in the frequency of a carrier signal about the mean frequency.

frequency, natural *np*
Also: resonant frequency
The object's natural frequency of vibration, i.e., it will vibrate with the greatest amplitude and with the least effort or applied energy at a certain frequency. The specific frequency depends upon the physical properties of the vibrating body.

frequency, Nyquist *np* Named after Harry Nyquist (1912–1976), a Swedish-American engineer, who investigated the mathematics of sampling.
Also: Nyquist limit
The highest frequency that can be coded at a given sampling rate so that the signal can be fully reconstructed. The Nyquist frequency is equal to half of the sampling rate.

frequencies, reference test *np*
The frequencies used in standard performance tests of hearing aids. Generally, the average of the decibel values at 1 kHz, 1.6 kHz, and 2.5 kHz, known as the high frequency average (HFA), but may be the average of three alternative fre-

quencies, known as the special purpose average (SPA), for hearing aids that are designed to deliver a different frequency range.

frequency resolution *np*
Also: frequency selectivity
The ability to differentiate frequency components, usually presented simultaneously. This is important to the ability to separate noise from the desired signal.

frequency response *np*
A graph of the amplitude of a device or system, plotted against frequency.

frequency selectivity *np*
Also: frequency resolution
The ability to differentiate frequency components, usually presented simultaneously; important to the ability to separate noise from desired signal.

frequency spectrum *np*
A signal represented as a plot of the distribution of the intensity of frequency components.

frequency-to-electrode map *np*
Also: cochlear implant map
A table or set of tables containing the parameters used for programming the speech processor of a cochlear implant, i.e., to set threshold (T-levels) and uncomfortable loudness levels (C-levels) for electrical stimuli.

frequency transposition *np*
The shifting of frequency information, generally a high-frequency input to that of a lower frequency, e.g., a frequency transposition hearing aid.

frequency weighting *np*
Standardized filtering in a sound level meter that can be applied to a signal being measured to emphasize or suppress selected frequencies, e.g., A-weighting.

fricative *n* [Lat *fricare* to rub]
A voiceless consonant formed by the turbulent escape of air through a narrow

opening between two articulators in the mouth, e.g., /z/ and /s/.

Friedreich ataxia *np* Named after Nikolaus Friedreich (1825–1882), a German doctor, who first described the condition in the 1860s.
A progressive nervous system disorder resulting from degenerating nerve tissue in the spinal cord and characterized by impaired muscle coordination (ataxia), muscle weakness in the arms and legs, visual impairments, nystagmus and/or saccadic eye movements, dysarthria, and sensorineural hearing loss of late onset.

frontal section *np* [Lat *frons* forehead; Lat *sectio* a cutting]
A part of the head or body sliced into anterior or posterior portions.

front end *np*
The initial signal processing stage in a hearing aid or cochlear implant (consisting of filtering, compression, etc.) that occurs before the signal is passed to the amplifier, or the electrode array in the case of a cochlear implant.

frontoproximal midline *np* [Lat *frons* forehead + Lat *proximus* nearest]
An electrode location on the forehead.

fugal *suffix* ˈfyūgəl [Lat *fuga* flight from]
Away from, e.g., ampullofugal, utriculofugal.

full-on *adj*
With the volume control (of a hearing aid) at maximum.

full shell *np*
An earmold or a custom hearing aid that fills the complete concha.

functional *adj* [Lat *fungere* to perform]
Also: 2. nonorganic
1. Pertaining to function. 2. A disorder without any known organic cause, most commonly due to malingering.

functional gain *np*
The difference in dB between the unaided and aided threshold.

fundamental frequency/tone *np* [Lat *fundamentum* the foundation]
Also: basic frequency
1. The frequency corresponding to the repetition rate. 2. The lowest frequency component, which is also the first harmonic in the acoustic spectrum of a complex sound (f0).

fundus *n* [Lat *fundus* base, bottom]
The bottom of a hollow, the furthest part from the opening.

furosemide/frusemide *n*
An ototoxic loop diuretic used mainly in the treatment of edema (oedema) and high blood pressure.

furuncle *n* [Lat *furunculus* a little thief, a knob on a vine that steals the sap]
A spot or boil. A painful skin infection in a hair follicle.

fusiform cells *np* [Lat *fusus* spindle]
1. Elongated cells that taper at each end. 2. Cells of the fusiform gyrus, part of the temporal lobe of the cerebral cortex.

fusion *n* [Lat *fundere* to pour forth]
The action of blending different inputs as one.

fusion, binaural *np*
The process involving the combination of different sounds presented to each ear to create a complete auditory image at the level of the brainstem.

fusion frequency *np*
The rate at which a succession of brief sounds are no longer perceived as separate events.

G

gabapentin *n*
An anticonvulscent drug used to treat symptoms caused by epilepsy, nerve pain, and chronic tinnitus. It can be ototoxic.

gain *n*
The difference between the input level and the amplified output level of a system, expressed in decibels.

gain control *np*
Volume control.

gain, coupler *np*
The gain provided by a hearing aid measured in a hearing aid test box, usually using a 2 cc coupler.

gain, effective *np*
The difference in decibels between the unaided and aided thresholds.

gain, full on *np*
Also: maximum gain
The gain of a hearing aid with the volume control turned to maximum, usually measured with 50 dBSPL input.

gain, functional *np*
The difference in dB between the unaided and aided threshold.

gain, insertion *np*
Also: etymotic gain; real ear gain; transmission gain
The mathematical difference in dB between the sound pressure level in the ear canal without and with a hearing aid.

gain, maximum *np*
Also: full on gain (FOG)
The most gain possible from a hearing aid. The hearing aid is set to give maximum output and the volume control is turned to maximum. Maximum gain is measured with 50 dBSPL input.

gain, real ear *np*
The amount of gain provided by a hearing aid when positioned in the ear, as opposed to a measurement of gain taken in a hearing aid test box.

gain, reference test *np*
A standard gain level that is generally measured with an input of 60 dBSPL and the volume control set so that the output is 17 dB (UK: 15 dB) below its maximum at the reference test position. This is intended to give more of a "user" volume setting than the maximum gain setting.

gain, reserve *np*
The amount of gain available to the hearing aid user to turn the hearing aid volume up or down from where it has been set by the audiologist.

gamete *n* [Gk *gamete/gametes* wife/husband]
A reproductive cell whose nucleus unites with that of another to form a new cell, known as a zygote. A gamete contains only a single set of chromosomes.
Deriv: –adj gametic

ganglia, basal *np* [Gk *ganglion* tumor near sinews or tendons; Gk *basis* base]
A mass of nerve tissue containing the cell nuclei situated deep within the cerebral hemispheres of the brain.

ganglia, spiral *np*
A mass of nerve tissue containing the cell nuclei that spirals through the cochlea and sends a representation of sound from the cochlea to the brain.

ganglion *n pl* ganglia [Gk *ganglion* tumor near sinews or tendons]
A mass of nerve cell bodies.

gap *n*
A space or breach in something otherwise continuous.

gap, air-bone *np*
The difference between air conduction and bone conduction readings on an audiogram symptomatic of conductive hearing loss.

gap detection *np*
The ability to discern the presence or absence of a short gap in a signal. A healthy human ear can detect a gap of as little as 8 ms between two identical stimuli.

gating signal *np* ˈgātĭng
A digital signal or pulse that provides a delay in order for another signal to be selected, disregarded, or eliminated.

Gaussian model *np* ˈgowsĭan Named for Karl Friedrich Gauss (1777–1855), a German mathematician, who developed many brilliant mathematical theories.
A statistical curve or frequency distribution showing a normal distribution of events.

Gaussian noise *np*
Also: white noise
Noise that contains equal power per unit of bandwidth.

gaze *n*
Also: gaze evoked nystagmus; gaze-paretic nystagmus
Fixation of the eyes on a steady target.

gaze nystagmus *np* [Gk *nustagmos* drowsiness, nodding, blinking]
Nystagmus evoked by attempting to maintain an extreme eye position.

gaze-paretic nystagmus *np* [Gk *paretos* relaxed; Gk *nustagmos* drowsiness, nodding, blinking]
A jerk nystagmus that appears when the eyes gaze away from straight ahead.

Gellé's test *np* ˈgĕlāz Named after Marie Ernst Gellé (1834–1923), a French otologist and author of *L'Audition et ses Organes* (1899).
A tuning fork test that was developed to test the mobility of the ossicular chain. The tuning fork is placed on the mastoid, while the air pressure is altered in the ear canal. A change in the loudness of the sound should be heard but if the ossicular chain cannot move, the loudness will not be altered.

gene *n* [Gk *genos* race, offspring]
The basic hereditary unit, each gene is found in a specific location on the chromosome. Genes consist of segments of deoxyribonucleic acid (DNA), which directs protein synthesis.

genetic *adj*
Pertaining to genetics or genes.
Deriv: –*adv* genetically

genetic code *np*
The system by which nucleic acid molecules store genetic information.

genetic counseling *np*
Counseling of parents or potential parents regarding the possible transmission of genetic abnormalities to their offspring.

genetic profile *np*
A list of an individual's significant genetic characteristics used in establishing the likelihood of transmitting certain inherited disorders.

genetic relationship *np*
A relationship formed from a common origin.

genetics *n*
The study of heredity dealing with the distribution, structure, and function of genes and patterns of inheritance.

geniculate *adj* [Lat *geniculus* small knee, joint in a plant]
Bent at a sharp angle, resembling a knee joint, e.g., the knee-shaped medial geniculate body.

genome *n* [Gk *genos* race, offspring + Gk *soma* body]
The entirety of genetic information in the chromosomes of an organism, encoded in the DNA and divided into discrete units called genes.

genotype *n*
The genetic makeup of an individual.
Deriv: –*adj* genotypical –*adv* genotypically

gentamicin/gentamycin *n*
A broad-spectrum antibiotic used in the treatment of a variety of infections. It is ototoxic and can affect both the cochlear and vestibular organs.

geriatric *adj* [Gk *geras* old age + Gk *iatros* doctor]
Pertaining to the process of aging and to the health and welfare of elderly people.

geriatrics *n*
Branch of medicine or social science dealing with geriatric problems.

German measles *np*
Also: rubella
A congenital viral infection passed from the mother to the fetus, can result in sensorineural deafness that is often severe to profound. Other characteristics may include conductive hearing loss, heart disease, learning difficulties, cataracts or glaucoma, and "salt and pepper" retinal pigmentation.

gerontologist *n* [Gk *geron* old man + Gk *-logia* study of]
A health professional who specializes in working with the elderly.

gerontology *n* [Gk *geron* old man + Gk *-logia* study of]
The study of the aging process, especially conditions affecting the health of the elderly.
Deriv: -*adj* gerontological

gestational age *np* [Lat *gestare* carry (in the womb)]
The age of an embryo from the time of fertilization.

gland *n*
A cell group that secretes substances.

gland, endocrine *np*
A cell group that secretes directly into the blood, e.g., hormones.

gland, exocrine *np*
A cell group that secretes through ducts opening in the skin, e.g., cerumenous glands.

glia *n* glīa/glēa [Gk *glia* glue]
Also: neuroglia
A fine web of connective tissue that supports the neurons in the central nervous system.

glide *n*
In phonetics, a transitional sound as the speech organs pass from the position of one speech sound to another, e.g., any diphthong or semivowel.

glioblastoma *n* [Gk *glia* glue + Gk *blastos* sprout, germ + Gk *-oma* denoting tumor, swelling]
A malignant tumor of the central nervous system. The most aggressive type of brain tumor.

glioma *n* [Gk *glia* glue + Gk *-oma* denoting tumor, swelling]
A tumor in the brain tissue. So-called because it arises from glial cells that surround and support the nerve cells.

globoid cell leukodystrophy *np* [Gk *globos* a globe + Gk *eidos* a shape; Gk *leukos* white + Gk *dus-* bad + Gk *trophe* nourishment]
Also: Krabbe disease
A very rare genetic disorder of the nervous system where the body lacks the substance required to produce myelin, the material that surrounds and protects nerve fibers. Symptoms are variable, but may include deafness with sensitivity to loud sounds. The condition is most common in persons of Scandinavian descent.

glomus tumor *np* 'glōmus [Lat *glomus* ball of thread; Lat *tumor* a swelling]
A painful tumor that can occur in the middle ear. Pain tends to be linked with the pulsation of blood.

glossopharyngeal nerve *n* [Gk *glossa* tongue + Gk *pharynx* pharynx]
The ninth cranial nerve which carries general sensory information from the middle ear, upper pharynx, and the posterior one-third of the tongue (including taste sensation) and supplies the muscles of the pharynx, tongue, middle ear, and soft palate.

glottal *adj* [Gk *glotta* tongue]
Formed at the level of the vocal folds, where the air is impeded, but not enough

to produce vocal fold vibration, as in the speech sound "h."

glottal stop *np* [Gk *glotta* tongue]
Closure of the glottis causing a brief stoppage of the airstream. Used in some dialects, often as a replacement for "t," e.g., "bo(tt)le" (bo◌l).

glottis *n* [Gk *glotta* tongue]
The air channel between the vocal cords.

glucocorticoid *n*
A steroid hormone produced by the adrenal cortex in response to serious injury or stress and having antiinflammatory properties, e.g., hydrocortisone. May be ototoxic in large doses.

glue ear *np*
Also: otitis media with effusion
Accumulation of a thick sticky fluid in the middle ear, common in children.

goblet cells *np*
Mucus secreting cells in the respiratory and intestinal tracts.

go game *np colloq*
A method of pediatric hearing testing using conditioning to the word "go."

goiter (goitre) *n*
A swelling in neck as a result of an enlargement of the thyroid gland.

Goldenhar syndrome *n* Named after Maurice Goldenhar (1924–2001), an American physician, who first described the condition in 1952.
Also: hemifacial microsomia; first and second branchial arch syndrome; facioauricular vertebral spectrum; oculoauricular vertebral dysphasia
A congenital disorder, prevalent in males, associated with abnormal development of the first and second branchial arches. This leads to incomplete development of the ear, nose, soft palate, lip, and mandible. Characteristics include severe conductive hearing loss, microtia and atresia, vision defects, marked facial asymmetry, skeletal malformations, colobomas

(clefts) of the upper eyelid, and occasionally mild to moderate learning difficulty.

gonadal dysgenesis *np* [Gk *gonades* gonads; Gk *dus-* bad + Gk *genesis* growth]
Also: Turner syndrome; XO syndrome
A chromosomal disorder in which there is not the usual pair of X chromosomes. Affects only females. characterized by small stature, broad flat chest, absent or incomplete puberty, infertility, webbing of the neck, kidney and heart defects, and hearing loss, which may be conductive and/or sensorineural.

gout *n*
Also: endosteal hyperostosis; hyperostosis corticalis generalisata; hyperphosphatasemia tarda
Inflammatory arthritis, a metabolic condition in which there is a build-up of uric acid in the blood (hyperuricemia). Renal problems occur together with late-onset progressive ataxia and progressive high-frequency sensorineural hearing loss. Deafness may become profound and be accompanied by vestibular abnormalities.

Gradenigo syndrome *np* grădĕ́nēgō
Named after Giuseppe Conte Gradenigo (1859–1926), an Italian otolaryngologist and professor of otolaryngology at the University of Napoli, who first described the syndrome in 1904.
Also: Gradenigo-Lannois syndrome; petrous apicitis
Ipsilateral paralysis of the abducens nerve (sixth cranial nerve) that supplies the lateral rectus muscle of the eyes, characterized by frontal headache, acute otitis media, and persistent double vision.

gradient *n* [Lat *gradiri* to step]
The degree of slope, usually expressed as a ratio or percentage of vertical distance to horizontal distance, e.g., the slope of a tympanogram. Not commonly used for tympanogram analysis.

gradually sloping audiogram *np*
The graph of a hearing loss that falls with increasing frequency by approximately 10 dB per octave.

grammar *n* [Gk *grammata* letters (of the alphabet)]
The rules of language, e.g., tenses, gender, and how words are arranged in sentences.

granulation tissue *n* [Lat *granulum* a little grain]
Vascular connective tissue that develops during the healing of injuries and which helps to prevent infection and to break down damaged tissue. It often leaves a scar and if it forms inside the ear canal it may also cause narrowing or stenosis (closure) of the canal.

granuloma *n* [Lat *granulum* a little grain + Gk *–oma* denoting tumor, swelling]
A nodular mass of granulation tissue associated with chronic infection or inflammation.

grapheme *n* [Gk *graphos* written + Gk *-eme* (from morpheme)]
A letter or letter combination that represents a phoneme.

graphic equalizer (equaliser) *np*
An electronic filter that is used to alter the frequency response of an audio system.

gray (grey) matter *np*
The part of the brain that appears dark in color and contains the nerve cell bodies and dendrites.

grommet *n*
Also: tympanostomy tube
A ventilation tube that is surgically inserted into the eardrum to resolve otitis media.

ground electrode *np*
An electrode whose potential is not affected by the current passing through it and which is used as a ground contact in a voltage-measuring circuit, e.g., the ground electrode in evoked response audiometry, which may be placed anywhere on the scalp.

group hearing aid *np*
An auditory training system that consists of a number of amplifying units, used in the education of groups of hearing impaired children, e.g., in special schools or units. The term is generally used to refer to hard-wired systems.

group therapy *np*
The practice of carrying out therapy, e.g., for tinnitus in groups rather than individually.

gun microphone *np*
A directional microphone on a long arm.

gusher *n colloq*
A gush of perilymph from the oval window of the cochlea, which is a possible complication of stapes surgery.

gyrus *n* ˈjīrus *pl* gyri [Gk *guros* a circle]
A convolution or fold of the cerebral hemispheres.

Haas effect *np* ˈhahs Named after Helmut Haas, a German scientist, who described the effect in his doctoral thesis in 1946.
Also: precedence effect
The condition in which two brief sounds in close succession from different distances are perceived as coming from the nearest source rather than from both.

habenulae perforatae *np sg* habenula perforata [Lat *habenula perforata* perforated strip of flesh]
Perforations running along the lip of the spiral lamina through which the cochlear nerves pass.

habilitation *n*
To make fit or capable.

habituation *n*
A reduced response to a constant or repeated stimulus.

HAIC gain *np*
A standard method (now superseded) of calculating the average gain at 500 Hz, 1 kHz, and 2 kHz that was developed by the Hearing Aid Industry Conference (now known as the Hearing Industries Association).

hair cell, inner *np*
The main sensory receptors of the cochlea that encode frequency information and convert it into nerve impulses.

hair cell, outer *np*
Electromotile cells in the organ of Corti that actively amplify low-level sounds to increase hearing sensitivity and frequency selectivity.

hair cells *np*
Receptor cells, which are end organs for hearing (found in the organ of Corti) and balance (found in the vestibule).

half concha *np*
Also: half shell
A small in-the-ear hearing aid designed to sit in the lower half of the concha area of the pinna.

half gain rule *np* Developed in 1944 by Samuel F. Lybarger (1909–2000), a hearing instrument engineer.
A hearing aid prescription rule that states that the required gain for a sensorineural hearing loss is predicted to be equal to half of the average hearing loss. This rule forms the basis of many hearing aid prescriptions.

half peak level (HPL) *np*
The intensity level of the speech signal at which the individual under test obtains half of their maximum speech discrimination score.

half peak level elevation (HPLE) *np*
The difference between the half peak level of the listener and half of the reference maximum speech recognition score on a speech audiogram.

half shell *np*
Also: half concha
A small in-the-ear hearing aid designed to sit in the lower half of the concha area of the pinna.

half skeleton *np*
A version of a skeleton earmold with more of the framework cut away making it less visible and easier to insert.

Hallgren syndrome *np* Named after Bertil Hallgren (1918–1960), a Swedish geneticist and pediatric psychiatrist at the Karolinska University Hospital Unit for Child and Adolescent Psychiatry. Hallgren recognized additional features that were part of a syndrome that he and his co-worker Carl-Henry Alström (1907–1993) had described in 1959.
Also: Usher-Hallgren syndrome
A rare autosomal recessive disorder. Characteristics include retinitis pigmentosa, atrophy of the optic nerve, unsteadiness, nystagmus, congenital severe sensorineural hearing loss, heart disease, obesity, and type 2 diabetes, combined with neurologic and psychiatric symptoms.

Hallpike maneuver (manoeuvre) *np*
Named after Charles Skinner Hallpike (1900–1979), an English otologist, who developed a bithermal caloric test and positional tests used in the evaluation of individuals with vertigo.
A test to elicit evidence for benign paroxysmal positional vertigo.

hammer *n colloq*
Also: malleus
The first and largest of the ossicles (bones) of the middle ear, connected to the tympanic membrane by the handle or manubrium.
Deriv: -adj malleolar

hand-hearing syndrome *np*
A syndrome characterized by wasting of the finger muscles with contraction of the digits and sensorineural hearing loss.

handicap *n*
A condition that limits activity or makes achievement difficult.

handle of malleus *np*
Also: manubrium; long process of the malleus
The long part of the malleus (the first bone in the middle ear) that extends from its head.

Harboyan syndrome *np* Named after Garbis Harboyan, a Lebanese otolaryngologist, who reported the syndrome in three siblings in 1971.
Congenital corneal dystrophy, usually detected during primary school age, which leads to blindness by about age 40, together with progressive sensorineural hearing loss of late onset.

hard failure *np*
The complete failure of a cochlear implant.

hard of hearing *adj*
1. Partial hearing loss, partially hearing impaired. 2. An individual with a hearing loss who has sufficient residual hearing to process linguistic information using audition.

hard wired *np*
A term indicating that one system is connected to another by a wire, e.g., a direct audio input connecting a hearing aid system to a radio or television.

harmonic *n* [Lat *harmonia* joining, concord (from Gk *harmos* joint)]
Also: overtone
A tone that is a component of a complex sound, whose frequency is a whole number (or integer) multiple of the fundamental frequency. The first harmonic is the fundamental frequency (f0). The second harmonic (f1 or 2f0) is the first overtone.

harmonic distortion *np*
Additional harmonic components at the output that are not present in the input.

harmonic motion, simple *np*
A repetitive pendulum-like motion back and forth across the equilibrium that traces out a sinusoidal pattern as a function of time. It occurs when acceleration is directed toward the midpoint or equilibrium and is proportional to the displacement away from the equilibrium.

head and torso simulator *np*
A device that replicates the effect of an average head and torso on the sound field at the ear.

head baffle effect *np*
An increase in the sound intensity of low frequencies and a roll-off of high frequencies at one side of the head, when the signal is being delivered from that same side.

headphones *n*
A pair of supra-aural earphones attached together by a headband.

head room *np*
The gain remaining between the measured sound pressure level (SPL) level at the patient's volume control setting and the maximum undistorted capability of the hearing aid.

headset *np*
A pair of supra-aural earphones attached together by a headband and linked to a microphone.

head shadow *np*
An area in which sound from the opposite side of the head is reduced when it reaches the ear shielded by the head. Head shadow is the effect of the head blocking the passage of short-wave high-frequency sounds. If the head is 20 cm wide (an approximate average), any sound wave shorter than 20 cm will not be heard as well on the opposite side. There is no significant attenuation under 1.5 kHz but the high frequencies of speech are particularly affected.

hearing *n*
The perception of sound.

hearing acuity *np*
Sharpness, clearness, keenness of hearing, e.g., being able to detect differences between sounds.

hearing aid *np*
Also: hearing instrument
A device that amplifies sound and delivers it to the ear of a person with hearing loss.

hearing aid audiologist/dispenser *np*
An individual qualified and registered or licensed to sell hearing aids.

Hearing Aid Industry Conference (HAIC) *np obs*
Previous name of the Association for Hearing Aid Manufacturers and Distributors in the USA, which is now called the Hearing Industries Association (HIA).

hearing aid test box *np*
An enclosure or box that attenuates ambient noise and generates sounds of varying frequency and intensity for testing the output of hearing aids.

hearing conservation *np*
A program for the prevention or reduction of hearing loss, usually in industry; including, e.g., reducing noise, monitoring hearing, and providing ear protection and education.

hearing dog *np*
A dog trained to assist a deaf individual by alerting the person to the presence of sounds in the environment, e.g., traffic, telephone, or doorbell ringing.

hearing instrument *np*
Also: hearing aid
A device that amplifies sound and delivers it to the ear of a person with hearing loss.

hearing level (HL) *np*
The level of a signal using audiometric zero as reference, i.e., the reference standard of normal hearing.

hearing loss *np*
1. The number of decibels a tone must be raised above the normal average threshold value for the tone to be detected. 2. A reduction in hearing sensitivity. Hearing loss may be described as mild, moderate, moderately severe, severe, or profound based on an individual's thresholds averaged over a specified range of frequencies, i.e., 250 Hz to 4 kHz (five frequency average), 500 Hz to 4 kHz (four frequency average), 1 kHz to 4 kHz (three frequency average). The World Health Organization (WHO) suggest classifying according to the hearing in the better ear using the four frequency average, but a diversity of methods continue to be used.

hearing loss, mild *np*
1. A subjective description of a minor hearing loss. 2. An average hearing level of 26 dBHL (UK: 2 dBHL) to 40 dBHL of 26 dBHL to 40 dBHL (UK: 21-40 dBHL; WHO: 26-40 dBHL).

hearing loss, moderate *np*
1. A subjective description of a medium level of hearing loss. 2. An average hearing of 41 dBHL to 55 dBHL (UK: 41-70 dBHL; WHO: 41-60 dBHL).

hearing loss, moderately severe *np*
An average hearing level of 56 dBHL to 70 dBHL (UK: not applicable).

hearing loss, profound *np*
An average hearing level in excess of 90 dBHL (UK: > 95 dBHL; WHO: > 80 dBHL).

hearing loss, severe *np*
1. A subjective description of a severe to profound level of hearing loss. 2. Average hearing level between 71 dBHL to 90 dBHL (UK: 71-95 dBHL; WHO: 61-80 dBHL).

hearing protection *np*
Earplugs or earmuffs to protect the ears from noise damage. These may be active (electronic) or passive.

hearing protection, double *np*
The use of both earplugs and earmuffs together, which increases the protection by 3 dB over single usage and which may be used in very high levels of noise.

hearing therapist *np* [Gk *therapeuein* to heal]
A professional with training to undertake rehabilitation of adults with impaired hearing.

hearing threshold level (HTL) *np*
The amount by which a person's hearing threshold exceeds the reference standard of normal hearing, i.e., a person's hearing loss as shown on an audiogram.

heel *n*
The part of an earmold that is between the tragus and the antitragus.

helicotrema *n* [Gk *helix* spiral + Gk *trema* hole]
The narrow connection in the cochlea between the scala vestibuli and the scala tympani.

helix *n* [Gk *helix* spiral]
1. The rolled edge of the pinna. 2. The part of the earmold that extends up to the helix of the pinna.

Helmholtz's theory of resonance *np*
Named after Hermann Ludwig Ferdinand von Helmholtz (1821–1894), a German physician and physicist, who proposed this theory and made significant contributions to the understanding of sound perception and the sensation of tone.
The theory, advanced in 1857, that the hair cells in the organ of Corti each vibrate to one particular frequency.

hema-/hemo- (haema-/haemo-) *prefix*
[Gk *haima* blood]
Blood.

hematoma (haematoma) *n* [Gk *haima* blood + Gk *–oma* denoting tumor, swelling]
An accumulation of blood.

hemifacial microsomia *np* [Gk *hemi-* half + Lat *facies* face; Gk *mikros* small + Gk *soma* body]
Also: Goldenhar syndrome; first and second branchial arch syndrome; facioauricular vertebral spectrum; oculoauricular vertebral dysphasia
A craniofacial disorder; characteristics are unilateral and include facial abnormalities, preauricular tags and pinna malformations, eye abnormalities, and unilateral conductive hearing loss.

hemotympanum (haemotympanum) *n*
[Gk *haima* blood + Gk *tumpanon* a drum]
A collection of blood in the middle ear space, usually due to head trauma.

hemorrhage (haemorrhage) *n* [Gk *haima* blood + Gk *rhegnunai* to burst]
Profuse bleeding from a damaged blood vessel.

Hennebert sign *np* ĕn'beα Named after Camille Hennebert (1867–1958), a Belgian otologist, who first described in 1909 the "fistula sign" (i.e., without a fistula) that occurs in hereditary syphilis.
Nystagmus induced by increasing pressure inside the ear canal.

Hensen canal *np* Named after Viktor Hensen (1835–1924), a German physiologist and professor of physiology at Kiel University, who described the organ of Corti including the cells now known as the cells of Hensen in 1863.
Also: Reichert's canal; reuniens canal/duct

113

The small channel that joins the cochlea to the saccule of the vestibular system.

Hensen cells *np* Named after Christian Andreas Viktor Hensen (1835–1924), a German physiologist and professor of physiology at Kiel University, who described the organ of Corti including the cells now known as the cells of Hensen in 1863.

Supporting cells in the organ of Corti, between the outer hair cells and the cells of Claudius.

Hensen stripe *np* Named after Christian Andreas Viktor Hensen (1835–1924), a German zoologist and professor of physiology at the University of Kiel, who described the organ of Corti including the structures now associated with his name in 1863.

A longitudinal ridge on the surface of the tectorial membrane, located directly opposite the inner hair cells. The curvature of the Hensen stripe along the cochlea causes it to act as a topographic waveguide or filter that controls the dispersion of the energy as a function of frequency.

hereditary *adj* [Lat *hereditas* heredity]
Traits that are passed through families from parents to their offspring.

hereditary hyperphosphatasia *np*
Also: Paget disease, juvenile; hyperphosphatasia osteoectasia; familial idiopathic phostophasia
A genetic autosomal recessive mutation; characteristics may include progressive bone deformity with pain, small stature, enlarged skull, and possible sensorineural hearing loss due to compression of the nerve.

Herrmann syndrome *np* Named after Jurgen Herrmann (b 1941), a German geneticist and professor of pediatrics in Wisconsin, who reported the syndrome in 1974.

A nervous system disorder characterized by muscle convulsions in response to flashes of light, personality changes, dementia, ataxia, diabetes, renal disease, and progressive sensorineural hearing loss.

hermetic *adj* [Gk *hermetikos* sealed]
With an airtight seal.

herpes zoster *np* [Gk *herpes* shingles (from *herpein* to creep)]
Also: shingles
A viral infection (varicella zoster virus) characterized by skin spots and rashes and commonly seen in children and young adults as chickenpox, but in later life as shingles. The virus can lie dormant in the bodies of nerves for many years before breaking out again. The virus may cause shingles (herpes zoster), a painful skin rash above the affected nerve, with possible nerve pain even when the rash has disappeared. If the auditory nerve is affected, there may be sensorineural hearing loss with pain.

Hertz (Hz) *n* Named after Heinrich Hertz (1857–1894), a German physicist, who first demonstrated the existence of electromagnetic waves. Hertz was established as the standard international unit of frequency in his honor in 1930.
Also: cycle per second (cps)
A unit of frequency that is equal to one cycle per second.

Heschl gyri *np* ˈhĕshĕl [Gk *guros* circle] Named after Richard L. Heschl (1824–1881), an Austrian professor of pathological anatomy, who published a description of the convolution of the temporal lobe in 1855.

Small convolutions of the temporal lobe that contain the primary auditory cortex, which has tonotopic organization and is responsible for processing auditory signals.

heterozygote *n* [Gk *heteros* other + Gk *zugotos* yoked]
Also: carrier
An individual who has two different forms of a particular gene, one inherited from each parent.
Deriv: –adj heterozygous

hiatus *n* hī′āt*us* [Lat *hiatus* gaping]
An opening, tear or weakness in tissue.

high fidelity *np*
Also: colloq hi-fi
High-quality sound reproduction, amplification, or transmission having minimal distortion.

high frequency *np*
A high-pitched tone. Tones of 1 kHz and above are generally thought to sound high frequency.

high-frequency audiometry *np*
Audiometry that extends beyond 8 kHz, usually to 16 kHz.

high-frequency average *np*
An electroacoustic characteristic that assesses the average response values of a hearing aid in dB by measuring the maximum gain at three standard high frequencies, e.g., 1 kHz, 1.6 kHz, and 2.5 kHz.

high pass filter *np*
A filter that attenuates the low frequencies, but allows the frequencies above the cut-off frequency to pass.

hillocks of His *np* hĭs Named after Wilhelm His (1831–1904), a German embryologist, who produced an early account of stages of development of human embryos. He published his findings in the *Anatomie Menschlicher Embryonen,* 1880.
Also: auricular hillocks of His
Small buds or hillocks that arise along the first and second arches by the fifth week of gestation and which form the pinna (or auricle) by the 20th week of gestation. Each hillock develops into a structure of the pinna, e.g., the first hillock forms the tragus.

hindbrain *n*
Also: rhombencephalon
The rear area of the brain that contains the pons, cerebellum, and medulla oblongata.

Hi-pro *n*
A hearing instrument programmer, i.e., a device that acts as an interface to connect hearing aids to the programming computer.

histogram *n* [Gk *histos* mast + Gk *gramma* something written]
A graph of statistical distribution in which each category is represented by a rectangular column.

histology *n* [Gk *histos* tissue + Gk *-logia* study of]
The study of the microscopic structure of tissues.

histopathology *n* [Gk *histos* tissue + Gk *pathos* disease + Gk *-logia* study of]
The study of changes in the microscopic structure of tissues caused by disease.

holophrase *n* [Gk *holos* whole + Gk *phrasis* speaking]
A single word utterance used to carry the meaning of a sentence, characteristic of the language of very young children.

homeostasis *n* [Gk *homoios* like + Gk *stasis* stoppage]
The regulation and maintenance of an organism's internal conditions, e.g., the regulation of body temperature.

homogeneous *adj* [Gk *homos* same + Gk *genos* race, kind]
1. Of the same kind or nature, uniform, and not diversified. 2. Composed of parts or elements that are all of the same kind.

homophasic *adj* [Gk *homos* same + Gk *phasis* appearance]
Having the same phase.

homophemes *n* [Gk *homos* same + Gk *phemi* I speak]
Words that look alike on the lips.

homophone *n* [Gk *homos* same + Gk *phone* sound]
A word that sounds the same as another, but is spelled differently.

Hood plateau method *np* Named after John Derrick Hood, a British audiologic physician, neurootologist, and the first chairperson of the British Society of Audiology (1967-1971), who first published a description of the method in 1960.

A method of masking used to obtain true hearing thresholds by introducing noise in the nontest ear to prevent detection by the nontest ear of stimuli presented to the test ear. Masking noise is gradually increased in the nontest ear to establish a plateau, i.e., where several successive levels of masking yield identical (within 5 dB) results in the test ear.

horizontal plane *np*
The tranverse plane of the body (i.e., across from one side to the other), e.g., the horizontal semicircular canal.

horizontal section *np*
A slice through the brain parallel to the ground.

horn *n*
An earmold tubing modification in which the narrow bore of the tubing (coming from the earhook) is increased gradually to a larger diameter in the ear canal. This provides a better impedance match to the ear and therefore improved transmission of high frequencies.

Hotchkiss otoscope *np* Named after John E. Hotchkiss (1925–2007), an American otolaryngologist, whose long-time interest in optics and photography culminated in the invention of the Hotchkiss Otoscope, which was patented in 1968.
A handheld brightly illuminated magnifying device used for examining the ear, often during the removal of wax from the ear.

Hunter syndrome *np* Named after Charles A. Hunter (1873–1955), a Scottish-Canadian physician, who described the syndrome in 1917. The syndrome was first observed in 1900 when it was termed "gargoylism."
A recessive X-linked syndrome that can affect both sexes. Normal appearance at birth soon gives way to progressive abnormalities including poor growth, learning difficulty, coarse facial features, chronic nasal discharge, and middle ear effusions. Mixed hearing loss is also common.

Hurler syndrome *np* Named after Gertrud Hurler (1889–1965), a German pediatrician, who described the syndrome in 1919. Hurler was probably unaware of Hunter's description due to disrupted communications during WWI.
An autosomal recessive syndrome similar to Hunter syndrome, but less severe and affecting only males. Includes progressive hearing loss.

hydro- *prefix* [Gk *hudor* water]
Pertaining to water.

hydrocephalus *n* [Gk *hudor* water + Gk *kephale* head]
Accumulation of fluid on and around the brain.

hydrops *n* [Gk *hydrops* accumulation of water]
Accumulation of fluid.

hypacusis/hypocusis *n* [Gk *hupo* below + Gk *akousis* sense of hearing]
Hearing loss.

hyper- *prefix* [Gk *huper* above]
Above or increased.

hyperacusis *n* [Gk *huper* above + Gk *akousis* sense of hearing]
An oversensitivity to sound.

hyperbilirubinemia (hyperbilirubinaemia) *n* [Gk *huper* above + Gk *haima* blood]
Also: erythroblastosis fetalis
An abnormally large amount of bilirubin present at birth that results in jaundice.

hypermetric saccades *np* [Gk *huper* above + Gk *metron* measure; Fr *saccade* jerky motion]
An overshoot of the eyes to beyond the target that can occur in ENG testing, during calibration.

hyperostosis corticalis generalisata *np* [Gk *huper* above + Gk *osteon* bone + Gk

-osis denoting a diseased state; Lat *cortex* tree bark, outer layer]
Also: endosteal hyperostosis; hyperostosis corticalis generalisata; hyperphosphatasemia tarda; Van Buchem syndrome
A genetic bone disorder characterized by overgrowth of the mandible and thickening of the long bones and the forehead and brow area. The bone growth may trap cranial nerves, causing facial palsy, and sight and hearing problems.

hyperphosphatasia *n*
Also: juvenile Paget disease; hyperphosphatasia osteoectasia; familial idiopathic phostophasia
A genetic autosomal recessive mutation. Characteristics may include progressive bone deformity with pain, small stature, enlarged skull, and possible sensorineural hearing loss.

hyperprolinemia (prolinaemia) II *np*
An inherited metabolic abnormality. Sometimes associated with learning difficulty, convulsions, and late-onset progressive sensorineural hearing loss.

hypertension *n* [Gk *huper* above + Lat *tensio* tension]
High blood pressure; the measurement of force against the walls of the arteries.

hypertrophy *n* hī'pertrofē [Gk *huper* above + Gk *trophe* nourishment]
Also: macrotia
Enlargement of the pinna.

hyperuricemia neurologic ataxia, deafness *n* [Gk *huper* above + Lat *urina* urine + Gk *haima* blood]
Inflammatory arthritis, a metabolic condition in which there is a buildup of uric acid in the blood (hyperuricemia). Renal problems occur together with late-onset progressive ataxia and progressive high-frequency sensorineural hearing loss. Deafness may become profound and be accompanied by vestibular abnormalities.

hypo- *prefix* [Gk *hupo* below]
1. Less or below. 2. Deficiency, underdevelopment or lack of.

hypoacusis *n* [Gk *hupo* below + Gk *akousis* sense of hearing]
Hearing loss.

hypogenesis *n* [Gk *hupo* below + Gk *genesis* creation]
Underdevelopment of an embryo.

hypoglossal nerve *np* [Gk *hupo* below + Gk *glossa* tongue]
The twelfth cranial nerve (XII) which leads to the tongue and is responsible for tongue movements and swallowing.

hypoglycemic *adj* [Gk *hupo* below + Gk *glukus* sweet + Gk *haima* blood]
Having reduced glucose in the blood.

hypoplasia *n* [Gk *hupo* below + Gk *plasis* formation]
The underdevelopment of a tissue or organ.

hypothalamus *n* [Gk *hupo* below + Gk *thalamos* chamber]
A small structure at the base of the brain that controls core functions of the autonomic nervous system and the endocrine system.

hypothesis *n pl* hypotheses [Gk *hupothesis* foundation]
An idea or a statement made for testing its empirical or logical consequences.

hypotympanum *n* [Gk *hupo* below + Gk *tumpanon* drum]
Also: atrium
1. A cavity affording entrance to another structure. 2. The part of the middle ear below the malleus.

hypoxia *n* [Gk *hupo* below + Gk *oxus* sharp (acid)]
A condition in which the body or body tissues is deprived of oxygen.

hypoxia, cochlear *np*
Decreased oxygen to the cochlea, which is extremely sensitive to oxygen deprivation. Oxygen deprivation causes degenerative changes in the cochlea, first affect-

ing inner hair cells, but with outer hair cells also affected if the hypoxia is sustained.

hysteresis *n* [Gk *husteron* behind]
A change that lags behind the agent for the change, e.g., magnetization lags behind the magnetizing force.

hysterical deafness *np obs* [Gk *husterikos* of the womb]
Deafness of psychological cause.

iatrogenic *adj* ĭătrō'jĕnĭk [Gk *iatros* doctor + Gk *–genes* born of, arising from]
Unintentional damage or effect due to a medical or surgical treatment.

ichthyosiform erythroderma deafness keratitis *np* ĭkthēōsĭfawm [Gk *ickthus* a fish + Lat *forma* shape; Gk *eruthros* red + Gk *derma* skin]
Also: Senter syndrome; keratitis ichthyosiform/ichthyosis deafness (KID syndrome); Desmond syndrome; *colloq* fish-skin disease
A genetic abnormality of the ectodermal structures (hair, teeth, skin, craniofacial structure, etc.). Symptoms include red skin covered with white scales, gradual destruction of the lens and cornea of the eyes and sensorineural hearing. The skin abnormalities result in poor control of water loss and temperature and difficulty in fighting infection.

ICRA noise *np*
A type of speech spectrum-shaped noise that was developed for the International Collegium of Rehabilitative Audiology for use in hearing aid testing.

icterus *n* [Gk *ikteros* jaundice]
Also: jaundice
A yellowish discoloration of the skin and other tissues caused by an excessive amount of bilirubin (bile pigment) in the blood. Jaundice is one of the high-risk factors for hearing loss.

idio- *prefix* [Gk *idios* peculiar, distinct]
Personal, peculiar, or distinct.

idiom *n* [Gk *idioma* private property]
Phrase or expression characteristic of a particular group.

idiopathic *adj* [Gk *idios* peculiar, distinct + Gk *patheia* form of suffering]
Arising spontaneously from an unknown cause, e.g., idiopathic hydrops.

iminoglycinuria *n* [Gk *glukus* sweet + Gk *ouron* urine]

Also: iminoglycynurea; familial iminoglycinuria
A metabolic disorder that affects the renal (kidney) transport system and affects reabsorption of amino acids. It may be associated with deafness, blindness, and learning difficulty.

immittance *n* [Lat *immitere* to send in, urge on]
Also: oto-immittance
A generic term for the flow of energy through the middle ear, including impedance and admittance.

immittance audiometry *np*
The procedure for measuring the acoustic impedance or admittance of the middle ear. Used in the identification of middle ear conditions.

immittance bridge *np*
The original term used when a tympanometer was based on a bridge circuit.

immotile *adj* [Lat *in-* (negative) + Lat *motus* motion]
Lacking mobility.

immune *adj* [Lat *immunis* exempt from]
Having a high degree of resistance, especially to disease.

immunology *n* [Lat *immunis* exempt from + Gk *-logia* study of]
The science of immunity and its causes.
Deriv: –adj immunological

immunomodulator *n* [Lat *immunis* exempt from + Lat *modulari* to measure, modulate]
A drug or other substance that stimulates or suppresses the immune system.

immunotherapy *n* [Lat *immunis* exempt from + Gk *therapeia* healing, treatment]
Immunization to stimulate immune function or treatment by immunosuppression.

impact *n/v* [Lat *impactus* struck firmly]
–n A forceful strike. *–v* To have a direct effect on.

impacted *adj*
Being tightly packed or wedged, e.g., impacted wax.

impact noise *np*
High-intensity noise caused by mechanical force through a structure, e.g., hammering or footsteps on a hard floor.

impairment *n* [Old Fr *empeirier* make worse]
Damage or decrease of function.
Deriv: -adj impaired

impedance *n* [Lat *impedire* to shackle the feet, impede]
The difficulty or hindrance to a flow of energy due to the combined effect of resistance and reactance.

impedance, acoustic *np* [Lat *impedire* to shackle the feet, impede; Gk *akoustikos* pertaining to hearing]
The property of a medium that opposes its vibration. This is frequency dependent and related to the density of the medium and the speed of sound in the medium.

impedance matching *np*
A way of optimizing the transfer of power between two mediums so that energy can pass readily from one medium to another.

impedance mismatch *np*
A condition that occurs where sound travels from one medium into another that has a different impedance or resistance, e.g., air to fluid. Some of the acoustic energy is reflected and only some transmitted into the second medium.

impede *v* [Lat *impedire* to shackle the feet, impede]
To resist flow.

implant *v/n*
–*v* To surgically fix or permanently insert.
–*n* A device that is surgically inserted, e.g., a cochlear implant.

implosive sound *np*
A stop consonant caused by a sudden inhaling of air into the pharynx, e.g., such as found in Swahili.

impression *n*
A cast.

impression, ear *np*
A plastic cast of the concha and outer ear canal used to make an earmold or hearing aid shell.

impulse noise *np*
An explosive burst of transient noise, e.g., hammering, gunshot, or explosion.

inaudible *adj*
Below the threshold of hearing.

incidence *n* [Lat *incidere* to happen]
The number of new cases, e.g., of a disease, within a specified time, place, or group.

incident *n/adj*
–*n* A noteworthy occurrence, an event or happening. –*adj* Striking a surface.

incident wave *np*
The direct wave from a source.

incudectomy *n* [Lat *incus* anvil + Gk *ektome* excision]
Surgical removal of the incus.

incus *n* *pl* incudes [Lat *incus* anvil]
The middle bone of the ossicular chain, thought by early anatomists to be shaped like an anvil.
Deriv: –adj incudal

independent variable *np*
An aspect that is manipulated in an experiment or study to see if it causes a change in some other aspect, i.e., the dependent variable.

index *n* *pl* indexes; indices
An alphabetical or numerical list or system.

index, articulation *np*
A means of quantifying the amount of the speech signal available to the listener.

indifferent *adj*
Having no significant effect on the resulting record.

indifferent electrode *np*
A reference or dispersive electrode.

induce *v* [Lat *inducere* to lead in, bring on]
To produce or influence, e.g., noise-induced hearing loss.

induction *n*
1. A change in voltage across a conductor, caused by a changing magnetic field. 2. An orientation or introductory program.

induction loop *np*
A wire loop installed around a room or similar space. Hearing aid wearers within the specified area can pick up transmitted signals by electromagnetic induction.

industrial audiometry *np* [Lat *industria* industriousness]
Audiometric testing undertaken to monitor the effects of high noise levels in a work space.

inertia *n* [Lat *inertia* inaction]
The property of an object to resist change in the existing state. Retention of the state of rest or uniform motion in a straight line unless acted on by an external force.

infantile cochleosaccular degeneration *np* [Lat *infans* an infant; Lat *cochlea* snail shell, spiral + Lat *sacculus* a little sack]
Degeneration of the cochlea during infancy resulting in unilateral or bilateral profound sensorineural hearing loss.

infarction *n* [Lat *infarcire* to stuff into or with]
An obstruction to the local circulation of blood (e.g., a blood clot) leading to the death of an organ or area of tissue (usually the heart).

infection *n* [Lat *inficere* to taint]
Invasion and increase in microorganisms in body tissue causing disease.

inferior *adj* [Lat *inferior* lower]
Situated in the lower area of an object or organ.

inferior colliculus *n* [Lat *inferior* lower; Lat *colliculus* little hill]
One of two protuberances on the roof of the midbrain formed by masses of nerves. The auditory relay center of the midbrain that is tonotopically organized and detects and analyzes auditory stimuli from either ear.

inflammation *n* [Lat *inflammare* to inflame]
Localized redness, heat, pain, and swelling, indicative of injury or infection.

inflection *n* [Lat *inflectere* to bend into]
A change in loudness during speech.

informational counseling *np*
Counseling that provides factual information regarding hearing loss, hearing aids, intervention, etc.

informed consent *np*
An agreement to participate (e.g., in surgery, treatment, or supply of a hearing aid) that is made when the individual fully understands what is involved.

infra- *prefix* [Lat *infra* below]
Below.

infrared *n*
Invisible beams of electromagnetic radiation that have wavelengths shorter than radio waves, but longer than light waves. Infrared is used to transmit sound in some assistive listening devices, e.g., an infrared television listening system.

infrasonic *adj* [Lat *infra* below + Lat *sonus* sound]
Below the range of human hearing (i.e., below about 16 Hz).

inherent noise *np*
Normal circuit noise.

inhibition *n* [Lat *inhibere* to hinder]
Decrease or abolition of an action.

inhibition, neural *np*
The suppression of neural impulses resulting in reduced functioning of an organ, muscle, etc.

inner ear *np*
The labyrinth of the ear, i.e., the cochlea and the semicircular canals (of the vestibular system). The bony labyrinth is a perilymph-filled otic capsule that consists of the cochlea, the vestibule and the semicircular canals. Suspended in the

perilymph within the bony labyrinth is the endolymph-filled membranous labyrinth. This consists of the membranous cochlea (the scala media or cochlear duct), the saccule, the endolymphatic sac, the utricle, and the semicircular canals.

inner hair cells *np*
Sensory cells with hairlike projections (stereocilia) situated along the length of the organ of Corti. They are responsible for transforming the incoming vibrations into electrical impulses and sending them to the brain via cranial nerve VIII.

innervation *n*
1. The supply of nerves to an organ or part of the body. 2. The distribution of nerve impulses.
Deriv: -v innervate

inorganic *adj*
Being or composed of matter other than plant or animal.

in phase *np* [Gk *phasis* appearance]
Having the same phase at the same time, e.g., waves of the same frequency are in phase when their peaks and troughs occur at the same time.

input *n*
The act or process of putting information, power, or energy into a device or system.

input compression *np*
A type of compression in a hearing aid where, as the volume control changes, the gain and output levels are locked together and are shifted up and down simultaneously depending on the volume control setting. The compression threshold remains constant. The volume control setting of the hearing aid does not affect the compression threshold because the level detector is positioned before the gain control.

input/output graph *np*
A graph showing the relationship between the input and output of a hearing aid or other amplifying device; output is on the vertical axis.

insert earphone *np*
A small earphone designed to fit into the external ear.

insertion gain *np*
Also: etymotic gain; real ear gain; transmission gain
The mathematical difference in dB between the sound pressure level in the ear canal without and with a hearing aid.

insertion loss *np*
Any loss or alteration of the natural amplification provided by the head, pinna, and ear canal, e.g., by the insertion of an earmold or hearing aid.

in situ *adj/adv* [Lat *in situ* on site]
On site; a measurement of performance within the actual ear.

in situ gain *np*
The gain of a hearing aid measured on a manikin.

inspissation *n* [Lat *inspissare* to thicken]
The process of becoming thick or dense.

instantaneous *adj*
1. Ocurring without a perceptible time lapse. 2. Occuring at a point in time, e.g., instantaneous amplitude.

integrated circuit *np*
A complex of electrical components and connections produced on a slice of silicon or similar material.

integrating sound-level meter *np*
A sound-level meter that samples the sound environment.

integration *np* [Lat *integrare* make whole]
The act or process of integrating, e.g., the adding of multiple copies of a weak signal to produce one with increased intensity, or the inclusion of hearing-impaired children in mainstream classes.

integration time *np*
The time over which a sound is averaged or summed.

integrity test *np*
A test for the output from a cochlear implant, used when failure of the internal

device is suspected; using a similar procedure to normal evoked response audiometry but concerned with the response
of the device rather than the response of
the nerve.

integument *n* [Lat *integumentum* a cov-
ering]
A covering, e.g., skin.

intelligence quotient (IQ) *np* [Lat *intelle-
gere* to understand; Lat *quot* how many]
A method of comparing mental age with
chronological age. The mental age is divided by chronological age and multiplied
by 100. Average normal IQ at any age is
100.

intelligibility *n*
The degree to which speech is understood by the listener.

intensity *n*
The measure of the strength or magnitude of a stimulating agent. The power
transmitted through a given area. The
amount of acoustic power per unit area
measured in watts per square meter (W/
m2).

intensity coding *np*
The ability of the nervous system to code
intensity changes by altering the firing
rate of neurons.

intensity difference limen *np*
The smallest detectable variation of intensity.

inter- *prefix* [Lat *inter* between]
Between.

interaural *adj* [Lat *inter* between + Lat
auris ear]
Between the ears.

interaural attenuation *np*
The reduction in the intensity of a tone
as it travels from the test ear to the nontest ear. The signal attenuation is due to
the distance and mass between the ears
and is at least 40 dB for air conduction
and is minimal for bone conduction.

interaural intensity difference *np*
The difference in the intensity of a signal
arriving at the left and the right ears of
an individual.

interaural time difference *np*
The difference in time of arrival of a signal at the left and the right ears of an individual.

interdental *adj* [Lat *inter* between + Lat
dens tooth]
Formed with the tongue between the
teeth, e.g., as in the production of the
speech sounds "th" (θ and ð).

interface *n*
The place where two devices come into
contact.

interference *n*
1. Unintended noise. 2. Areas of reduced
sound pressure that occur when two or
more waves of the same frequency are
out of phase.

interference, constructive *np*
The condition that occurs when waves
are completely in phase, such that the resultant wave will be twice the amplitude
of the original.

interference, destructive *np*
Where waves of the same amplitude,
wavelength, and frequency are fully out
of phase, the interference between the
wave crests and troughs is such that they
cancel each other out and there is no
sound.

interferometry *n*
A technique that uses patterns of wave
interference to make accurate measurements. It is used to obtain high-resolu-
tion anatomic images.

interleave processing *np*
A process that allows separate data channels to be played back simultaneously.

intermittent *n*
Coming and going at intervals; not continuous.

intermittent sounds *np*
Sounds that have breaks interrupting a continuous signal.

intermodulation distortion *np*
Distortion that occurs when two or more signals are passed through a nonlinear system. Additional frequencies are present in the output that are equal to the sums and differences of those frequencies already present.

internal auditory/acoustic meatus/canal
np [Lat *internus* internal; Lat *auditorius* pertaining to hearing; Lat *meatus* passage]
Also: meatus acousticus internus
The canal in the petrous portion of the temporal bone that contains the vestibulocochlear nerve.

internal carotid artery *np* [Lat *internus* internal; Gk *karotis* drowsiness; Gk *arteria* blood vessel, artery]
Either of the two major arteries (left and right) that supply blood to the head and neck.

internal feedback *np*
1. Feedback that is due to electrical or mechanical causes within a hearing aid. 2. The information received from the body, e.g., heart rate, used to monitor one's own physical state.

international phonetic alphabet (IPA)
np
A set of standardized symbols used to represent the phonemes of speech.

interneuron *n* [Lat *inter* between + Gk *neuron* a string, nerve]
A neuron located entirely in the central nervous system.

interpeak *adj*
Pertaining to the difference between two wave peaks, e.g., interpeak latency.

interpolation *n* [Lat *interpolare* to refurbish, alter]
1. Data inserted between elements. 2. The determination of intermediate frequencies, which have not been measured, based on a set of measured frequencies.

interruptor *n*
The switch on an audiometer that presents or interrupts the signal being delivered to the individual being tested.

interstitial fluid *np* ĭnterˈstĭshəl [Lat *interstitium* a standing between]
Fluid that is found in intercellular spaces within an organ or tissue.

intertragic notch *np* ĭnterˈträjĭk [Gk *tragus* goat (from the characteristic tuft of hair that grow in old men, like a goat's beard)]
The small U-shaped notch at the bottom of the concha, between and below the tragus and antitragus.

interval *n*
1. An intervening gap between two points or units. 2. A period of cessation.

interval data *np*
Items measured on a scale, e.g., a 5-point scale, where each position is equidistant from the neighboring positions. Often used to assess benefit and residual disability after a hearing aid fitting.

interval, frequency *np*
The spacing in frequency between two sounds.

interval scale *np*
A quantitative scale that relates to a particular reference but is arbitrary and has no true or absolute zero. The scale compares differences in relative magnitude, e.g., rating scales, decibel scales.

intervention *n* [Lat *interventio* a coming between]
Action planned to hinder, improve or modify, e.g., early intervention for deaf children to help establish language.

intonation *n* [Lat *intonare* to chant]
The rising and falling pattern of pitch changes in connected speech which can convey differences in meaning, e.g., as a question or a statement.

intra- *prefix* [Lat *intra* within]
Within.

intraaural *adj*
Within the ear.

intraaural muscles *np* [Lat *intra* within + Lat *auris* ear]
Muscles found within the ear, i.e., the tensor tympani and stapedial muscles.

intraaxial *adj* [Lat *intra* within + Gk *axis* axis]
Within the brain or central nervous system.

intracellular *adj*
Contained inside cells.

intratympanic *np* [Lat *intra* within + Gk *tumpanon* a drum]
Within the middle ear or tympanic cavity.

in utero *np* [Lat *in utero* in the uterus]
Within the uterus, before birth.

inverse square law *np*
Also: Coulomb's law
A law that states that the intensity of a sound decreases in proportion to the square of the distance from the source. In practical terms, the amplitude of the wave reduces by 6 dB every time the distance from the sound source doubles.

in vitro *np* [Lat *in vitro* in glass (i.e., in a dish or test tube)]
Occurring outside the body, in an artificial environment.

in vivo *np* [Lat *in vivo* in the living body]
Occurring within a living body or in a real-life situation.

ion *n* [Gk *ion* going]
An atom or molecule that carries a positive or negative charge as a result of having lost or gained one or more electrons.

ion channel *n*
A specialized protein molecule that permits ions to enter or leave cells.

ion channel, voltage-dependent *np*
An ion channel that opens or closes de-

pending on the value of the membrane potential.

ipsilateral *adj* [Lat *ipse* the same + Lat *latus* side]
On the same side.

ipsilateral paralysis of the abducens nerve *np*
Also: Gradenigo syndrome
Ipsilateral paralysis of the abducens nerve (cranial nerve VI) that supplies the lateral rectus muscle of the eyes. Characterized by frontal headache, acute otitis media, and persistent double vision.

ipsilateral routing of signals (IROS) hearing aid *np*
A hearing aid system that delivers the signal to the same ear to which it is fitted.

irrigation, caloric *np* [Lat *irrigare* to water or irrigate; Lat *calor* heat]
Also: caloric stimulation
The method of introducing warm and cool water into the ear canal to test vestibular function.

ischemia *n* [Gk *ischemia* stopping the blood]
A deficiency in the blood supply to a body part due to an obstruction or narrowing of the arteries.

iso- *prefix* [Gk *isos* equal]
Equal.

isometric *adj* [Gk *isos* equal + Gk *metron* a measure]
Having equal dimensions.

isophonemic *adj* [Gk *isos* equal + Gk *phone* sound]
Having the same distribution of phonemes, i.e., each word list contains the same phonemes, but not necessarily having phonemic or phonetic balance.

isthmus *n* [Gk *isthmos* a narrow strip of land]
A narrow connection between two parts or larger structures, e.g., the isthmus of external auditory meatus is the narrow-

est part of the ear canal at the junction of its bony and cartilaginous part.

iterative *adj* [Lat *iterare* to repeat] Repeated.

-itis *suffix* [Gk *-ites* denoting disease of] Inflammation.

Iwashita syndrome *np* Named after Hiroshi Iwashita, a Japanese neurologist, who first reported the syndrome in 1971.
A rare hereditary syndrome, similar to Rosenberg-Chutorian syndrome, characterized by progressive loss of vision and hearing from birth, together with many other functional disturbances of the nervous system.

J

jack plug *np*
A female fitting in an audio or electrical circuit used with a (male) plug to make a connection.

Jacobson nerve *np* Named after Ludwig Levin Jacobson (1783–1843), a Danish anatomist, who published a detailed description of the anatomy of the mammalian ear in 1818.
Also: tympanic nerve
The tympanic branch of cranial nerve IX, the glossopharyngeal nerve. Provides the main sensory fibers to the middle ear and the Eustachian tube.

jargon *n*
1. The specialized language of a profession or group. 2. Prelinguistic vocalizations. The strings of syllables spoken by infants with adultlike intonation that is mostly incomprehensible.

jaundice *n* [Fr *jaune* yellow]
Also: icterus
A yellowish discoloration of the skin and other tissues is caused by an excessive amount of bilirubin (bile pigment) in the blood. Jaundice is one of the high-risk factors for hearing loss.

Jervell and Lange-Neilsen syndrome *np*
Named after Anton Jervell (1919–1989) and Fred Lange-Neilsen (1901–1987), Norwegian physicians, who first completely described the condition in 1957.
Also: cardioauditory syndrome
An autosomal recessive genetic syndrome that causes congenital profound deafness and an irregular heart rhythm.

Jewett sequence/waves *np colloq*
Named after Don L. Jewett, professor emeritus in the department of orthopedic surgery at the University of California–San Francisco, who was the co-discoverer (with J.S. Williston) of the auditory brainstem response in 1971.
The fast wave components of the auditory brainstem response

joint *n*
A point of articulation; the point of contact between elements of an animal skeleton and their supporting structures.

joule *n* Named in honor of James Prescott Joule (1818–1889), an English physicist, who established the basis of the law of conservation of energy.
A derived unit of energy, work, or amount of heat in the International System of Units. The unit of energy expended in 1 second by an electric current of 1 ampere against a resistance of 1 ohm.

just noticeable difference (JND) *np*
Also: difference limen; threshold difference; differential threshold
The differential threshold. The minimum detectable change in a stimulus, e.g., the smallest change in intensity of a pure tone.

K-amp *n* Introduced in 1989 by Mead Killion (b 1939), an American electronic engineer working in the hearing aid industry, who developed the K-amp in 1988.
An automatic signal processing hearing aid circuit.

Kabuki syndrome *np* Named after a type of Japanese theater as it was thought that the distinctive facial features of children with this syndrome resembled the characters in Kabuki theater.
A rare congenital disorder with very variable symptoms. These may include elongated eyelids, prominent earlobes, cleft palate, recurring ear infections in infancy, heart defects, hearing loss, and growth defects.

kanamycin *n*
A water-soluble broad spectrum aminoglycoside antibiotic used to treat severe infections, which can have a toxic effect on the outer hair cells of the cochlea and the striola (small stria) of the utricle.

karyotype *n* [Gk *karuon* nut kernal + Gk *tupos* form, type]
An organized visual profile of the chromosomes within the nucleus of a cell of an organism.

Kearns-Sayre syndrome (KSS) *np* Named after Thomas P. Kearns (1922–2011), an American neuroophthalmologist and George Pomeroy Sayre (1911–1992), an American ophthalmologist, who first described the syndrome in 1958.
A rare genetic progressive neuromuscular disorder due to abnormalities in the DNA of the mitochondria. Characteristics may include progressive immobility of the eyes, eyelid droop, pigmentary degeneration of the retina, hearing loss, cardiac defects, short stature, learning difficulty, and ataxia (inability to coordinate voluntary movements).

keloid *n/adj* ˈkēloid [Gk *khele* crab's claw + Gk *eidos* shape, form]

–n Thick scar resulting from excessive growth of fibrous tissue. *–adj* consisting of keloid scar tissue.
Deriv: –adj keloidal

keratin *n* [Gk *keras* horn, nail]
A tough fibrous protein substance that occurs in the outer layer of skin and forms the chief structural constituent of the hair and nails.

keratitis, ichthyosis, and deafness syndrome (KID) *np* [Gk *keras* horn, nail + Gk *-ites* denoting disease of; Gk *ikhthus* fish + Gk *-osis* denoting a diseased state]
A rare genetic syndrome in which there is congenital deafness, noninflammatory scaling of the skin, thin or absent hair, and gradual destruction of the cornea, which can lead to blindness. The condition is due to glycogen deposited in the skin and liver, which can also result in the need for a liver transplant.

keratoma *n* [Gk *keras* horn, nail + Gk *–oma* denoting tumor, swelling]
A localized thickening or enlargement of the outer layer of skin, often due to friction or pressure.

keratopachyderma *n* kĕˈrătōpăkīˈderma [Gk *keras* horn, nail + Gk *pakhus* thick + Gk *derma* skin]
A condition in which there is excessive development of the keratin (horny layer of the skin) of the palms, soles, knees, and elbows, which causes furrows on the fingers and toes, and may be accompanied by mild to severe congenital high-frequency hearing loss.

keratosis obturans *np* [Gk *keras* horn, nail + Gk *-osis* denoting a diseased state; Lat *obturare* stop up, block]
An abnormal accumulation of keratin that can block the ear canal and cause pain and temporary hearing loss.

kernicterus *n* [Gk *ikteros* jaundice]
An accumulation of bile pigment in the brain and other nerve tissue that causes yellow staining and tissue damage, e.g.,

neurosensory damage, including hearing loss.

ketoaciduria *n*
The excretion of large amounts of ketone bodies in the urine, e.g., in diabetes mellitus.

keyhole *adj*
Minimally invasive surgery, e.g., for cochlear implantation.

kilo- *prefix* [Gk *khilioi* thousand]
One thousand.

kiloHertz (kHz) *n* Named after Heinrich Hertz (1857–1894), a German physicist, who first demonstrated the existence of electromagnetic waves. The Hertz was established as the standard international unit of frequency in his honor in 1930.
A thousand Hertz, a unit of frequency

kineme *n* ˈkīnēm [Gk *kinein* to move]
A nonverbal signal, e.g., facial expression or gesture, used in nonverbal communication or to support lipreading.

kinesthesia (kinaesthesia) *n* [Gk *kinein* to move + Gk *aesthesis* sensation]
The sense that detects body position, weight, or muscle movement.
Deriv: –adj kinesthetic (kinaesthetic)

King-Kopetzky syndrome *np obs* Named after Samuel J. Kopetzky (1876–1950), a professor of otology at New York Polyclinic Medical School and Hospital, who first described the condition in 1948 and P.F. King (b 1922), an English otolaryngologist, who discussed its etiology in 1954.
Also: auditory processing disorder (APD); central auditory processing disorder; *obs* obscure auditory dysfunction
An impairment of neural function that does not solely result from a deficit in general attention, language, or other cognitive processes. It may be characterized by difficulty in understanding speech especially in background noise and poor recognition, discrimination, separation, grouping, localization or ordering of non-speech sounds.

kinocilium *n* ˈkīnōˈsīlēŭm [Gk *kinein* to move + Lat *cilium* hair]
A long single hair that appears on the apex of hair cells within the cochlea and the vestibular organ. Bending of the hair cells toward the kinocilium results in the depolarization of the hair cells and increased excitivity, bending of the hair cells away from the kinocilium results in hyperpolarization and reduced afferent activity.

Klinefelter syndrome *np* Named after Harry Fitch Klinefelter (1912–1990), an American endocrinologist, who described the syndrome in 1942.
Also: XXY syndrome
A syndrome in which males are born with an extra X chromosome. Characteristics include abnormal body proportions, female characteristics, underdeveloped male genitalia, and infertility. May be associated with hearing loss.

Klippel-Feil syndrome *np* ˈklĭpel-ˈfīel Named after Maurice Klippel (1858–1942) and André Feil (b 1884), French physicians, who gave a full description of the syndrome in 1912.
Also: brevicollis
A disorder that is characterized mainly by fusion of the upper cervical spine. Characteristics may include short neck, low hairline, decreased range of motion, and bilateral sensorineural hearing loss.

kneepoint/knee point, threshold (TK) *np*
The point at which a hearing aid circuit changes from linear to nonlinear amplification, i.e., the point at which the intensity of the input (or output) signal activates the compression circuit and begins to reduce the gain. On a graph, the change in angle looks like a knee joint.

Kniest syndrome *np* knēst Named after Wilhelm Kniest (b 1919), a German pediatrician, who first described the condition in 1952.
Also: Kniest dysplasia/disease
An autosomal dominant disorder of bone

growth. Characteristics are usually fully expressed by about age 3 and may include short stature, a barrel-shaped chest, short limbs, joint enlargement, and stiffness, visual problems, cleft palate, curvature of the spine, and a round face with a central depression. It may be associated with both sensorineural and conductive hearing loss with the conductive element secondary to otitis media.

Knowles electronic manikin for acoustic research (KEMAR) *np*
The trade name for a widely used version of a head and torso simulator which has occluded ear simulators fitted into the skull.

knuckle pads and leukonychia *np* lū-kō'nĭkē*a* [Gk *leukos* white + Gk *onux* nail, claw]
A pigmentary syndrome; characteristics may include thickening of finger and toe joints, progressive whitening of nails, and mild to moderate mixed hearing loss.

Kobrak caloric method *np* Named after Franz Kobrak, a German otolaryngologist, who investigated vestibular testing at University College Hospital, London and devised this minimal stimulation test in 1918 (published 1920).
A method of caloric irrigation in which the ear canal is syringed, usually with cold water while the head is supported on a head rest so that the lateral semicircular canal is approximately vertical. Nystagmus is then timed.

Kolliker organ *np* Named after Rudolph Albert von Kolliker (1817–1905), a Swiss physiologist, who wrote one of the earliest textbooks on embryology and carried out extensive research on the nervous system.
A thickened epithelial structure seen within the embryonic cochlea that develops into the inner sulcus (a groove in the floor of the cochlear duct between spiral limbus, tectorial membrane, and organ of Corti).

Krabbe disease *np* Named after Knud Haraldsen Krabbe (1885–1965), a Danish neurologist, professor of neurology in Copenhagen, and a major researcher in Nordic neurology.
Also: globoid cell leukodystrophy
A very rare genetic disorder of the nervous system where the body lacks the substance required to produce myelin, the material that surrounds and protects nerve fibers. Symptoms are variable, but may include deafness with sensitivity to loud sounds. The condition is most common in persons of Scandinavian descent.

L

labial *adj* ˈlābēəl [Lat *labium* lip]
Of or pertaining to the lips.

labio-dental *adj* [Lat *labium* lip + Lat *dens* tooth]
Formed with the lower lip contacting the upper teeth, e.g., as in the production of the speech sounds /f/ and /v/.

labyrinth *n* [Gk *laburinthos* labyrinth]
The passageways within the temporal bone that contain the cochlea and the vestibular system.
Deriv: –adj labyrinthine

labyrinth, cochlear *n* [Gk *laburinthos* labyrinth; Lat *cochlea* snail shell, spiral]
Also: canalis spiralis cochlea
The cochlear pathways in the petrous part of the temporal bone.

labyrinth, membranous *np* [Gk *laburinthos* labyrinth; Lat *membrana* partition]
The membranous sac filled with endolymph in the bony labyrinth of the inner ear that contains the receptor organs for hearing and vestibular senses.

labyrinth, osseous *np* [Gk *laburinthos* labyrinth; Lat *osseus* bony]
The bony labyrinth of the inner ear that consists of the cochlea and the vestibular system.

labyrinth, vestibular *np* [Gk *laburinthos* labyrinth; Lat *vestibulum* entrance hall]
The vestibular pathways in the petrous part of the temporal bone, which consist of the semicircular canals, the saccule, and the utricle.

labyrinthectomy *n*
Surgical removal of the labyrinth.

labyrinthitis *n*
Inflammation of the labyrinth or the inner ear.

laddergram *n*
A method of plotting results in which equal points on two vertical scales are joined to give the appearance of the rungs of a ladder. This method may be used for recording results from the alternate binaural loudness balance (ABLB) test in which points of equal loudness in the ears of an individual are joined. (With two normal ears the plot has the appearance of a ladder, but where one ear has recruitment the rungs are not horizontal.)

lamella *n* [Lat *lamella* a flat plate]
A flattened area.

lamina *n* [Lat *lamina* a layer]
A thin, flat layer of membrane or tissue that may be part of another structure

lamina, reticular *np* [Lat *lamina* a layer; Lat *reticulum* a small net]
A netlike structure of cells in the organ of Corti that constitutes its upper surface. The reticular lamina isolates the stereocilia of the hair cells from their cell bodies.

lamina, spiral *np*
The thin bony shelf in the cochlea that juts out from the modiolus in the cochlea and to which the inner edge of the basilar membrane is attached.

Landau-Kleffner syndrome *np* Named after William Landau and Frank Kleffner, American physicians, who first identified the syndrome in 1957.
A rare neurologic disorder in which a child, usually between 5 and 9 years old, suddenly or gradually develops aphasia and loses the ability to understand and express language. It may be due to epilepsy, but not all affected individuals have seizures.

landmark *n*
A distinctive feature.

Langer-Giedion syndrome *np* lănger-gī-dĭyon Named after Leonard O. Langer Jr. (b 1928), an American radiologist, and Andreas Giedion (b 1925), a Swiss radiologist, who each reported the condition in 1969.
Also: trichorhinophalangeal syndrome type 2 (TRPS)
An autosomal dominant deletion disorder characterized by a bulbous nose, a

high lipline, microcephaly (small head), protuberant ears, sparse hair, loose skin in infancy, small stature, multiple exostoses (bony projections) of long bones, hypotonia (low muscle tone/floppiness), and learning difficulty, and associated with progressive sensorineural hearing loss that is moderate to severe.

Langerhans, cells of *np* lăngerhănts
Named after Paul Langerhans (1847–1888), a German anatomist, who first described these cells in the late 1868.
A type of dendritic cells, in the skin and airways, that modulate the immune response.

language *n*
A set of symbols used to convey meaning between members of a cultural group.

language delay *np*
The acquisition of language at a later stage than normal.

language disorder *np*
A difficulty with the production or reception of language due to neurologic damage. This may vary from a minor problem with speech sounds to total lack of ability to generate or understand speech (aphasia).

laryngeal tone *np* [Gk *larunx* throat; Gk *tonos* tone]
The sound made by the vibration of the vocal folds in the larynx. The sound is similar to a low-frequency buzz, although the tone is modified within a certain range by the vocal tract.

laryngectomy *n* [Gk *larunx* throat + Gk *ektome* cutting out, excision]
Surgical removal of all or part of the larynx.

laryngitis *n* [Gk *larunx* throat + Gk *-ites* denoting disease of]
Inflammation of the larynx, which often causes temporary loss of voice.

laryngology *n* [Gk *larunx* throat + Gk *-logia* denoting study of]
The study of disorders of the larynx; a branch of medicine that studies the causes and treatments of vocal pathology.

laryngograph *n* [Gk *larunx* throat + Gk *graphia* writing]
Also: electroglottograph
An instrument that plots, as a waveform, the changes in the vocal fold contact area during voicing. This is achieved by measuring the current flow between two electrodes (placed on opposite sides of the thyroid cartilage), which falls as the vocal folds open and the contact area reduces.

larynx *n* [Gk *larunx* throat]
Also: colloq voice box
The cavity in the throat that connects the pharynx to the trachea and houses the vocal folds, which are vibrated to produce voiced sounds.

latency *n* [Lat *latere* to lie hidden]
The time interval between a stimulus and the response, e.g., between a stimulus and an evoked potential.

latency, absolute *np*
The time interval in milliseconds (ms) between the onset of a sound stimulus and the peak of a wave in evoked audiometry.

latency, delayed *np*
The difference between the latency in the left and right ears of an individual. A difference of over 4 ms in interaural latency may suggest a retrocochlear problem.

latency, interaural *np*
An abnormally long time interval between the onset of a sound stimulus and the peak of a wave in evoked audiometry, which may suggest a retrocochlear disorder.

lateral *adj* [Lat *latus* side]
1. A sound produced by the airstream passing along the sides of the tongue, e.g., /l/. 2. To the side, away from the midline.
Deriv: −n lateralization

lateral lemniscus *np* [Lat *latus* side; Gk *lemniskos* wad or bundle]
A bundle of afferent nerve fibers in the central auditory pathways responsible for the auropalpebral reflex. It carries auditory information from the cochlear nuclei in the brainstem to the inferior colliculus in the midbrain.

lateral semicircular canal *np*
Also: horizontal semicircular canal
One of the three semicircular canals; it joins the utricle at both ends and is involved in sensing movement in the horizontal plane.

lateral superior olive *np*
Part of the superior olivary complex. It receives auditory input from both ears and is involved in processing interaural intensity differences.

lavaliere/lavalier *n* lăvă'lĭer/lă'vălēā
A loop (e.g., of string) around the neck.

lavaliere/lavalier microphone *np*
A microphone attached to a cord worn around the neck.

lead *n*
A conductor attached to an electrical or electronic component, e.g., a wire between a microphone and an amplifier.

learned helplessness *np*
The tendency to give up trying when past attempts have been repeatedly unsuccessful.

left-beating nystagmus *np*
A horizontal nystagmus in which the fast phase is angled to the left.

lemniscus, lateral *np* [Gk *lemniskos* wad or bundle; Lat *latus* side]
A bundle of afferent nerve fibers in the central auditory pathways responsible for the auropalpebral reflex. It carries auditory information from the cochlear nuclei in the brainstem to the inferior colliculus in the midbrain.

lenticular process *np* [Lat *lentiscus* little lentil]
A knob at the inferior end of the incus that connects with the head of the stapes.

lentigines *n* lĕn'tĭgĭnēs [Lat *lens* a lentil + Gk *-genes* producing]
Dark pigmented spots that occur on the skin.

leopard syndrome/lentiginosis, cardiomyopathic multiple lentigines syndrome *np*
A dominant genetic syndrome characterized by cardiac changes associated with lentigines and sensorineural deafness. The name (leopard) is an acronym for the main characteristics of the syndrome, i.e., lentigines, electrocardiographic conduction abnormalities, ocular hypertelorism (eyes set wide apart), pulmonic stenosis, abnormal genitalia, retarded growth, and deafness.

Leri-Weill disease *np* Named after A. Leri and Jean Weill (1903–1997), French physicians, who described the syndrome in 1929.
Also: dyschondrosteosis; Madelung disease; multiple symmetric lipomatosis (MSL)
A bone dysplasia, characterized by an uncommon congenital wrist deformity (known as Madelung deformity), fat deposits at the neck, and short stature. Conductive hearing loss may also be present.

Lermoyez syndrome *np* Named after Marcel Emile Joseph Lermoyez (1858–1929), a French otologist, who was influential in founding otolaryngology in France.
A form of Ménière syndrome in which an attack of vertigo, usually rotary and commonly lasting several hours, is preceded by some days or months of progressive deafness and tinnitus. The hearing recovers after the attacks.

lesion *n* [Lat *laedere* to injure]
An abnormal change to an organ or part due to injury or disease.

Leudet's tinnitus *np* Named after Theodore E. Leudet (1825–1887), a French physician, who reported the condition in 1869.
Objective clicking tinnitus caused by the tensor palati muscle going into spasm.

levator veli palatini *np* [Lat *levator veli palatini* the raiser of the velum of the palate]
The muscle of the soft palate.

level *n*
A position on a rank or scale.

level-dependent *adj*
Based on the input level of the signal.

level-dependent frequency response *np*
A type of sound processing used in hearing aids, in which the frequency response changes constantly as the input level alters.

level, sensation *np*
The level of a tone above a person's threshold. It is measured in decibels and used as a reference point for presentation levels of speech perception testing.

level, sound pressure (SPL) *np*
A ratio (20 logP/Pref) between the measured sound pressure (P) and the standard audiologic reference pressure (Pref), which is 0.00002 (20 micropascals). 0 dB-SPL is based on the minimum pressure required to cause hearing in the mid-frequency region. The dB SPL scale is a logarithmic scale, but takes no account of the way hearing varies with frequency and is used, e.g., in audiometer calibration.

level, uncomfortable loudness (ULL) *np*
Also: uncomfortable level (UCL); loudness discomfort level (LDL); threshold of discomfort
The sound level at which the listener begins to experience discomfort.

lever *n*
A mechanism, usually a bar, which is fixed at a point known as the fulcrum and is acted upon by two forces; e.g., the

long process of the incus relative to the shorter manubrium of the malleus gives a lever effect, which forms a small part of the middle ear transformer action.

Libby horn *np* Named after Cy (E. Robert) Libby, an American hearing aid specialist working for Associated Hearing Instruments, who developed the Libby horn in 1979. He also introduced the colloquial term "earmold plumbing."
A stepped bore horn that may be used as a tube in the open ear or placed within the earmold. Its function is to preserve and extend the high-frequency response of a hearing aid.

lidocaine *n*
A local anesthetic, and less commonly also used as an antiarrhythmic medication. The side effects can include ototoxicity.

ligament *n* [Lat *ligare* to attach]
A thin elastic membrane that attaches bone (or cartilage) to bone (or cartilage).

ligament, annular *np* [Lat *ligare* to attach; Lat *annulus* ring or circle]
The ligament that attaches the stapes to the oval window; one of five ligaments that help to support the ossicular chain.

ligament, lateral malleolar *np* [Lat *ligare* to attach; Lat *latus* side; Lat *malleus* a hammer]
A ligament that connects the neck of the malleus to the lateral wall of the middle ear. One of five ligaments that help to support the ossicular chain.

ligament, malleolar *np* mă'lēola [Lat *ligare* to attach; Lat *malleus* a hammer]
A ligament that connects the malleus to the anterior wall of the middle ear. One of five ligaments that help to support the ossicular chain.

ligament, postincudal *np* [Lat *ligare* to attach; Lat *post* behind + Lat *incus* anvil]
A ligament that connects the short process of incus to the posterior wall of the middle ear. One of five ligaments that help to support the ossicular chain.

ligament, superior malleolar *np* [Lat *ligare* to attach; Lat *superior* upper; Lat *malleus* a hammer]
A ligament that connects the head of the malleus to the roof of the middle ear. One of five ligaments that help to support the ossicular chain.

light reflex *np*
The light reflected back from the eardrum when the ear is examined using an illuminated otoscope. The reflected light is normally approximately triangular in shape with the apex of the triangle extending from the umbo (at the middle of the eardrum). The light reflex follows the line of the jaw such that in the right ear the reflex appears at the 5 o'clock position and in the left ear it appears at the 11 o'clock position.

lignocaine *np*
A drug used as a local anesthetic and an antiarrhythmic medication (used to resolve irregular or rapid heartbeats).

limbus, spiral *np* [Lat *limbus* border or edge]
A mass of connective tissue that lies on the osseous or bony spiral lamina (which extends from the bony core of the cochlea, the modiolus) and to which the tectorial membrane is attached.

limen *n* ˈlīmĕn [Lat *limen* threshold]
Also: threshold
The minimum amount of stimulation required to produce sensation.
Deriv: -adj liminal

limen, difference *np*
Also: differential threshold
The minimum detectable change in a stimulus, e.g., the smallest change in intensity of a pure tone.

limit *n*
A restriction that serves as a boundary, e.g., the maximum output (OSPL90) of a hearing aid.

line amplifier *np* [Lat *linea* line]
An amplifier used to feed audio signals to a number of receivers.

line microphone *np* [Lat *linea* line]
A directional microphone that is a single straight line element or an array of small tubes each leading to a microphone.

line spectrum *np* [Lat *linea* line]
A graph in which amplitude is displayed as a function of frequency.

linear *adj* [Lat *linea* line]
1. Pertaining to a line. 2. Where a response is directly proportional to an input.

linear amplification *np* [Lat *linea* line]
1:1 sound processing, i.e., increases in output levels are proportional to increases in input levels (up to the maximum output of an amplification device).

Ling sounds *np* Named after Daniel Ling (1926–2003), a Canadian teacher of speech to deaf children and professor of graduate studies in aural habilitation at McGill University, who developed the Ling sounds in 1976 as a simple speech test that teachers could use.
A range of familiar speech sounds that represent low-, mid-, and high-frequency speech sounds across the same frequency range as tested in audiometry (250 Hz to 8 kHz), which is used to give a basic indication of a deaf child's ability to detect and identify a range of speech stimuli. Phonemes included are /ah/, /ē/, /ū/, /aw/, /s/, /sh/, and /m/.

linguistic deprivation *np*
Inadequate exposure to (verbal) language to facilitate normal language development.

linguistics *n*
The study of language.

lipids *n, pl* [Gk *lipos* fat]
The fats that are found in living organisms.

lipreading/lip-reading *n*
The ability to obtain meaning from watching a speaker's lips. This usually includes facial expression and other cues in

addition to lip-reading, therefore speech-reading is a generally preferred term.

liquid *n*
1. A substance whose particles move freely but do not tend to disperse. 2. A consonant with a smooth flowing sound, i.e., made without friction and capable of being prolonged like a vowel, that is made by obstructing the airstream and allowing it to flow around the obstruction (e.g., the tongue), as in /l/ and /r/.

listen *v*
To pay attention to what is being heard.

listening check *np*
A simple assessment of whether a hearing aid or other amplification device is working appropriately, carried out by listening to the device.

listening strategies *np*
Plans or methods devised to improve comprehension of auditory signals.

live *adj*
Active, having life or containing energy.

live room *np*
An enclosure that is highly reflective, i.e., has very poor sound absorption properties.

live voice *np*
The use of the tester's own voice to present words or sentences in speech audiometry.

live voice, monitored *np*
The monitoring of the tester's voice level by means of a volume unit (VU) meter during speech audiometry.

lobe/lobule *np* [Gk *lobos* lobe, pod]
1. A rounded projection. 2. The four divisions of the cerebral cortex, named after the bones that cover them: frontal, parietal, temporal, and occipital.

lobe, ear *np*
The small lobule at the bottom of the pinna that contains fat but no cartilage.

lobe, frontal *np*
The largest lobe of the brain, which is lo-

cated behind the forehead and is involved in executive functioning.

lobe, occipital *np* [Gk *lobos* lobe, pod; Lat *ob* up against + Lat *caput* the head]
The lobe of the brain that is positioned at the back of the head and that is the visual processing center.

lobe, parietal *np* pa'rīetal [Gk *lobos* lobe, pod; Lat *paries* wall]
The lobe of the brain that is positioned above the occipital lobe and behind the frontal lobe. Its functions include visual-spatial processing and the integration of sensory information.

lobe, temporal *np* [Gk *lobos* lobe, pod; Lat *temporalis* pertaining to the temple (side of forehead)]
The lobe that is located at the base of the brain and that juts forward from the occipital lobe toward the frontal lobe. Its functions include auditory processing (in the primary auditory cortex) and memory.

lobster-claw syndrome *np*
Also: Marshall syndrome; ectodermal dysplasia; saddle nose; and myopia
A rare genetic pigmentary disorder characterized by distinctive facial features that include a flattened nasal bridge, upturned nose, and widely spaced eyes, also lobster-claw deformity of hands and feet, nearsightedness, cataracts, and congenital progressive moderate-to-severe sensorineural, conductive or mixed hearing loss, and poor vestibular function.

localization (localisation) *n* [Lat *locus* a place]
The determination of the direction from which a sound is coming, based on interaural differences in sound signal in terms of the time of arrival and intensity.

locus *n* *pl* loci [Lat *locus* a place]
The specific location on a chromosome of a gene or deoxyribonucleic acid (DNA) sequence.

logarithm *n* [Gk *logos* proportion + Gk *arithmos* number]

Also: –colloq abbr log

The power to which a base number has to be raised to equal a given number, e.g., 2 is the logarithm of 100 to base 10 ($10^2 = 10 \times 10 = 100$). Hearing is considered to be logarithmic and a logarithmic scale is used to represent it.

logatom *n*
A nonsense syllable or sound.

Lombard effect *np* Named after Etienne Lombard (1869–1920), a French physician, who first described the effect in 1911.
An automatic raising of the voice in the presence of background noise.

long arm 18 deletion syndrome *np*
Also: chromosome 18q- syndrome
A rare condition in which the long arm (q) of chromosome 18 is missing. Characteristics are variable but may include short stature; learning difficulties; malformation of hands, feet, and skull; underdeveloped midface; prominent ears; and hearing loss.

long latency auditory evoked potential *np*
Also: auditory late response
Evoked potentials that have wave peaks that occur between approximately 90 and 200 milliseconds.

long process *np*
An extension from a bone.

long process of the incus *np*
The part of the incus that extends toward the stapes.

long process of the malleus *np*
Also: manubrium; handle of the malleus
The part of the malleus that extends from its head.

long-term average speech spectrum (LTASS) *np*
Also: colloq speech banana
A graphic representation of the average normal level and frequency distribution of everyday speech.

longitudinal *adj* [Lat *longitudo* length]
Pertaining to length.

longitudinal fracture *np* [Lat *longitudo* length]
A fracture that follows the long axis of the bone, e.g., fracture of the temporal bone that may result in hearing loss.

longitudinal wave *np*
A pressure wave that moves in the medium in the same direction as the wave is traveling, i.e., wave movement is parallel to the initial vibratory movement.

loop (system) *n*
A wire loop fitted around a room or other required area. A sound source fed into an amplifier attached to the loop will create a fluctuating signal that can be picked up by a suitable receiver. Hearing aid wearers within the specified area can pick up transmitted signals by switching to the loop or T setting. Background noise is cut out as the required sound is transmitted directly to the hearing aid using the principle of electromagnetic induction.

loop diuretic *np* [Gk *diouretikos* pertaining to the flow of urine]
A diuretic (a drug that reduces reabsorption of water and increases urine production) that acts on the ascending loop of Henle in the kidneys. Many loop diuretics are ototoxic, e.g., ethacrynic acid and furosemide. These act on the stria vascularis and can cause a temporary or permanent hearing loss.

lop ear *np*
Also: constricted ear; cup ear
An autosomal dominant genetic disorder that is characterized by an underdeveloped jaw, overfolded ears with large ear lobes, ossicular abnormalities, and conductive hearing loss.

loudness *n*
1. The subjective impression of the volume (intensity) of sound. 2. A standardized measure in sones based on the ratio of perceived sound to a reference sound, i.e., 1 sone that is judged on aver-

age to be equally loud as 1 kHz at 40 dBSPL, 2 sones is a sound judged to be twice as loud, etc.

loudness balance *np*
Also: Fowler's loudness balance test
The state in which sound stimuli are perceived to be of equal loudness across the frequency range.

loudness balance test, alternate binaural (ABLB) *np*
A method of assessing the loudness growth of a unilaterally impaired ear by comparing it with the loudness growth of the normal ear.

loudness contours *np*
Also: phon curves
Lines on a graph that join points of equal loudness.

loudness discomfort level (LDL) *np*
Also: uncomfortable level (UCL); threshold of discomfort (TD); uncomfortable loudness level (ULL/UCL)
The sound level at which the listener begins to experience discomfort.

loudness growth *np*
Perceived increases in loudness as a function of increases in stimulus intensity.

loudness level *np*
A standardized measure in phons, judged against a pure tone at 1 kHz, e.g., the 60 phon curve represents pure tones across the frequency range that are judged to be equally loud as the 1 kHz tone at 60 dBSPL.

loudness level contour *np*
A line on a graph that joins the intensities at different frequencies that are perceived as being of the same loudness level.

loudness matching *np*
A method of matching the loudness of a given signal with a reference signal of known intensity used, e.g., when assessing the patient's perception of the loudness.

loudness recruitment *np*
An abnormally rapid increase in the rate of loudness growth, associated with cochlear hearing loss.

loudness scaling *np*
The action of relating subjective loudness to its intensity.

loudspeaker *n*
An output transducer that converts amplified electrical signals to sound.

low fence *np*
The accepted lower limit of hearing impairment, i.e., the slight hearing loss in comparison to average normal hearing that is no longer considered to be within the normal range. This is lower for children than for adults because children are still developing language and learning skills. The low fence is approximately 15 dB for children and 20-25 dB for adults.

low frequency *np*
1. Sound with a frequency below 1 kHz.
2. Radio waves with a long wavelength, used for long-range communication.

low-pass *adj*
Pertaining to a filter that attenuates high frequencies but allows the low frequencies below a given cutoff frequency, to pass.

lucite *n*
A type of transparent plastic material used in earmolds.

luetic *adj* [Lat *lues* plague]
Pertaining to syphilis, e.g., luetic deafness results from a syphilis infection.

lumen *n* [Lat *lumen* light]
1. An opening. 2. A light.

lupus *n* [Lat *lupus* wolf] The name may refer to the likeness of the facial rash to the scarring around the muzzle that develops in wolves due to the snarling and biting that occurs during feeding.
Lupus is an autoimmune disease that causes inflammation throughout the body.

lupus erythematosus *np* [Lat *lupus* wolf; Gk *eruthros* red + Gk *haima* blood]
A skin disease that causes scaly red patches mostly on the face. It may occur in a systemic form that also involves connective tissue and is accompanied by fever.

lupus pernio *np* [Lat *lupus* wolf; Lat *pernio* chilblain]
A disorder in which disfiguring purple skin lesions, resembling frostbite, affect the ears and face. It may occur in conjunction with flu-like symptoms, sinusitis, or otitis.

lupus vulgaris *np* [Lat *lupus* wolf; Lat *vulgaris* common]
Also: tuberculosis luposa
A progressive form of skin tuberculosis in which there are raised brownish lesions on the skin, especially on the face.

Lybarger earmold (earmould) *np*
Named after Samuel F. Lybarger (1909–2000), an American hearing instrument engineer, who designed early hearing aids and studied earmold acoustics including the effects of venting in solid earmolds.
An earmold that has a tube that is stepped to enhance transmission of high frequencies above 4 kHz.

Lyme disease *np* Named after the town Lyme in Connecticut, where a cluster of more than 50 cases of mainly pediatric arthritis was noted in 1975. The condition was called Lyme arthritis but was changed to Lyme disease in 1979 when additional neurologic symptoms were discovered.
An inflammatory disease that is spread through the bite of a tick. There may be a rash and initial flu-like symptoms followed by the development of widespread itching, joint inflammation, stiff neck, severe fatigue, and unusual behavior. Lyme disease can affect the brain, nervous system, skin, muscles, bone, and cartilage. Symptoms may also include hearing loss, earache, hyperacusis, and tinnitus.

lymph *n* [Gk *lumpha* water]
A colorless or slightly yellow watery fluid containing white blood cells that bathes the tissues and drains from the lymphatic system into the blood.
Deriv: –adj lymphoid

lymphokinesis *n* [Gk *lumpha* water + Gk *kinesis* movement]
The movement of endolymph in the semicircular canals.

lysosomes *n, pl* [Gk *luein* to release + Gk *soma* body]
Vesicles that hold and release enzymes that break down complex molecules and remove waste.

macro- *prefix* [Gk *makros* large]
Being large, thick, or very prominent.

macrocephaly *n* [Gk *makros* large + Gk *kephale* head]
A congenital condition in which the head is abnormally large.

macroglossia *n* [Gk *makros* large + Gk *glossa* tongue]
Protruding or enlarged tongue.

macrolide *n*
A group of antibiotics that are similar to penicillin, e.g., erythromycin, which prevent bacteria from multiplying but that can be ototoxic, causing tinnitus and hearing loss.

macromolecule *n*
A very large molecule made up of a collection of smaller structural units linked together, e.g., a protein.

macrotia *n* mă̆krōshēa [Gk *makros* large + Gk *ous* ear]
Also: hypertrophy
Enlargement of the pinna.

macula *n* *pl* maculae [Lat *macula* spot]
1. A patch of sensory cells found in the utricle and saccule. The macula is sensitive to linear acceleration (i.e., motion along a line) and is used to maintain posture (position), e.g., detecting body lean. 2. The macula lutea, a yellow spot in the retina where vision is sharpest. 3. A small spot or blemish usually on the skin.

Madelung disease *np* mahdelung Named after Otto Wilhelm Madelung (1846–1926), a German surgeon, who first reported cases of Uber den Fetthals "About fat neck" in 1888.
Also: dyschondrosteosis; Leri-Weill syndrome; multiple symmetric lipomatosis (MSL)
A bone dysplasia, characterized by an uncommon congenital wrist deformity (known as Madelung deformity), fat deposits in the neck, and short stature. Conductive hearing loss may also be present.

magnetic resonance imaging (MRI) *np*
A scan that uses a magnetic field and radio wave pulses to produce very clear images of body tissues, including tissues that are surrounded by bone.

mainstream *n/v*
–*n* Regular normal school. –*v* To be placed in a regular normal school, e.g., when deaf children are educated alongside their hearing peers.

Makaton *n* Devised in 1972, the name Makaton is made up from the first names of those involved in its development (Margaret Walker, Kathy Johnston, and Tony Cornforth).
A simplified sign language designed to help children and adults with learning and communication difficulties.

malformation *n* [Lat *malus* bad + Lat *formare* to form]
Bad or imperfect formation of a structure.
Deriv: -v malform

malformed low-set ears syndrome *np*
A craniofacial syndrome characterized by conductive hearing loss and low-set ears.

malignant *adj* [Lat *malignare* to contrive maliciously]
1. Tending toward deterioration or death; 2. Rapidly growing or of extreme virulence and able to invade other parts of an organism.

malingerer *n*
An individual who feigns hearing loss for personal reward.

malleoincudal joint *np* [Lat *malleus* hammer + Lat *incus* anvil]
The joint between the malleus and incus, which tends to move as one mass, therefore there is little movement in this joint.

malleolar *adj* mă 'lēola [Lat *malleus* hammer]
Pertaining to the malleus.

malleolar folds *np*
Two folds, anterior and posterior, on the surface of the tympanic membrane that

extend from the notch of Rivinus to the lateral process of the malleus. The pars flaccida lies above these folds.

malleolar stripe *np*
A white area that may be seen where the manubrium of the malleus is positioned on the tympanic membrane.

malleus *n* mă lēŭs [Lat *malleus* hammer]
The first and largest of the ossicles of the middle ear, which is connected to the tympanic membrane by the handle or manubrium.
Deriv: colloq hammer

malleus, handle of *np*
Also: long process of the malleus; manubrium; handle of the malleus
The part of the malleus that extends from its head.

mandible *n* [Lat *mandibula* jaw bone]
The lower jaw bone. It is the largest, strongest, and only movable facial bone. The mandible articulates with the temporal bone at the temporomandibular joint (TMJ).

mandibular dysostosis *np* [Lat *mandibula* jaw bone; Gk *dus-* bad + Gk *osteon* bone]
Also: Treacher-Collins syndrome; first arch syndrome
A syndrome characterized by craniofacial deformities including downward sloping eyelid fissures, depressed cheek bones, receding chin, large fish-like mouth, and abnormalities of the external and middle ear, e.g., pinna abnormalities, atresia and middle ear deformities. Hearing loss is usually severe conductive, but may be mixed if there is also inner ear deformity.

manikin *n*
A dummy that simulates the human head and torso. It can be used with an ear simulator to demonstrate how sound is affected by the head and body.

manner of articulation *np*
The degree of constriction as the consonants initiate or terminate a syllable. Speech sounds may be classified according to the specific condition (manner) of constriction of the vocal tract.

mannosidosis *n*
A metabolic disorder due to an enzyme (mannosidase) deficiency, which affects glycoprotein (proteins containing sugar) storage and causes the accumulation of mannose (a type of sugar). It is characterized by facial and skeletal deformities and learning difficulty and is associated with sensorineural and conductive hearing loss.

manometer *n* [Gk *manos* thin + Gk *metron* measure]
A device that measures the pressure of gases and vapors, e.g., air.

manual *adj/n* [Lat *manus* hand]
-adj Pertaining to or involving the hands.
-n An instruction booklet

manual alphabet *np* [Lat *manus* hand]
An alphabet represented by finger positions, designed for use by deaf people.

manual audiometer *np* [Lat *manus* hand]
An audiometer where the tester manually selects the frequency, level, and signal type for presentation, and manually presents the signals and records the results.

manual communication *np* [Lat *manus* hand]
A visual communication method involving the use of signs and fingerspelling; sign language.

manubrium *n* [Lat *manubrium* handle]
Also: long process of the malleus; handle of the malleus
The part of the malleus that extends from its head.

map *n/v*
-v To represent or to plan in detail. *-n* A representation of the settings programmed into a cochlear implant. Threshold and comfort levels (electrical stimulation limits) are set for each electrode during the mapping process.

map, cochlear implant *np*
A table or set of tables containing the parameters used for programming the speech processor of a cochlear implant, i.e., to set threshold (T-levels) and uncomfortable loudness levels (C-levels) for electrical stimuli.

map, neural *np*
The information obtained from intracochlear evoked audiometry that may be used in setting the features, such as rate and intensity, for cochlear implant stimulation.

Marfan syndrome *np* Named after Antonin B.J. Marfan (1858–1942), a French physician, who first described the condition in 1896.
A genetic disorder of connective tissue. Individuals usually appear tall with long arms, legs, fingers, and toes; slim; and loose jointed. Areas affected may include the skeleton, heart, blood, eyes, nervous system, skin, and lungs. Hearing loss has been reported, but is poorly documented.

marginal perforation *np*
A perforation of the tympanic membrane that involves the annular ligament.

Marshall syndrome *np* Named after Don Marshall (1905–1965), an ophthalmologist, who described the syndrome in an article published in the *American Journal of Ophthalmology* in 1958.
Also: ectodermal dysplasia; lobster-claw syndrome; saddle nose and myopia
A rare genetic pigmentary disorder characterized by distinctive facial features that include a flattened nasal bridge, upturned nose and widely spaced eyes, also lobster-claw deformity of hands and feet, nearsightedness, cataracts, and congenital progressive moderate to severe sensorineural, conductive, or mixed hearing loss and poor vestibular function.

masker *n*
Any acoustic signal that produces masking.

masker, tinnitus *np*
Also: sound generator
A sound-generating device that emits sound intended to mask tinnitus (fully or partially).

masking *n*
1. The ability of one acoustic signal to obscure the presence of another acoustic signal so that it cannot be detected. 2. The process in which the threshold of one sound is shifted due to the presence of another sound. 3. Suppression.

masking, backward *np*
Masking that appears to happen fractionally before the masker has been presented.

masking, central *np*
A threshold elevation in the test ear in the order of 5 dB due to interactions in the central nervous system when masking is introduced in the nontest ear.

masking, cross/crossover *np*
Masking in which sound delivered to the nontest ear is audible in the test ear.

masking, dilemma *np*
The inability to obtain a reliable masked threshold because successive increases in the masking level in the nontest ear raise the threshold in the test ear due to crossover. This is most likely to occur in individuals with moderate to severe bilateral conductive hearing loss.

masking, effective (EM) *np*
The ability of the masking noise to shift a pure tone or speech threshold by a value equal to an increase in the value of the masking noise. Most modern audiometers have masking that is calibrated in terms of dB EM.

masking level difference *np*
Also: release from masking
A method of comparison between threshold responses with masking noise that is presented in phase and out of phase with the test signal. Normal release from masking indicates an intact

auditory pathway at the level of the brainstem.

masking, upward spread of *np*
The ability of a sound to mask frequencies that are higher than the masking sound. As the intensity of the masker increases the range of frequencies that it will mask becomes wider and extends upward in frequency.

Maslow's hierarchy of needs *np* Named after Abraham Harold Maslow (1908–1970), an American humanistic psychologist, who created the theory of hierarchical needs.
A theory proposing that physiologic needs, e.g., biologic needs, must be met before higher needs, e.g., self esteem, can be achieved.

mass *n*
1. The measure of the amount of matter contained in a physical body. In most general situations, mass and weight are equal. Mass does not change but weight is affected by gravity. The SI unit of mass is the kilogram (kg). 2. A (large) body of matter with no particular shape.

master hearing aid *np*
A device or computer-generated program capable of producing a wide variety of gain/frequency response curves and other amplification options intended to simulate the performance of a hearing instrument. It can be used to assist in the initial fitting and fine tuning of the patient's hearing instrument.

mastoid *n* [Gk *mastoeides* breast-shaped]
The part of the temporal bone behind the pinna.

mastoid airspaces/air cells *np*
Highly irregular air cells in the mastoid. The mastoid airspaces reduce the mass of the bone. The largest space is the mastoid antrum. In some ears it may be the only air space, but most mastoids are pneumatized. The arrangement of cells may appear haphazard but is really in seven well-defined groups: the zygomatic root, periantrum, subdural, sinodural angle, perisinus, tip, and retrofacial.

mastoid cavity *np*
A cavity formed when diseased tissue extending into the mastoid bone has been surgically removed between the ear canal and the middle ear. The ear canal widens out into this cavity.

mastoidectomy *n* [Gk *mastoeides* breast-shaped + Gk *ektome* excision]
A procedure to remove infected bone from the mastoid area.

mastoidectomy, modified (radical) *np*
Surgical removal of the mastoid with minimal possible removal of the middle ear structures.

mastoidectomy, radical *np*
A mastoidectomy in which the mastoid and the middle ear are converted into a common cavity that is easily accessible through the external auditory meatus. This is done by removing the tympanic membrane, the ossicles, and the posterior and superior walls of the external auditory meatus.

mastoidectomy, simple *np*
A mastoidectomy in which infected bone from the mastoid is removed.

maternal reflective method *np* The method was developed by Father Anton J. Van Uden (1912–2008), a Dutch educational psychologist at St Michielgestel, a school for deaf children in Holland.
An oral-aural approach to teaching speech and language to deaf children that involves using texts written by the teacher based on conversations held in the class.

matrix *np* *pl* matrices [Lat *matrix* womb]
1. A grid of symbols or quantities. 2. A method of specifying parameters from the audiogram traditionally used by manufacturers for custom hearing aids. The matrix specifies parameters, e.g., desired levels of maximum output, gain, and frequency response (slope).

matrix, confusion *np*
A symmetric matrix for analyzing phonemic errors. The stimuli are listed down the side and the responses across the top of the matrix.

maxilla *n* [Lat *maxilla* upper jaw]
Upper jaw.
Deriv: –*adj* maxillary

maximum level (M-level) *np*
Also: comfort level (C-level)
The maximum level of electrical current in a cochlear implant that is comfortably loud.

maximum power output (MPO) *np*
Also: saturation sound pressure level (SSPL); output sound pressure level (OSPL)
The highest value of sound pressure level that a hearing aid can produce. An input of 90 dBSPL is used when testing maximum output.

mean *n*
A measure of central tendency; the values in a list are added and the total is divided by the number of items/values in the list.

measles *n*
A severe contagious viral infection of the respiratory system. Possible complications include blindness, encephalitis, respiratory infections, hearing loss, and ear infections.

measles, German *np*
Also: rubella
A viral infection passed from the mother to the fetus, which can result in sensorineural deafness that is often severe to profound. Other characteristics may include conductive hearing loss, heart disease, learning difficulties, cataracts, glaucoma, and "salt and pepper" retinal pigmentation.

meatal tip *np*
An earmold that consists only of a tip to insert in the ear canal.

meatus *n* [Lat *meatus* passage]
A passageway or canal.
Deriv: -*adj* meatal

mechanical *adj* [Gk *mekhane* a machine]
Concerned with machines.

mechanical coupler *np*
A device that acts as an artificial mastoid for testing bone conduction vibrators. Designed to present a specified mechanical impedance to the vibrator.

mechanical feedback *np*
1. Noise that occurs when mechanical vibrations from the receiver assembly in a hearing aid are detected by the microphone and amplified. 2. The mechanical amplification of sound-induced vibrations, e.g., by outer hair cells in the cochlea.

medial *adj* [Lat *medius* middle]
1. Occupying a middle position; toward the midline. 2. Relating to an average or mean.

medial geniculate body *np* [Lat *medius* middle; Lat *geniculatus* bent (from *geniculum* small knee, joint of plant)]
The part of the posterior thalamus that contains the major nuclei in the central auditory system.

medial superior olivary body *np* [Lat *medius* middle; Lat *superior* upper]
The nucleus of the superior olivary complex that is involved in processing interaural time differences.

median *n* [Lat *medius* middle]
The median is the middle number in a list of numbers sorted in value order.

median plane *np*
Also: midsagittal plane
The vertical plane through the body midline, i.e., dividing the body into right and left halves.

medical *adj/n* [Lat *medicus* doctor]
-*adj* 1. Pertaining to medical not surgical treatment. 2. Pertaining to the study or practice of medicine. -*n* An examination

of the health of an individual; a physical examination.

medical model *np*
A model in which the physician/professional focuses on the defect or dysfunction within the patient, using a problem-solving approach. A history, examination, and diagnostic tests provide the basis for the identification and treatment of the issue.

medicolegal *adj*
Concerned with the law and medicine.

medium *n/adj* [Lat *medius* middle]
–*n* An intervening substance through which sound travels, e.g., air or water. –*adj* Middle sized

medulla oblongata *np* [Lat *medulla* bone marrow; Lat *oblongatus* oblong]
The lowest part of the brainstem that controls autonomic functions, e.g., breathing, heart rate.

mega- *prefix* [Gk *megas* great]
1. Very large. 2. One million, e.g., 1 megahertz (1 MHz) equates to one million cycles per second.

Meige syndrome *np* māj Named after Henri Meige (1866–1940), a French physician and professor at the école de Beaux-Arts, who studied motor disturbances.
A disorder of movement characterized by excessive blinking and involuntary movements of the jaw, chin, lips, and tongue.

mel *n* [Shortened form of melody from Gk *melos* song + Gk *ode* singing]
A unit of pitch. A 1 kHz tone at 40 dBSPL has a pitch of 1000 mels. A tone of 2000 mels is twice as high in pitch as 1000 mels.

melanin *n* [Gk *melas* black]
Black or dark brown pigment that occurs in the hair, skin, and the iris and choroid layer of the eye.

melanoma *n* *pl* melanomas [Gk *melas* black + Gk *–oma* denoting tumor, swelling]
The most serious type of skin cancer arising in the pigment cells of the skin. Most commonly it appears as an irregular black or brown area or as a mole that has changed appearance and is sometimes found on the upper part of the helix of the pinna.

melanophore cell *np* [Gk *melas* black + Gk *phoros* carrying]
Also: branchio-oto-renal (BOR) syndrome
A cell containing melanin.

Melnick-Fraser syndrome *np* Named after Michael Melnick, an American medical geneticist, who published an article on the syndrome in 1975 and Frank Clarke Fraser (b 1920), a Canadian medical geneticist, who added to the knowledge of this syndrome.
An autosomal dominant syndrome that includes underdeveloped or absent kidneys and resultant renal failure. Ear abnormalities may include malformations of the outer and middle ear, and deafness that may be conductive, sensorineural, or mixed.

melotia *n* měl'ōshēa [Gk *melon* cheek + Gk *ous* ear]
Congenital displacement of the pinna onto the cheek.

membrane *n* [Lat *membrana* partition]
A thin flexible sheet-like tissue of plant or animal origin, e.g., the tympanic membrane.

membranous labyrinth *np* [Lat *membrana* partition; Gk *laburinthos* labyrinth]
The membranous sac filled with endolymph in the bony labyrinth of the inner ear that contains the receptor organs for the hearing and vestibular senses.

Ménière syndrome/disease/disorder *np*
Named after Prosper Ménière (1799–1862), a French physician, who first described the condition in 1861.
Also: endolymphatic hydrops
A disorder in which there is excessive endolymph within the inner ear, character-

ized by recurrent episodes of spontaneous vertigo, aural fullness, tinnitus, and fluctuating low frequency or flat sensorineural hearing loss.

meninges *n, pl* měˈnĭnjēz *sg* meninx [Gk *meninx* membrane]
The three membranes that cover and protect the brain and spinal cord, made up of the dura mater (the outer layer), the arachnoid membrane (the middle layer), and the pia mater (the inner layer).

meningioma *n* měˈnĭnjēōmа [Gk *meninx* membrane + Gk *-oma* denoting tumor, swelling]
A tumor that occurs in the meninges.

meningitis *n* ˈměnĭnjītĭs [Gk *meninx* membrane + Gk *-ites* denoting disease of]
Inflammation of the meninges. May be viral or bacterial. Bacterial meningitis can result in hearing loss, brain damage, or even death. Viral meningitis is less severe.
Deriv: –adj meningitic

meningitis, otic *np*
Meningitis that occurs as a result of mastoiditis, labyrinthitis, or otitis media.

meniscus *n* [Gk *meniskos* crescent]
1. A curved upper surface of a liquid. 2. A crescent moon-shaped body. 3. A line sometimes seen through the eardrum when there is fluid in the middle ear.

mental age (MA) *np* [Lat *mens* mind]
An equivalent age based upon the ability to perform intellectual tasks appropriate to chronological age.

mercury battery *np*
A nonrechargeable primary cell containing mercury, previously used to power hearing aids but now banned due to environmental concerns and replaced by a zinc-air battery.

mesencephalon *n* mězěnˈsěfаlŏn [Gk *mesos* middle + Gk *enkephalon* brain]
Also: midbrain
The part of the brainstem that connects the hindbrain and the forebrain. It is situated between the diencephalon, which includes the thalamus and hypothalamus, and the metencephalon, which includes the pons and medulla, and contains nuclei for auditory and visual reflexes.

mesenchyme *n* mězĭnˈkīm [Gk *mesos* middle + Gk *enkhuma* infusion]
Embryonic connective tissue that is undifferentiated and can therefore develop into any type of mature cell.

mesial *adj* [Gk *mesos* middle]
Situated in or toward the midline.

mes(o)- *prefix* ˈmēzō- [Gk *mesos* middle]
Middle.

mesoderm *n* [Gk *mesos* middle + Gk *derma* skin]
The middle of the three primary germ layers in the embryo, which differentiates into various tissues, e.g., connective tissue and the middle layer of the skin.

mesotympanum *n* [Gk *mesos* middle + Gk *tumpanon* drum]
The upper part of the tympanic cavity that contains the ossicles.

messenger ribonucleic acid (MRA) *np*
A macromolecule that carries genetic information for protein synthesis and delivers this from a chromosome to a ribosome.

meta- *prefix* [Gk *meta* after]
Higher or transcending.

metabolism *n* [Gk *metabole* change]
The processes and activities by which substances are managed in a living organism.

metalinguistic *adj*
With thought and attention to the use of language.

metastasis *n* měˈtăstаsĭs *pl* metastases [Gk *metastasis* removal, change]
The transference of pain, disease, or tumor from one body part to another.

meter *n* [Gk *metron* measure]
1. A measuring device, e.g., sound-level meter. 2. The standard metric unit of linear measurement.

methylprednisolone *n* mĕth'ĭlprĕd'nĭsolōn (mĕth'elprĕd'nĭsolōn)
A corticosteroid drug with antiinflammatory properties that may be used to reduce dizziness after cochlear implantation.

Metz test *np* Named after Otto Metz, a Danish physician, who investigated acoustic impedance (1946) and reflex contractions and recruitment (1952). He produced the first electro-acoustic impedance bridge in 1957.
Also: acoustic reflex test
A test that measures the acoustic reflex threshold and compares it with the behavioral pure tone threshold. It is used to indicate possible recruitment.

mexiletine hydrochloride *np*
An orally administered local anesthetic and antiarrhythmic drug similar to lidocaine. Its side effects may include dizziness and tinnitus.

Michel aplasia/dysplasia *np* Named after E.M. Michel, a French physician, who described this condition in 1863.
A condition in which the inner ear does not develop, although the outer and middle ears may be normal. Hearing loss (unilateral or bilateral) is total.

micin (mycin) *suffix* 'mĭsĭn [Gk *mukes* mushroom, fungus]
Fungus-based drugs.

micro- *prefix* [Gk *mikros* small]
1. Very small. 2. One millionth (μ).

microbiologic *adj* [Gk *mikros* small]
Pertaining to the isolation and identification of disease-causing microorganisms.

microcephaly *n* mĭkrō'sĕfalē [Gk *mikros* small + Gk *kephale* head]
An abnormally small head due to reduced growth of the brain.

microglia *n* [Gk *mikros* small]
The smallest of neuroglia cells that act as phagocytes and protect the brain from invading microorganisms.

microglossia *n* [Gk *mikros* small + Gk *glossa* tongue]
An abnormally small tongue.

micrognathia *n* mĭkrō'nāthēa (mĭkrō'nă-thēa) [Gk *mikros* small + Gk *gnathos* jaw]
Underdevelopment of the jaw.

micropascal (μPa) *n* 'mĭkrōpăskăl [Gk *mikros* small]
A unit of pressure equivalent to 1 newton per square meter.

microphone *n* [Gk *mikros* small + Gk *phone* sound]
A transducer that converts acoustic signals into electrical signals.
Deriv: -adj microphonic

microphone, boom *np*
A microphone fixed to a pole in order to position it some distance away.

microphone, carbon *np*
A microphone in which carbon granules are disturbed when sounds cause the diaphragm to move. This causes changes in resistance between the granules.

microphone, ceramic *np*
A microphone in which a thin ceramic plate is attached to the diaphragm for transducing acoustic to electric signals.

microphone, condenser *np*
Also: capacitor microphone; electrostatic microphone
A microphone that uses a capacitor to convert acoustic energy into electrical energy.

microphone, directional *np*
A microphone in which the sensitivity varies unequally according to the angle of sound incidence. The sensitivity variations are usually represented by a polar directivity pattern.

microphone, electret *np*
A type of condenser microphone that utilizes permanently polarized dielectric

material and that is widely used in hearing aids.

microphone, omnidirectional *np*
A microphone that is equally sensitive to sounds from all directions.

microphone, piezoelectric *np* pēāzōe'lĕk-trĭk (pēātzōe'lĕktrĭk)
A microphone in which the electroacoustic conversion is carried out by a piezoelectric element.

microphone, probe *np*
A microphone attached to a small tube that can be placed in the ear canal to facilitate measurement of sound pressure levels in the ear canal.

microphone, reference *np*
A monitoring microphone.

microphonic, cochlear *np*
An electrical potential from the outer hair cells of the cochlea that resembles the waveform of the input signal.

microtia *n* mĭ'krōshēa [Gk *mikros* small + Gk *ous* ear]
A congenital small and underdeveloped pinna that may appear as a bump of tissue or a partially formed ear.

microvilli *n, pl* mĭkrō'vĭlī *sg* microvillus [Gk *mikros* small + Lat *villus* hair]
Hairlike protrusions that increase the surface area of cells. Stereocilia in the cochlea are specialized microvilli.

midbrain *n*
Also: mesencephalon
The part of the brainstem that connects the hindbrain and the forebrain and is situated between the diencephalon (which includes the thalamus and hypothalamus) and the metencephalon (which includes the pons and medulla). It contains nuclei for auditory and visual reflexes.

middle ear *np*
Also: tympanic cavity
The portion of the ear between the eardrum and the cochlea. An irregular air-filled space in the temporal bone that contains the ossicles and is ventilated by the Eustachian tube. The ossicles connect the lateral and medial walls of the tympanic cavity and convey sound vibrations to the oval window of the cochlea.

middle ear cavity *np*
The air-filled space in the temporal bone that contains the ossicles.

middle ear implant *np*
An amplifying device that is attached to the ossicular chain or eardrum.

middle ear pressure *np*
Static pressure in the middle ear relative to the atmospheric pressure. The pressure in the middle ear is equalized via the Eustachian tube and is normally the same as atmospheric pressure. Middle ear pressure that is equal to atmospheric pressure is important in achieving the efficient transfer of acoustic energy to the cochlea.

middle latency *np*
An auditory evoked potential from the thalamus to the cortex and the primary auditory cortex that occurs between 12 and 80 ms.

midsagittal plane *np* [mid- + Lat *sagitta* arrow]
Also: median plane
The vertical plane through the body midline, i.e., dividing the body into right and left halves.

mike *n colloq*
Short for microphone: a transducer that converts acoustic signals into electrical signals.

milia *n* *sg* milium [Lat *millium* millet (seed)]
Also: postaxial acrofacial dysostosis
Small pimple-like lesions found in the ears in oral-facial-digital syndrome.

mild hearing loss *np*
1. A subjective description of a small degree of hearing loss. 2. A hearing level between 25 dBHL (UK: 20 dBHL) and 40

dBHL of 26 dBHL to 40 dBHL (UK: 21–40 dBHL; WHO: 26–40 dBHL).

Miller syndrome *np* Named after Robert W. Miller (1922–2006), an American birth defects epidemiologist.
Also: postaxial acrofacial dysostosis
An autosomal recessive condition characterized by drooping lower eyelids, small jaw, cleft palate and lip, small cup-shaped pinnae, limb abnormalities, missing digits, external and middle ear anomalies, and possible conductive hearing loss.

milli- *prefix* [Lat *mille* a thousand]
One thousandth.

minimal pair *np*
Words that sound alike except for a single phonetic feature, e.g., "soon" and "moon."

minimum audible angle (MAA) *np*
The smallest difference in localization that can be determined when two successive adjacent sounds are presented.

minimum audible field (MAF) *np*
The sound pressure level that relates to average normal binaural threshold of hearing measured in a free field.

minimum audible pressure (MAP) *np*
Normal average monaural threshold of hearing under headphones expressed as the sound pressure level within the external ear and measured at the eardrum.

minimum masking level (MML) *np*
The lowest intensity level of a masking noise that effectively masks the nontest ear.

minocycline hydrochloride *np*
A broad spectrum tetracycline antibiotic, commonly used for treating acne and bacterial infections, which can be ototoxic.

misarticulation *n*
Mispronunciation of a speech sound or sounds.

mismatch, impedance *np*
Occurs where sound travels from one medium into another that has a different impedance or resistance, e.g., air to fluid. Some of the acoustic energy is reflected and only some transmitted into the second medium.

misophonia *n* [Gk *misos* hatred + Gk *phone* sound] A term devised by Arthur Guy Lee (1919–2005), a Fellow of St John's College at the University of Cambridge.
An aversion to sound. A disorder of sensitivity to sound that involves the dislike of a sound or group of sounds.

missing fundamental *np*
Also: pitch periodicity; virtual pitch
A low-frequency tone that is not in the original stimulus, but that is perceived to be the pitch of the tone because the brain can recognize the missing fundamental tone from the pattern of the harmonics present.

mitochondrion *n* mīto'kŏndrēon *pl* mitochondria [Gk *mitos* thread + Gk *khondrion* small granule]
The main energy source of the cell. Each mitochondrion has a chromosome containing 37 genes, inherited from the mother. Mutations in mitochondrial DNA may cause hearing loss.
Deriv: –adj mitochondrial

mitomycin *n* mīto'mīsin [Gk *mitos* thread + Gk *mukes* fungus]
An ototoxic anthracycline antibiotic that inhibits cancer cells. It may also be given topically to reduce scarring and the formation of granulation tissue in the ear.

mixed hearing loss *np*
Hearing loss due to a combination of conductive and sensorineural causes.

mnemonics *n* ne'mŏnĭks [Gk *mnemonikos* bringing to mind]
A way of improving memory for a list of events that is difficult to recall, e.g., making a sentence using the first letter of each referable condition.

mobilization (mobilisation) *np*
A surgical procedure to free up or mobilize, e.g., mobilization of the stapes.

mode *n* [Lat *modus* measure]
1. The most frequently occurring value in a list of numbers. 2. A distinct or characteristic pattern, e.g., mode of vibration.

moderate hearing loss *np*
1. A subjective description of a medium level of hearing loss. 2. A hearing level between 41 dBHL and 55 dBHL (UK: 41 dBHL and 70 dBHL; WHO: 41–60 dBHL).

moderately severe hearing loss *np*
A hearing level between 56 dBHL and 70 dBHL (UK and WHO: not applicable).

modification *n*
An adjustment.
Deriv: *–adj* modified

modification, earmold *np* [Lat *modificare* to change]
Changes made to an earmold to alter its shape; the changes may modify the acoustic properties of the amplified signal.

modified (radical) mastoidectomy *np* [Lat *modificare* to change; Gk *mastoeides* breast-shaped + Gk *ektome* excision]
Surgical removal of the mastoid with the minimal possible removal of the middle ear structures.

modiolus *n* [Lat *modiolus* hub (of axle)]
The central bony core of the cochlea from which the spiral lamina projects. The basilar membrane and the Reissner membrane are attached to the spiral lamina.

modular hearing aid *np*
In-the-ear hearing aids having uniform shape and performance that can be coupled to a custom earmold.

modulate *v* [Lat *modulare* to change]
1. To pass gradually from one state to another. 2. To vary the frequency, amplitude or phase of a carrier signal for transmission of information.

modulation rate *np*
Also: symbol rate; Baud rate
The rate at which a carrier signal is varied to represent the information in a digital signal.

Moebius syndrome/Möbius syndrome *np* ˈmɜːbēus Named after Paul Julius Möbius (1853–1907), a German neurologist, who reported 44 cases of the condition, which he called "nuclear atrophy," in 1892.
Also: facial dysplagia
A rare congenital craniofacial nervous system syndrome affecting cranial nerves VI and VII although it may also affect other cranial nerves. It is characterized by facial paralysis including an inability to suck, frown, smile, blink, or move the eyes laterally. About one-third of children with this syndrome have some degree of autism. Congenital sensorineural hearing loss is present if cranial nerve VIII is involved.

Mohr syndrome *np* maw Named after Otto Lous Mohr (1886–1967), a Norwegian geneticist, who published the first case report describing the combination of symptoms in 1941.
Also: orodigitofacial dysostosis; oral-facial-digital syndrome
An autosomal recessive disorder of the oral cavity, face, and hands. Often accompanied by hearing loss, usually conductive in nature.

mold (mould) *n*
Also: earmold (earmould)
A device fitted within the outer ear and connected to a behind the ear hearing aid by means of tubing that channels amplified sound into the ear.

monaural *adj* [Gk *monos* single + Lat *auris* ear]
The use of only one ear, e.g., stimuli presented to one ear at a time.

Mondini dysplasia *np* mŏnˈdēnē [Gk *dus-* bad + Gk *plasis* formation] Named after Carlo Mondini (1729–1803), an Italian anatomist, who described the condition in 1791.

A congenital condition in which the cochlea develops only 1.5 turns instead of the normal 2.5. The basal turn of the cochlea is present, but the septum between the middle and apical segments fails to form so that the middle and apical turns occupy a common space. Low- and mid-frequency sensorineural hearing loss are present.

monitored live voice *np*
The monitoring, usually by means of a VU meter, of the intensity level of a speech signal.

mono- *prefix* [Gk *monos* single]
Single.

monomeric eardrum *np* [Gk *monos* single + Gk *meros* part]
An eardrum having a healed perforation where the fibrous layer of the tympanic membrane has not grown back and the area therefore remains thin and flaccid.

monophonic *adj* [Gk *monos* single + Gk *phone* sound]
A single sound channel, such that all sounds appear from the one source.

monopolar *adj* [Gk *monos* single + Gk *polos* sky, axis]
An electrode arrangement where one electrode is detecting the response and the second electrode is inactive.

monosyllable *n* [Gk *monos* single + Gk *sullabos* (from *sullambanein* to take together)]
A single syllable.

monothermal *adj* [Gk *monos* single + Gk *therme* heat]
Use of only one temperature, e.g., a monothermal caloric test uses either warm or cool water.

monotic *adj* [Gk *monos* single + Gk *ous* ear
Presented to one ear.

monotone *n* [Gk *monos* single + Gk *tonos* tone]
A single tone, without change.

monozygotic *adj* [Gk *monos* single + Gk *zugotos* yoked]
Identical twins formed when a single egg, fertilized by a single sperm, divides into two. The twins therefore share the same DNA.

morbid *adj* [Lat *morbidus* diseased]
Indicative of disease.
Deriv: -n morbidity

Moro reflex *np* ˈmawrō Named after Ernst Moro (1874–1951), a German pediatrician, who discovered the reflex.
A baby's normal startle response that involves extending the arms, hands, and fingers. This is present at birth and disappears after about 3 to 4 months. Absence of the reflex in babies may indicate central nervous system damage, whereas presence of the reflex in older children and adults may suggest cortical damage.

morpheme *n* [Gk *morphe* form]
The smallest meaningful unit of language.

morphology *n* [Gk *morphe* form + Gk *-logia* study of]
1. The study of the form and content of words. 2. The study of the form and structure of an entity.
Deriv: -adj morphological

Morquio syndrome *np* ˈmawkēō Named after Luis Morquio, (1867–1935), a Uruguayan physician, who first described the syndrome.
A type of mucopolysaccharidosis, an autosomal recessive inherited disease of carbohydrate metabolism, characterized by severe skeletal deformity, slow growth, a thick and dense skull, coarse facial features, clouding of the eyes, and hearing loss.

most comfortable loudness level/most comfortable level (MCL) *np*
Also: most comfortable listening level
The intensity of sound that the listener

chooses as most comfortable for listening. The MCL may not be the level that provides the best speech understanding.

motherese *n*
Also: baby talk
A simplified manner of speech used by an adult when speaking to a young child, which may include use of raised pitch, short sentences, simplified grammar and vocabulary, slower speech, longer pauses, and some nonsense sounds.

motility *n* [Lat *motus* motion]
The capacity to move.

motor *adj*
Pertaining to muscular action.

motor nerve *np*
Nerves that carry impulses from the brain to the muscles, causing them to contract.

motor neuron *np*
A nerve cell that releases chemicals that stimulate muscle contraction.

moving coil *np*
A coil of wire suspended in a stationary magnetic field. When current is sent through the coil, a magnetic field is induced around it; the coil moves according to the strengths and directions of the permanent and induced magnetic fields.

MRI *np abbr*
Short for magnetic resonance imaging: a scan that uses a magnetic field and radio wave pulses to produce very clear images of body tissues, including tissues that are surrounded by bone.

Muckle-Wells syndrome *np* Named after Thomas James Muckle (b 1938) and Michael Vernon Wells (b 1932), medical researchers, who first described the syndrome in 1962.
Also: amyloidosis
A syndrome in which a starch-like substance known as amyloid is deposited in the kidneys and other tissues. Characteristics include a recurrent rash, limb pain, renal failure, and progressive sensorineu-

ral deafness. The organ of Corti may be absent and the cochlear nerve atrophied.

mucoid *adj* ˈmyūkoid [Lat *mucus* mucus + Gk suffix *-oides* resembling]
Resembling mucus.

mucopolysaccharidosis *n* ˈmyūkōpŏlēsăkarĭˈdōsĭs [Lat *mucus* mucus + Gk *polus* many + Lat *saccharum* sugar + *-ide* + Gk *-osis* denoting a diseased state]
A group of inherited metabolic disorders caused by lack or malfunction of lysomal enzyme, required to break down glycosaminoglycans (long chain of sugar needed for connective tissue, e.g., bone and cartilage). Characteristics, which develop after a period of normal growth, include abnormal facial features, abnormal bone size and shape, progressive cellular damage, organ dysfunction and learning difficulty. Abnormal bone size and shape may press on organs and compress nerves, leading to associated disorders, e.g., hearing loss.

mucosa *n* *pl* mucosae/mucosas [Lat *mucosus* pertaining to mucus]
Also: mucous membrane
The tissue that lines many internal parts of the body that are involved in secretion and absorption, e.g., the mucous membrane lining the middle ear.

mucosal cobblestoning *np*
Multiple mucosal nodules that give the appearance of a cobbled street, e.g., cobblestoning of the oropharynx. It is usually a sign of chronic inflammation.

mucus *n* ˈmyūkus [Lat *mucus* mucus]
A thick slippery fluid secreted by the goblet cells in the mucous membranes.
Deriv: -adj mucous

Muller-Zeman syndrome *np* Named after Jans Muller and Wolfgang Zeman, American neuropathologists, who described the syndrome in 1965.
An autosomal recessive disorder characterized by severe learning difficulty and psychomotor problems, progressive visu-

al impairment, and sensorineural hearing loss.

multiband compression *np*
A form of speech processing in which the input is split into frequency bands, each subject to compression before being recombined.

multichannel *adj*
A term pertaining to the splitting of a signal into frequency channels or bands, each of which has separate processing. "Multichannel" may be used to refer to the chain of devices through which the band of signals pass or it may be used interchangeably with "multiband."

multiple lentigines syndrome *np* [Lat *lens* lentil + Gk *-genes* produced]
Also: Capute-Rimoin-Konigsmark syndrome; leopard syndrome
A disorder whose characteristics include lentigenes or freckles on the head and neck, dwarfism, and sensorineural deafness.

multiple memory *np*
Amplifying programs, each with different performance characteristics, that are stored in a hearing aid for access by the wearer according to need.

multiple sclerosis (MS) *np* [Gk *sklerosis* hardening]
An autoimmune disease that affects the central nervous system. Caused by inflammation of the myelin sheath that covers the nerves. Symptoms include muscle weakness, incontinence, numbness, vision loss, slurred speech, hearing loss, nystagmus, and balance problems.

multiple symmetric lipomatosis (MSL) *np* [Gk *lipos* fat + Gk *–oma* denoting tumor, swelling]
Also: Madelung disease; dyschondrosteosis; Leri-Weill syndrome
A bone dysplasia, characterized by an uncommon congenital wrist deformity (known as Madelung deformity), fat deposits in the neck, and short stature. Conductive hearing loss may also be present.

multisensory *adj*
Using more than one of the senses, e.g., vision, hearing, and touch.

mumps *n*
A contagious viral disease that can result in painful inflammation and swelling of the salivary glands (parotitis). It may also infect the central nervous system, pancreas, and testes. Complications can include sudden-onset hearing loss that is usually unilateral and profound.

muscle *n*
A contractile fibrous tissue that facilitates movement.

muscular dystrophy *np* [Gk *dus-* bad + Gk *trophe* nourishment]
A group of genetic degenerative disorders that involves muscle weakness and loss of muscle tissue and possible sensorineural hearing loss.

musician's earplugs *np*
Filtered earplugs designed to provide approximately uniform attenuation across frequency.

mutate *v* [Lat *mutare* to change]
To undergo relatively permanent significant alteration.
Deriv: –*n* mutation

mute *adj/n/v* [Lat *mutus* mute]
–*adj* Silent or unable to emit an articulate sound. –*n* A person who is silent or who is unable to emit an articulate sound. -*v* To make silent.

mycomyringitis *n* mīkōmīrĭnj'ītis [Gk *mukes* fungus + Gk *myrinx* membrane + Gk *-ites* denoting disease of]
Fungal inflammation of the eardrum.

mycosis *n* mīk'ōsĭs [Gk *mukes* fungus + + Gk *-osis* denoting a diseased state]
Fungal infection.

myelin sheath *np* [Gk *muelos* bone marrow]
The fatty layer that covers the axons of nerve cells.

myiasis *n* mīˈīāsĭs *pl* myiases [Gk *muia* a fly]
An infestation of tissue, e.g., in the outer, middle, or inner ear, by fly larvae.

myoclonic epilepsy *np* [Gk *mus* muscle + Gk *klonos* turmoil; Gk *epilepsia* seizure]
A syndrome characterized by seizures with jerking movements and late-onset sensorineural hearing loss.

myoclonus *n* [Gk *mus* muscle + Gk *klonos* turmoil]
A type of objective tinnitus, e.g., clicking, snapping, or fluttering sounds caused by muscle spasm of the soft palate or middle ear muscles.

myogenic *adj* mīˈōˈjĕnĭk [Gk *mus* muscle + Gk *-genes* produced]
Produced by the muscles' activity.

myopia *n* mīˈōpēa [Gk *muein* to shut + Gk *ops* eye]
Nearsightedness or shortsightedness; defective vision of distant objects. This can occur as a syndrome in conjunction with congenital sensorineural hearing loss and possible learning difficulty.

myositis ossificans *np* [Gk *mus* muscle + Gk *-ites* denoting disease of; Lat *ossificans* bone-making]
A condition in which bone forms in connective tissue and muscles. Calcification of the labyrinth may occur following injury or disease, e.g., following bacterial meningitis.

myringitis *n* [Gk *myrinx* membrane + Gk *-ites* denoting disease of]
Inflammation of the eardrum.

myringoplasty *n* [Gk *myrinx* membrane + Gk *plastos* formed]
An operation to repair the eardrum.

myringotomy *n* [Gk *myrinx* membrane + Gk *–tomia* cutting]
An operation in which an incision is made in the eardrum.

myrinx *n* [Gk *myrinx* membrane]
Also: tympanic membrane; eardrum

The elastic membrane between the external auditory canal and the middle ear. The normal color is pearly gray and a cone-shaped light reflex should be seen during otoscopic examination.

myxodema/myxedema (myxoedema) *np* [Gk *muxa* slime + Gk *oedema* swelling]
A condition in which there is an accumulation of fluid under the skin, resulting from hypothyroidism (caused by reduced activity of the thyroid gland), which releases hormones that control metabolism. Characteristics may include swelling of the face and hands, migraines, extreme sensitivity to heat and cold, slow reactions, and impaired memory.
Deriv: -adj myxedemic (myxoedemic)

N

Nager syndrome *np* ˈnăger Named after Felix Robert Nager (1877–1959), a Swiss otorhinolaryngologist and professor of otorhinolaryngology at the University of Zurich.

A rare autosomal recessive disorder with numerous characteristics including underdeveloped cheeks and jaw; defects of the toes, thumbs, and soft palate; small or poorly developed outer and middle ears; and conductive hearing loss, which may be due to stapes fixation.

Nance-Sweeney syndrome *np* Named after Walter Elmore Nance (b 1933) and Anne Sweeney, American geneticists, who described the syndrome in 1970.

Also: chondrodysplasia/chondrodystrophy/chondrodystrophia

A genetic disorder affecting the development of cartilage mainly in the long bones, leading to arrested growth and associated with sensorineural hearing loss.

nanoparticles *n* [Gk *nanos* dwarf]

Microscopic particles that have one or more dimensions that are 100 nanometers (nm) or less in size. The properties of many conventional materials change when they are composed of nanoparticles, e.g., nanoparticles are used in waterproofing hearing aids and to improve magnetic resonance images.

naproxen *n*

A nonsteroidal antiinflammatory drug, often used in the treatment of arthritis and other musculoskeletal inflammation, and which may cause tinnitus and sensorineural hearing loss.

narrow-band *adj*

Restricted to a bandwidth of half an octave or less, e.g., a narrow-band filter.

nasal *adj/n* [Lat *nasus* nose]

-adj Pertaining to the nose. *-n* A consonant formed by closing the mouth and passing sound through the nose, e.g., /m/ and /n/.

nasion *n* ˈnāzēon [Lat *nasus* nose]

A point between the eyebrows or on the bridge of the nose where the frontal and nasal bones meet. (The ground electrode may be placed here in evoked response audiometry.)

nasolacrimal duct *np* [Lat *nasus* nose + Lat *lacrima* tear]

A tear duct.

nasopharynx *n* [Lat *nasus* nose + Gk *pharunx* pharynx]

The back of the throat above and behind the soft palate, continuous with the nasal passages; the area is connected to the middle ear by the Eustachian tube.

natal *adj* [Lat *natalis* relating to birth]

Relating to birth.

natural resonant frequency *np*

The frequency of free oscillation, i.e., where no external force has been applied.

near (sound) field *np*

The part of the sound field that is close to the source and where sound does not decrease in accordance with the inverse square law, as it does in the far field. The near field generally extends to a distance of not more than one wavelength from the sound source and is a region in which the sound pressure and acoustic particle velocity are not in phase.

neck loop *np*

A personal assistive listening device, worn around the neck, that transmits signals via electromagnetic induction to a device, usually a hearing aid, worn by the listener.

necro- *prefix* [Gk *nekros* corpse]

Death.

necrosis *n* neˈkrōsis [Gk *nekros* corpse + Gk *-osis* denoting a diseased state]

Tissue death.

negative *n/adj*

-n The absence of positive attributes. *-adj* Having an absence of positive attributes.

negative correlation *np*
A situation in which increases in the values of one variable are associated with decreases in the values of another variable, e.g., the use of ear plugs is negatively correlated with the incidence of noise induced hearing loss.

negative middle ear pressure *np*
The condition in which the air pressure in the middle ear is below atmospheric pressure, which is usually due to Eustachian tube dysfunction.

neomycin *n* [Gk *neos* new + Gk *mukes* mushroom, fungus]
A broad-spectrum antibiotic often used as an intestinal antiseptic in surgery, which can be ototoxic.

neonate *n* [Gk *neos* new + Lat *natus* born]
A newborn child, up to 28 days after term.
Deriv: –adj neonatal

neoplasm *n* *pl* neoplasia [Gk *neos* new + Gk *plasis* shape, form]
An abnormal new growth of benign or malignant tissue, a tumor.

neper *n* ˈnāpər (ˈnēpər) Named in honor of John Napier (1550–1617), also known as John Neper, a Scottish physicist and mathematician, who invented logarithms.
An uncommon unit of level, where 1 neper = 8.7 dB.

nephritis *n* [Gk *nephros* kidney + Gk *-ites* denoting disease of]
Also: Bright syndrome
Kidney inflammation.

nephrosis deafness urinary tract digital malformations *np* [Gk *nephros* kidney + Gk *-osis* denoting a diseased state]
A rare genetic renal disorder that is associated with congenital conductive hearing loss. Characteristics include kidney disease, deafness, and abnormalities of the fingers and toes and of the urinary tract.

nerve *n* [Gk *neuron* string or nerve]
A cord-like bundle of conducting nerve fibers (axons/and or dendrites), enclosed in a myelin sheath, within the peripheral nervous system. Sensory stimuli and motor impulses are passed along the nerves to the brain and to and from other parts of the central nervous system.

nerve, afferent *np* [Gk *neuron* string or nerve; Lat *afferens* taking to]
Conducts signals from sensory neurons to the central nervous system.

nerve, auditory *np* [Gk *neuron* string or nerve; Lat *auditorius* pertaining to hearing]
One branch of the eighth cranial nerve (the vestibulocochlear nerve) that carries impulses from the inner ear to the brain. The second branch is the vestibular nerve, concerned with balance information.

nerve, cranial *np* [Gk *neuron* string or nerve; Lat *cranium* skull]
One of 12 pairs of nerves that emerge from the brainstem. Cranial nerves (CN) that are important in audiology include the trigeminal nerve (CNV), facial nerve (CNVII), and the acoustic or vestibulocochlear nerve (CNVIII).

nerve deafness *np colloq*
Also: sensorineural hearing loss; *obs* perceptive deafness
A hearing loss that involves the sensory and/or neural cells of the cochlea and their connections, or occasionally cranial nerve VIII or brainstem lesions.

nerve, efferent *np* [Gk *neuron* string or nerve; Lat *efferens* taking away]
Conducts signals from the central nervous system to target muscles and glands.

nervous system *np*
The system of nerves and organs that regulate the body's responses to stimuli.

nervous system, central *np*
The brain and spinal cord, which integrate sensory impulses from all parts of the body.

nervous system, parasympathetic *np*
One of the main divisions of the autonomic (self-regulating) nervous system, part of the peripheral nervous system that controls the internal environment of the body. Its effects include bronchiole and pupil constriction, alimentary canal and smooth muscle contraction, heart rate moderation, increases in saliva and mucus production and some glandular secretion.

netilmicin (netilmycin) *n* [Gk *mukes* mushroom, fungus]
One of the aminoglycoside group of broad spectrum antibiotics. It can be ototoxic, causing balance problems and hearing loss, which may occur even after the drug has been stopped.

neural *adj* [Gk *neuron* string, nerve]
Relating to nerves or the nervous system.

neural hearing loss *np*
A retrocochlear hearing loss relating to a lesion of the auditory nerve, between the cochlea and the brain, e.g., a tumor on the auditory nerve.

neural plasticity *np*
The ability of the central nervous system to reorganize the neural pathways, e.g., for learning and memory and as an adaptive mechanism for recovery after brain injury.

neural potential *np*
A difference in electrical charge that represents the work involved or energy released in the transfer of a quantity of electricity from one point to another, e.g., between two electrodes or across cell membranes.

neural response telemetry (NRT) *np*
[Gk *tele* far off + Gk *metria* measuring]
Also: neural response imaging (NRI); auditory nerve telemetry (ART)
The measurement of the evoked auditory nerve response via a cochlear implant, e.g., used in cochlear implant fitting during surgery.

neuralgia *n* n(y)urăljēa [Gk *neuron* string, nerve + Gk *algos* pain]
Pain along the course of a nerve with no apparent change in nerve structure.

neuraxis *n* [Gk *neuron* string, nerve + Lat *axis* axle, pivot]
An imaginary line through the center of the length of the nervous system from the bottom of the spine to the front of the forebrain.

neuritis *n* [Gk *neuron* string, nerve + Gk *-ites* denoting disease of]
Inflammation of a nerve or group of nerves.

neurofibromatosis *n* [Gk *neuron* string, nerve + Lat *fibra* fiber + Gk *oma* denoting tumor, swelling + *osis* denoting a diseased state]
A genetic disorder associated with growth of benign tumors on nerves, sometimes accompanied by bone deformity and a predisposition to cancer. There are three types of neurofibromatosis: type 1 (which involves multiple café au lait spots and fibromas of the peripheral nervous system), type 2 (which involves tumors on the auditory and vestibular branches of cranial nerve VIII) and a rare form, known as schwannomatosis (which involves multiple schwannomas on cranial, spinal and peripheral nerves, accompanied by pain). Type 2 causes hearing loss, tinnitus and balance problems. Tumors may occur bilaterally. Other problems may include facial weakness, headache, numbness, limb weakness, cataracts, and possible brain tumors.

neuroglia *n* n(y)u'rōglēa (n(y)u'rŏglēa) [Gk *neuron* nerve + Gk *glia* glue]
Also: glia
A fine web of connective tissue that supports the neurons in the central nervous system.
Deriv: -*adj* glial

neurolinguistic programming *np*
A way of thinking that focuses on helping individuals to overcome their psychological problems.

neuroma *n* n(y)uˈrōmɑ [Gk *neuron* string, nerve + Gk *-oma* denoting tumor, swelling]
A tumor composed of nerve tissue.

neuron (neurone) *n* [Gk *neuron* string, nerve]
The basic functional unit of the nervous system. A neuron is a cell body with an axon and dendrites extending from it. Neurons do not touch each other but at the synapse (junction) between them, an electrochemical reaction occurs when they are close. Nerve impulses are transmitted across the synapse to the next neuron.

neuron (neurone), motor *np*
A neuron in the central nervous system that controls muscle contraction or gland secretion.

neuron (neurone), sensory *np*
A neuron that detects changes in the external or internal environment and transmits this information to the central nervous system.

neuronal transmission *np*
The process by which a nerve impulse passes along the neuron. Each neuron has a semipermeable covering that allows electrically charged particles to pass. In the resting state, the membrane is polarized, being positively charged on the outside but negatively charged on the inside, with a difference of -70 mv. When the situation is reversed, the neuron is depolarized and the change can become an action potential that passes to affect the next neuron. Another action potential can only be generated once the cell has returned to its resting position.

neurootology *n* [Gk *neuron* string, nerve + Gk *ous* ear + Gk *-logia* study of]
The study of the neurology of the auditory and vestibular systems.

neuropathy, auditory (AN) *np* [Gk *neuron* string, nerve + Gk *patheia* suffering, disease]
Also: auditory dyssynchrony (AD)
A disorder in which responses to non-speech sounds are normal but the ability to decode speech and language is impaired.

neurotransmitter *n* [Gk *neuron* string, nerve]
A chemical released by the neuron that crosses the synapse to be received by the next neuron.

newton (N) *n* Named after Sir Isaac Newton (1642–1727), an English mathematician, who identified gravity as the fundamental force that controls the movement of celestial bodies.
A unit of force, where one Newton over one square meter is equivalent to a pressure of one pascal (Pa).

niche *n* nĭtch (nēsh)
A shallow recess or hollow, e.g., the round window niche is the recess in which the round window of the cochlea is located.

nitrogen mustard *np*
An ototoxic antineoplastic drug used in the treatment of cancer.

Noah *n* Named after Noah and his ark because it includes all types, as in the ark. Audiologic software used to store patient details and audiometric test results. Also the platform used to link to individual programming software developed by hearing aid manufacturers.

node *n* nōd [Lat *nodus* knot]
A point in a standing wave that has zero amplitude.

Nodes of Ranvier *np* rŏnˈvīā
A natural constriction or narrowing in the myelin sheath, which occurs at intervals along the length of the nerve fiber.

noise n
Also: distortion
1. Undesired or interfering sound. 2. Random, irregular oscillation. 3. A type of sound used in certain audiometric tests to mask the test tone in the nontest ear.

noise, background np
Extraneous noise which, if excessive, may mask the signal of interest.

noise, broadband np
Complex noise that is distributed across a wide range of frequencies.

noise, colored (coloured) np
A group of noises that are known by their colors, e.g., black noise (spikes of noise), purple noise (contains more energy with increasing frequency), etc.

noise, composite np
The noise from all sources present.

noise dose np
The amount of sound energy/noise that an individual receives is calculated from the noise level and the duration of exposure. An equal noise dose is accepted as causing an equal degree of hearing loss regardless of variation in the level and time of exposure, i.e., short exposure at high levels or long exposure at lesser levels.

noise emission level np
A measure of the total (cumulative) level of noise exposure over time, e.g., over a working life. It is a function of the level of noise and the number of years of exposure.

noise exposure np
A representation of the total sound energy heard by the ear during a stated time period.

noise exposure level np
The total sound energy from a single event expressed in decibels.

noise floor np
The internal noise of an electrical or acoustic device, e.g., a hearing aid.

noise, Gaussian np ˈgowsēan Named after Carl Friedrich Gauss (1777–1855), a German mathematician and astronomer, who pioneered the application of mathematics to electricity and magnetism.
Noise in which the amplitudes follow a gaussian distribution (i.e., a statistical normal distribution), e.g., gaussian white noise.

noise-induced hearing loss (NIHL) np
A hearing loss associated with exposure to high or prolonged levels of sound. Hearing loss often starts as a temporary reduction in hearing that recovers after a relatively short period. With repeated exposure (or with single exposure to very high sound levels) the hearing loss becomes permanent. The hearing loss due to excessive noise is mainly in the high frequencies with the worst hearing in or around the 4 kHz region, which gives the audiogram a characteristic "noise notch."

noise-induced permanent threshold shift np
Permanent hearing loss caused by exposure to excessive noise, most often in the workplace.

noise, masking np
Noise that is used in audiometry to prevent hearing in the nontest ear.

noise, narrow band np
Contains frequencies of equal intensity within a restricted band.

noise notch np
A dip in the hearing thresholds shown on an audiogram, e.g., the 4 kHz notch found in many cases of noise-induced hearing loss.

noise, notched np
Noise from which narrow bands (notches) of frequencies have been removed.

noise, pink np
A random noise where amplitude decreases by one half with each doubling of frequency, i.e., 3 dB per octave.

noise, random *np*
A complex sound wave whose instantaneous amplitude varies over time in a random manner.

noise, saw-toothed *np*
A complex noise whose zigzag waveform resembles the teeth of a saw with equal amplitude of all harmonics of the fundamental frequency (most commonly 60 or 120 Hz.)

noise, speech-weighted *np*
Noise that has a sound pressure level which is constant from 125 Hz to 1 kHz and falls by 12 dB per octave from 1 kHz to 6 kHz. This corresponds to the long-term average speech spectrum.

noise, white *np*
1. Noise in which all frequencies within a specified range are present, without regard to phase, and where the average power over the frequency range is constant. 2. Noise that contains equal power per unit of bandwidth, i.e., equal sound energy at all frequencies.

noise, wide band *np*
Any complex noise that is contained within a wide frequency range.

nominal *n/adj* [Lat *nomen* name]
–*n* A word or words that function as a noun. -*adj* Pertaining to names.

nominal data *np*
Items in a category that are differentiated by name. They can be counted but not ordered or measured.

nominal value *np*
A given value, e.g., the value of a hearing aid's performance characteristic as specified by the manufacturer.

non- *prefix* [Lat *non* not]
Not.

noninvasive *adj*
Not penetrating the body, e.g., noninvasive surgery.

noninverting electrode *np*
A primary or active electrode, e.g., the vertex electrode in auditory evoked response measurements.

nonlinear *adj*
1. Not having a one-to-one correspondence, e.g., between input levels and output levels. 2. Occurring as a result of an operation that is not linear, e.g., nonlinear compression in hearing aids, where the amount of amplification varies depending on the input levels and the maximum power output settings.

nonoccluding *adj* [Lat *non* not + Lat *occludere* to shut up]
An open earmold that reduces low-frequency amplification and that is therefore used with high-frequency hearing losses where the low frequency hearing is relatively good.

nonorganic hearing loss *np* [Lat *non* not + Gk *organikos* pertaining to life]
Also: malingering; functional hearing loss; pseudohypacusis/pseudohypoacusis
Deafness that is not of the body, but that is feigned (malingering). Nonorganic hearing loss in children is usually related to emotional problems and is not normally considered malingering.

nonparametric *adj* [Lat *non* not + Gk *para* beside + Gk *metron* measure]
A statistical quantity that does not assume any particular distribution, e.g., nominal or ordinal data.

nonsense syllable *np*
A meaningless monosyllable, i.e., a consonant and vowel combination that has no meaning; sometimes used in speech audiometry.

nonsuppurative *adj* [Lat *non* not + Lat *suppurare* to suppurate]
Inflammation without the production of pus, e.g., serous otitis media.

nonsyndromic hearing loss *np* [Lat *non* not + Gk *sundrome* a running together, syndrome]
A genetic hearing loss that is not accompanied by other associated abnormalities, e.g., nonsyndromic mitochondrial hear-

ing loss is characterized by moderate to profound hearing loss only.

nontest ear *np*
The ear that it is not intended to test. The nontest ear will be the ear to receive masking noise where masking is required.

nonverbal *adj*
Facial expression, gesture, movements, or posture used to convey information.

Noonan syndrome *np* Named after Jacqueline Anne Noonan (b 1921), an American pediatric cardiologist, who described the syndrome in 1963.
An autosomal dominant condition similar to Turner syndrome, but with no chromosomal defect and affecting both sexes. Characteristics include small stature, cognitive impairment, webbed neck, vertebral abnormalities, and down-slanting eyes. It may also be associated with cleft palate and conductive and/or sensorineural hearing loss.

norm *n* [Lat *norma* a carpenter's square, rule]
A generalized understanding of what is considered normal or appropriate for a homogeneous group.

normal distribution *np*
A symmetrical frequency graph where measures are evenly distributed on both sides of the mean; this results in a bell-shaped curve.

normal hearing *np*
The range of frequencies and intensities that can be heard by a listener who has undamaged hearing. Average normal hearing is taken as 0 dBHL but "normal hearing" is generally accepted as hearing levels that are better than 25 (UK: 20) dBHL across the frequency range under test (usually 250 Hz to 8 kHz).

normalized (normalised) hearing level (nHL) *np*
A decibel level (dBnHL) that uses a behaviorally determined normative reference

level, where no standardized reference level exists.

normative data *np*
Statistical information regarding average normal characteristics. The data can be used to differentiate normal from abnormal results, e.g., to differentiate individuals with central auditory dysfunction from those without.

Norrie syndrome *np* Named after Gordon Norrie (1855–1941), a Danish surgeon and ophthalmologist, who is recognized for his work with the blind.
Also: oculoacousticocerebral degeneration
A recessive X-linked disorder, i.e., it generally affects only males, and characterized by progressive blindness, often associated with learning difficulty and late onset progressive bilateral sensorineural hearing loss.

nosoacusis *np* nōsōak(y)ūsĭs [Gk *nosos* disease + Gk *akousis* sense of hearing]
A subclinical hearing loss that occurs following disease or general ill-health.

notch *np*
1. An indentation. 2. A V-shaped dip in the audiogram, e.g., Carhart notch, which occurs in the bone conduction thresholds at about 2 kHz and is considered indicative of otosclerosis.

notch filter *np*
Also: band-reject filter, band-stop filter, band elimination filter
A filter that stops the passage of a band of frequencies, but allows frequencies to pass in a band both above and below the range of frequencies that have been filtered out.

notched noise *np*
Noise from which narrow bands (notches) of frequencies have been removed.

not-masked *adj*
Without the use of masking noise.

notochord *n* nōtōkawd [Gk *noton* back + Lat *chorda* rope]
A strip of mesodermal cells in the early embryo that is incorporated into the spinal column as part of the intervertebral disks.

noy *n* *pl* noys The unit was conceived by Karl D. Krypter, an American engineer, in 1959. The term was chosen because the plural is pronounced "noise."
A unit of perceived noisiness, equal to a 40 dBSPL one-third octave band centered on 1 kHz.

nucleate *adj*
Having a nucleus.

nucleolus *n* [Lat *nucleolus* a little kernal]
A structure in the nucleus that is responsible for the production of ribosomes.

nucleus *n* *pl* nuclei [Lat *nucleus* kernel]
1. The positively charged center of an atom. 2. The part of a cell that carries genetic material.

nucleus, cochlear *np*
The first relay station in the brainstem of the auditory system. Information arrives at the cochlear nucleus via cranial nerve VIII.

null hypothesis *n*
The hypothesis that is to be tested. Statistical analysis will consider the probability of the results occurring if the null hypothesis should be true. The null hypothesis will then be accepted or rejected.

null zero *n*
Nothing, i.e., a set having no magnitude.

Nyquist frequency/limit *np* ˈnīkwĭst
Named after Harry Nyquist (1912–1976), a Swedish-American engineer, who investigated the mathematics of sampling.
Also: Nyquist limit
The highest frequency that can be coded at a given sampling rate so that the signal can be fully reconstructed. The Nyquist frequency is equal to half of the sampling rate.

Nyquist rate *np* Named after Harry Nyquist (1912–1976), a Swedish-American engineer, who investigated the mathematics of sampling.
The minimum rate that an analog signal must be sampled to avoid loss of information and subsequent distortion. The minimum rate that must be sampled is equal to or greater than twice the bandwidth of the signal.

Nyssen-van Bogaert-Meyer syndrome *np* Named after Rene Nyssen (1891–1972), a Belgian neurologist, and Ludo van Bogaert (1897–1989), a Belgian neuropathologist, who together first described the condition in 1934, also Joachim-Ernst Meyer (1917–1998), a German psychiatrist, who further expanded the description in 1949.
Also: opticochleodentate degeneration
A rare genetic condition in which there is progressive degeneration of the central nervous system, characterized by progressive vision loss, hearing loss, and quadriplegia. There may also be microcephaly and mental deterioration. Death usually occurs in childhood.

nystagmography *n* [Gk *nustagmos* drowsiness, nodding, blinking + Gk *graphia* writing]
The recording of the features, e.g., amplitude and time, of nystagmus.

nystagmus *n* nĭsˈtăgmus [Gk *nustagmos* drowsiness, nodding, blinking]
Involuntary eye movements.

nystagmus, downbeat *np*
Nystagmus in which the fast phase beats in a downward direction.

nystagmus, endpoint *np*
Nystagmus evoked by maintaining an eye position in extremes of the range of movement.

nystagmus, gaze *np*
Nystagmus evoked by attempting to maintain an eye position away from the center.

nystagmus, gaze-paretic *np*
A form of gaze nystagmus found during recovery from gaze palsy. When the eyes look in the direction of the previously affected side, jerk nystagmus occurs in the direction of gaze.

nystagmus, jerk *np*
A nystagmus in which the movements are slow in one phase and fast in the other. The direction of the jerk nystagmus (i. e., which way it "beats") is defined by the fast phase, which is the corrective saccade. Nystagmus arising from vestibular dysfunction is of this type.

nystagmus, optokinetic *np* [Gk *nustagmos* drowsiness, nodding, blinking; Gk *optos* seen + Gk *kinetikos* moving]
Nystagmus with alternating fast saccadic eye movements in one direction followed by slower smooth movements in the opposite direction. This occurs when the eyes track a moving visual field.

nystagmus, pendular *np*
Nystagmus with an equal velocity in each direction (i.e., horizontal, vertical, circular, elliptical) often with marked asymmetry between the eyes, which may reflect brainstem or cerebellar dysfunction.

nystagmus, periodic alternating *np*
A horizontal jerk nystagmus with the fast phase beating in one direction and then in the opposite direction.

nystagmus, positional *np*
Nystagmus that occurs in specific head positions with respect to gravity. Positional nystagmus of short duration may be due to a benign lesion of the posterior semicircular canal. It may also be found sometimes in serious brainstem and cerebellum lesions.

nystagmus, rotary *np*
Also: torsional nystagmus
Nystagmus with a rotary movement. Most nystagmus resulting from vestibular dysfunction has a rotary component.

nystagmus, upbeat *np*
Nystagmus in which the fast phase beats in an upward direction.

objective *adj*
1. Without allowing personal interpretation or bias to have an influence. 2. Having behaviors that are observable/measurable and independent of an individual's subjective behavioral response.

objective audiometry *np*
A method of testing hearing function that does not rely upon the individual's subjective behavioral responses, e.g., tympanometry.

objective tinnitus *np*
Tinnitus that is due to internally generated sound or vibration that may be heard or measured by an external observer.

obliterate *v*
To cause to disappear; to completely remove.
Deriv: -*adj* obliterative

obliterative otosclerosis *np*
Otosclerosis in which the growth of bone has filled the basal turn of the cochlea and obliterated the round window.

oblique *adj*
Having a slanting or sloping direction or position, e.g., the eardrum lies at an oblique angle with reference to the ear canal floor.

obscure auditory dysfunction (OAD) *np*
obs
Also: auditory processing disorder (APD); central auditory processing disorder; King-Kopetzky syndrome
An impairment of neural function that does not solely result from a deficit in general attention, language, or other cognitive processes. It may be characterized by difficulty in understanding speech especially in background noise and poor recognition, discrimination, separation, grouping, localization, or ordering of nonspeech sounds.

observer bias *np*
Error introduced into experiments or measurements by unintended/unconscious manipulation of the results by the experimenter. This is a confounding variable in observational research that can be controlled, e.g., by double-blind studies.

obstruent *adj* [Lat *obstruere* to obstruct, block]
A sound produced with the flow of breath partially or fully obstructed, e.g., /b/.

occipital *adj* ŏkˈsĭpĭtal [Lat *ob* against + Lat *caput* head]
1. Pertaining to the the occiput or back of the head. 2. Located near the occipital bone, e.g., the occipital lobe of the brain.

occipital bone *np*
A curved bone at the rear and base of the skull that supports the back of the head. It is joined to the parietal bones by the lambdoidal suture (an immovable joint of connective tissue).

occluded *adj* [Lat *occludere* to shut up]
Blocked, e.g., an ear canal can be occluded by wax.

occluded ear simulator *np*
Also: Zwislocki coupler
A device for measuring hearing aid performance that has a complex shape and a cavity size of 1.2 cc that approximates the acoustic impedance of the average adult ear.

occlusion effect *np*
An increase in sound level that occurs when the ear canal is occluded. This causes an apparent improvement in hearing by bone conduction when the ear canal is blocked, e.g., by earplugs, earmolds, hearing aids, or wax. Occlusion is a low-frequency phenomenon (mainly below 1 kHz) and has no effect at frequencies over 2 kHz.

octave *n* [Lat *octavus* an eighth]
The interval between two frequencies which is a ratio of 2:1, i.e., doubling the

frequency equates to one octave, e.g., 125 Hz–250 Hz and 2 kHz–4 kHz.

oculo- *prefix* [Lat *oculus* eye]
Pertaining to the eyes.

oculoacousticocerebral   degeneration *np* [Lat *oculus* eye + Gk *akousis* sense of hearing + Lat *cerebrum* brain]
Also: Norrie syndrome
A recessive X-linked disorder, i.e., generally affecting only males, that is characterized by progressive blindness, often associated with learning difficulty and late-onset progressive bilateral sensorineural hearing loss.

oculocutaneous albinism *np* [Lat *oculus* eye + Lat *cutis* skin; Lat *albus* white]
Also: Tietz syndrome
An autosomal dominant genetic syndrome of hypopigmentation and deafness, characterized by a white forelock; white spots on the arms, legs and abdomen; blue eyes; and bilateral profound congenital sensorineural deafness.

odorant *n*
An odorous substance.

odynacusis *n* [Gk *odune* pain + Gk *akousis* sense of hearing]
Painful sensitivity to noise.

offset *n/adj*
-*n* The termination of an acoustic stimulus. -*adj* In response to an offset stimulus.

ohm (Ω) *n* Named after George Simon Ohm (1787–1854), a German physicist, who formulated the law now called Ohm's law.
The standard international unit of electrical resistance equal to the electrical resistance between two points on a conductor, when a constant potential difference of 1 volt produces a current of 1 ampere in the conductor.

Ohm's acoustical law *np* Named after George Simon Ohm (1787–1854), a German physicist, who formulated the law.
A law that states that a listener can perceive the individual frequency components of a complex sound. This analysis is not generally possible, but the listener can be trained to perceive individual harmonics.

Ohm's law *np* Named after George Simon Ohm (1787–1854), a German physicist, who formulated the law.
The strength of electric current flowing through a conductor is directly proportional to the potential difference, and inversely proportional to the resistance of the circuit, i.e., V = IR, where V is the voltage, I is the current and R is the resistance.

olfaction *n* [Lat *olfactus* a smell]
The sense of smell.

oligodendroglia *n* ŏlĭgŏdĕn'drŏglēa [Gk *oligos* little + Gk *dendron* tree + Gk *glia* glue]
Branched cells that are associated with the formation of the myelin sheath around nerve fibers. One oligodendroglia can myelinate several axons.

olivary complex, superior *np*
A collection of nerve cells in the lower portion (medulla oblongata) of the brainstem in the central auditory system that is involved in sound processing. It is the first place where binaural stimulation occurs and the functions include the detection of interaural differences (i.e., differences between sounds received by the right and left ears), e.g., of time and intensity, which are important for localization. The two main nuclei are the lateral superior olive, which compares high-frequency differences in amplitude, and the medial superior olive, which compares low frequency differences in time delay.

olivocochlear bundle *np*
Also: bundle of Rasmussen
Efferent auditory nerve fibers that originate from the superior olivary complex and innervate the hair cells in the cochlea.

omnidirectional *adj*
Equally sensitive to sounds from all directions, e.g., an omnidirectional microphone.

on effect *n*
The vigorous initial response of the sensory system to a stimulus when it is first presented.

one-tailed test *np*
A statistical test of significance that is used only when the researcher is certain that results can only go in one direction.

on–off cycle *np*
The time that an intermittent signal is on compared with the time it is off as it repeats itself.

onset *n*
The initiation of an acoustic stimulus.

on-time *n*
The length of time for which a sound is present.

onychodystrophy *n* ŏnĭkō'dĭstrŏfē [Gk *onux* nail, claw + Gk *dus-* bad + Gk *trophe* nourishment]
A disorder in which there are triphalangeal thumbs, i.e., that have three phalanges similar to the fingers, and rudimentary nails on the fingers and toes. Onychodystrophy can appear as a syndrome with hereditary severe congenital sensorineural hearing loss and there may also be skeletal abnormalities, epilepsy, and learning difficulty.

open *adj*
Also: unoccluded
A position that permits passage.

open circuit *np*
1. An electrical circuit in which there is a break such that the current cannot flow.
2. In a cochlear implant, a break in the wire leading to an electrode.

open earmold *np*
An earmold that does not occlude the ear.

open jaw impression *np*
An ear impression taken with the mouth propped open so that the canal is at its widest position. It is often used where there is feedback from the hearing aid during chewing or talking and also for small completely-in-the-ear hearing aids to ensure a tight fit.

open platform *np*
A silicone chip that provides general purpose programmability, e.g., the chip in a digital hearing aid that is capable of using many different algorithms.

open set *np*
Having no restriction in the range of possible answers.

open syllable *np*
A syllable that ends in a vowel.

open question *np*
A question that cannot be answered simply by yes or no but which requires more depth and insight, e.g., questions starting with "why?" or "how?"

operant behavior *np*
A change in behavior as a result of providing reinforcement for the desired behavior; used in pediatric audiometry.

optic atrophy polyneuropathy deafness *np* [Gk *optos* seen; Gk *a-* negative + Gk *trophe* nourishment; Gk *polus* many + Gk *neuron* string, nerve + Gk *patheia* suffering]
Also: Rosenberg-Chutorian syndrome
A rare X-linked genetic syndrome. Characterics include progressive visual deterioration, progressive severe high-frequency sensorineural hearing loss, and polyneuropathy, especially affecting the arms and legs.

opticochleodentate degeneration *np* [Gk *optos* seen + Lat *cochlea* snail shell, spiral + Lat *dentatus* having teeth]
Also: Nyssen-van Bogaert-Meyer syndrome
A rare genetic condition in which there is progressive degeneration of the central nervous system, characterized by pro-

gressive vision loss, hearing loss, and quadriplegia. There may also be microcephaly and mental deterioration. Death usually occurs in childhood.

optimum speech level *np*
The lowest speech intensity level at which maximum speech recognition score occurs.

optokinetic *adj* [Gk *optos* seen + Gk *kinetikos* moving]
Pertaining to involuntary movement or twitching of the eyes when viewing moving objects.

optokinetic nystagmus *np*
Nystagmus with alternating fast saccadic eye movements in one direction followed by slower smooth movements in the opposite direction. This occurs during head rotation or when a visual stimulus moves past.

oral *adj* [Lat *os* mouth]
1. Taken through, applied, or pertaining to the mouth. 2. Spoken or relating to speech.

oral-aural approach *np* [Lat *os* mouth + Lat *auris* ear]
An approach to teaching deaf children through the use of speech, utilizing residual hearing.

oralism *n*
A method of teaching based on auditory and speechreading cues without the use of manual communication.

oralist *n*
Someone who believes in an oral approach for deaf children and does not accept the use of signs in education and habilitation.

order effect *np*
The tendency to perform differently because of the order in which things are done or tried, e.g., the magnitude of the effect of hearing aid A may be altered depending whether it precedes or follows hearing aid B.

ordinal *adj*
Of a specified order or rank in a sequence or series.

ordinate *n*
The vertical or y axis of a graph.

organ *n* [Gk *organon* sense organ]
A collection of bodily parts or tissues that fulfils or performs a specific function.

organic *adj*
Having the characteristics of an organism.

organ of Corti *np* Named after Alfonso Giacomo Gaspare Corti (1822–1876), an Italian anatomist, who described the structure of the organ situated on the basilar membrane.
The spiral ribbon-like sense organ of hearing that is situated along the entire length of the basilar membrane in the scala media of the cochlea. It contains the inner and outer hair cells that convert sound pressure waves into the electrical impulses that are transmitted via cranial nerve VIII, to the brain. The frequency of the sound activates a particular area along the organ of Corti, e.g., high frequencies near the base and low frequencies near the apex.

orienting reflex *np*
Also: orienting response
An unconditioned response to a change in the environment, e.g., a sound stimulus that results in an immediate turning of the head toward the direction of the sound.

orodigitofacial dysostosis *np* [Lat *os* mouth + Lat *digitus* finger + Lat *facies* face; Gk *dus-* bad + Gk *osteon* bone + Gk *-osis* denoting a diseased state]
Also: Mohr syndrome; oral-facial-digital syndrome
An autosomal recessive disorder of the oral cavity, face, and hands, which is often accompanied by hearing loss, usually conductive in nature.

oscillation *n* ŏsĭlāshun [Lat *oscillare* to swing]
A repetitive variation around a mean value that occurs when a system is disturbed from its state of rest, e.g., the back and forth movement of a pendulum.

oscillogram *n* [Lat *oscillare* to swing + Gk *gramma* written thing]
A trace or graph from an oscilloscope.

oscillopsia *n* ŏsĭ'ŏpsēa [Lat *oscillare* to swing + Gk *ops* eye]
A visual disturbance in which objects appear to move back and forth, when the head is moved, which usually indicates a bilateral vestibular disorder, e.g., oscillopsia is one of the symptoms that may occur after taking the ototoxic drug, gentamicin.

oscilloscope *n* ŏsĭ' loʹskōp [Lat *oscillare* to swing + Gk *skopein* to look]
An electronic instrument that facilitates measurement of the amplitude, frequency, or temporal characteristics of a signal. It displays a visual representation of variations in voltage across time.

osseointegration *n*
The direct anchoring or growing in of an implant into living bone, e.g., for attachment of a bone-anchored hearing aid.

osseous *adj* ŏsēus [Lat *osseus* bony]
Also: bony
Pertaining to bone.

osseous labyrinth *np*
Also: bony labyrinth
The bony labyrinth of the inner ear that consists of the cochlea and the vestibular system.

osseous spiral lamina *np*
A bony ledge that projects from the modiolus (throughout the spiral cochlea) to which the basilar membrane is attached.

ossicle *n* 'ŏsĭkul [Lat *ossiculum* small bone]
A small bone, e.g., one of the three ossicles that make up the ossicular chain in the middle ear.
Deriv: -adj ossicular

ossicular chain *np* [Lat *ossiculum* small bone]
The incus, malleus, and stapes, three small linked bones within the middle ear cavity that transmit sound from the tympanic membrane to the oval window.

ossicular disarticulation/discontinuity *np*
Damage or fracture of the ossicular chain, such that the chain of bones is no longer continuous; this results in a conductive hearing loss.

ossicular fixation *np*
Immobilization of the ossicular chain, which prevents the efficient passage of vibrations and causes a conductive hearing loss.

ossiculoplasty *n* [Lat *ossiculum* small bone + Gk *plastos* formed]
Repair or reconstruction of the ossicular chain.

ossification *n* [Lat *os* bone + Lat *facere* to make]
1. The process of new bone formation. 2. The calcification of soft tissue into a bone-like material.

osteitis deformans *np* ŏstēïtis [Gk *osteon* bone + Gk *-ites* denoting disease of; Lat *deformare* to deform]
Also: Paget disease; Beethoven deafness
A skeletal condition in which there is excessive bone absorption followed by excessive poor abnormal bone formation, such that new bone is weak and bulky and liable to deformation and fracture. Bones affected can include the skull, and can lead to tinnitus, vertigo, and sensorineural hearing loss related to loss of bone mineral density in the cochlear capsule.

osteo- *prefix* ŏstēō [Gk *osteon* bone]
Pertaining to bone.

osteoblast *n* [Gk *osteon* bone + Gk *blastos* sprout]
Bone forming cells that deposit new tissue as the bone grows or is reshaped.

osteoclast *n* [Gk *osteon* bone + Gk *klastos* broken]
The largest of the bone cells. A large multinucleate cell that absorbs bone.

osteoclastogenesis *n* [Gk *osteon* bone + Gk *klastos* broken + Gk *genesis* generation, creation]
The development of osteoclasts.

osteodental dysplasia *np* [Gk *osteon* bone + Lat *dens* tooth; Gk *–dus* bad + Gk *plasis* formation]
A disorder of bone development in the skull and clavicle (collar bone) with associated conductive and sensorineural hearing loss and a susceptibility to sinus and ear infections.

osteogenesis imperfecta *np* [Gk *osteon* bone + Gk *genesis* generation, creation; Lat *imperfectus* imperfect]
Also: brittle bones
An autosomal dominant congenital disorder of variable severity. Characteristics include brittle bones causing multiple fractures, short stature, blueish whites of the eyes (sclera), and a conductive hearing loss that resembles otosclerosis.

osteolysis *n* [Gk *osteon* bone + Gk *lusis* loosening]
Degeneration or disappearance of bone tissue due to inflammation or disease.

osteoma *n* [Gk *osteon* bone + Gk *–oma* denoting tumor, swelling]
A slow-growing benign tumor composed of bone or bone-like tissue and usually having a narrow base. It may occur in the ear canal and most commonly at the joint between the tympanic and mastoid portions of the temporal bone.

osteomyelitis *n* [Lat *osteon* bone + Gk *muelos* bone marrow]
Inflammation of the bone marrow generally due to infection.

osteopetrosis *n* [Gk *osteon* bone + Gk *petros* rock + Gk *-osis* denoting a diseased state]
Also: Albers-Schönberg disease; chalk bone disease; marble bone disease
A craniofacial and skeletal disorder with brittle but hardened and thickened bones. Characteristics include enlarged head, learning difficulty, visual problems, and moderate progressive conductive, or sensorineural hearing loss.

ostium *n* ˈŏstēum *pl* ostia [Lat *ostium* door, opening]
An opening, e.g., the tympanic ostium of the Eustachian tube.

ot-/oto- *prefix* ˈŏt-/ˈōtō- (ˈōto-) [Gk *ous* ear (*ota* ears)]
A combining form relating to the ear.

otalgia *n* [Gk *ous* ear + Gk *algos* pain]
Also: earache
Pain in the ear.

otapostasis *n* [Gk *ous* ear + Gk *apostasis* a standing out]
Also: (2.) *colloq* bat ears
1. Surgical repair of the pinna, usually for cosmetic purposes. 2. Abnormally protruding or prominent ears.

otic *adj* [Gk *ous* ear]
Having a relationship to the ear.

otic capsule *np*
The membranous sac that contains the inner ear.

otitis *n* [Gk *ous* ear + Gk *-ites* denoting disease of]
Inflammation of the ear.
Deriv: -adj otitic

otitis externa *np* [Gk *ous* ear + Gk *-ites* denoting disease of; Lat *externa* external]
Also: colloq swimmer's ear
Inflammation of the external ear.

otitis media *np* [Gk *ous* ear + Gk *-ites* denoting disease of; Lat *media* middle]
Inflammation of the middle ear.

otoacoustic emissions (OAE) *np* [Gk *ous* ear + Gk *akousis* sense of hearing]
Also: colloq cochlear echoes; Kemp echoes
A sound generated by the outer hair cells of the cochlea that can be recorded in the ear canal of normal ears and which is used in hearing screening, especially of

neonates. The presence of these emissions was first hypothesized in 1948 by Thomas Gold and experimentally proved by Kemp in 1978.

otoacoustic emissions, distortion product (DPOAE) *np*
Emissions evoked when two tones of different frequency are presented simultaneously to the ear.

otoacoustic emissions, evoked *np*
Emissions that occur when the ear is presented with a sound stimulus and that are used as a test of cochlear function.

otoacoustic emissions, spontaneous (SOAE) *np*
Normal emissions that occur in the absence of auditory stimulation.

otoacoustic emissions, sustained frequency (SFOAE) *np*
Emissions in response to a continuous tone.

otoacoustic emissions, transient evoked (TEOAE)/transient evoked otoacoustic emissions (TOAE) *np*
Emissions evoked by very brief sounds, usually clicks, but can be tone bursts.

otoadmittance *np*
Also: immittance
The flow of energy through the middle ear, including impedance and admittance.

otoblock *n*
A block, usually of foam, inserted into the ear canal to impede the flow of ear impression material to the eardrum.

otocephaly *n* [Gk *ous* ear + Gk *kephale* head]
A condition in which the main feature is agnathia, i.e., all or part of the lower jaw is missing due to maldevelopment of the first branchial arch. Ears are usually misplaced (e.g., to the cheek) and the mouth is abnormally small (microstomia). Death usually occurs soon after birth.

otocleisis *n* [Gk *ous* ear + Gk *kleisis* closing]

1. Complete closure of the ear canal, e.g., by wax or a growth. 2. Obstruction of the Eustachian tube. 3. Surgery to correct protruding ears.

otoconia *n, pl sg* otoconium [Gk *ous* ear + Gk *konos* cone]
Also: otoliths
Minute granules of calcium carbonate in the gelatinous otolithic membrane of the vestibular system. Cilia are embedded in the membrane and movement of these stimulate sensory cells to pass positional information to the brain, which is important in the maintenance of the body's upright position in respect to gravity.

otofaciocervical dysmorphia *np* [Gk *ous* ear + Lat *facies* face + Lat *cervix* neck; Gk *dus-* bad + Gk *morphe* shape]
Also: cervicooculoacoustic syndrome; Wildervanck syndrome
A syndrome where two or more cervical vertebrae are fused; it is similar to Klippel-Feil syndrome. Characteristics include narrow elongated face, short webbed neck, poorly developed neck muscles, facial asymmetry, deafness that may be total, prominent ears, preauricular fistulas, eyeball retraction, and nystagmus.

otogenic *adj* [Gk *ous* ear + Gk *-genes* produced by]
Originating in the ear, e.g., otogenic pain.

otolaryngology *n* [Gk *ous* ear + Gk *larunx* larynx + Gk *-logia* study of]
The branch of medicine dealing with diseases of the ear, nose, and throat.

otolight *n*
Also: otoprobe; ear light
An illuminated hand-held probe used for insertion and inspection of an otoblock in the ear canal.

otoliths *n, pl* [Gk *ous* ear + Gk *lithos* stone]
Also: otoconia
Minute granules of calcium carbonate in the gelatinous otolithic membrane of the vestibular system. Cilia are embedded in

the membrane. Movement of these stimulate sensory cells to pass positional information to the brain, which is important in the maintenance of the body's upright position in respect to gravity.

otolithic catastrophe *np* [Gk *ous* ear + Gk *lithos* stone]
Also: Tumarkin otolith crisis
A drop attack without warning. The sudden fall may be due to inappropriate stimulation of the saccule, causing the interpretation of gravity having changed, before visual and proprioceptive input can be asssessed for accuracy of the situation.

otologist *n*
A specialist in otology.

otology *n* [Gk *ous* ear + Gk *-logia* study of]
The study of the anatomy, physiology, and pathology of the ear.

otomycosis *n* [Gk *ous* ear + Gk *mukes* mushroom, fungus + Gk *-osis* denoting a diseased state]
A fungal infection of the ear canal; a fungal form of otitis externa.

otoneuralgia *n* [Gk *ous* ear + Gk *neuron* a string, nerve + Gk *algos* pain]
Also: reflex otalgia
Referred pain in the ear.

otopalatodigital syndrome (OPD) *np* [Gk *ous* ear + Lat *palatum* palate + Lat *digitus* finger]
A sex-linked recessive hereditary condition. Characteristics may include cleft palate, widely spaced fingers and toes, small low-set ears, downturned mouth and eyes, mild learning difficulty, and conductive hearing loss due to ossicular deformities.

otoplasty *n* [Gk *ous* ear + Gk *plastos* formed, molded]
Surgical repair of the pinna, usually for cosmetic purposes.

otoprobe *n* [Gk *ous* ear + Lat *probare* to test]
Also: otolight
An illuminated hand-held probe used for insertion and inspection of an otoblock in the ear canal.

otorhinolaryngology *n* [Gk *ous* ear + Gk *rhis* nose + Gk *larunx* larynx + Gk *-logia* study of]
The branch of medicine dealing with diseases of the ear, nose, and throat.

otorrhagia *n* [Gk *ous* ear + Gk *rhegnunai* to burst out]
Bleeding from the ear.

otorrhea/otorrhoea *n* [Gk *ous* ear + Gk *rhoia* flow, flux]
A discharge of pus from the ear canal.

otosclerosis *n* [Gk *ous* ear + Gk *skleros* hard + Gk *-osis* denoting a diseased state]
Also: otospongiosis
An abnormal growth of spongy bone around the stapes, which progressively hardens causing conductive hearing loss.

otoscope *n* [Gk *ous* ear + Gk *skopein* to look]
A hand-held torch-like device with a magnifying lens, used for inspection of the ear canal and eardrum.

otoscopy *n* [Gk *ous* ear + Gk *skopein* to look]
The inspection of the ear canal and eardrum using an otoscope.

otoscopy, pneumatic *np* [Gk *ous* ear + Gk *skopein* to look; Gk *pneuma* air]
An otoscopic examination performed using an otoscope equipped with an air-filled bulb that releases pressure into the ear canal to visualize tympanic membrane movement.

otospondylomegaepiphyseal dysplasia (OSMED) *np* ˈōtōspŏndĭlōmĕga ĕpĭfsēal dĭs ˈplāzēa [Gk *ous* ear + Gk *spondulos* vertebra + Gk *megas* large + Gk *epiphusis* additional growth; Gk *dus-* bad + Gk *plasis* formation]
A rare autosomal recessive disorder of bone growth that results in skeletal and facial deformities and in which severe high frequency hearing loss is common.

otosteal *adj* 'ōt'ostēal [Gk *ous* ear + Lat *ostium* door, opening]
Pertaining to the bones of the middle ear.

otostop *n* [Gk *ous* ear]
A block, usually of foam, inserted into the ear canal to impede the flow of ear impression material to the eardrum.

otosyphilis *n* [Gk *ous* ear + *Syphilus* name of the supposed first sufferer from syphilis, cited in a poem of 1530]
A form of neurosyphilis (a bacterial infection generally spread through sexual contact) that causes hearing loss and vertigo and which may include other neurologic symptoms.

ototoxic *adj* [Gk *ous* ear + Gk *toxikos* poisonous]
Poisonous to the ear, i.e., producing temporary or permanent hearing loss, tinnitus and/or balance problems.

outcome measure *np*
A measure of the results of an experiment relative to its aim.

outer ear *np*
The external ear, which consists of the pinna and external ear canal and ends at the eardrum.

outer hair cells *np*
Cells with fine hair-like projections (cilia) that are embedded in the tectorial membrane, within the organ of Corti. Movement of these cells causes them to act as a nonlinear mechanical amplifier, improving the cochlea's response to quiet sounds, i.e., those that are less than about 50 dB SPL.

out-of-phase *adj*
The condition when the movement of two sound waves have the opposite direction of movement and speed. If they are fully out of phase the sound will be canceled out and there will be an area of silence. If two waves are fully out of phase, they are said to be 180° out of phase. If two waves are out of phase by a quarter of a wavelength, they are said to be 90° out of phase.

output *np*
The exiting signal from a hearing aid or other device

output compression *np*
A type of compression circuit where gain is increased as the volume control is reduced, and vice versa. The compression threshold varies according to volume control setting, while the output signal remains at a fixed level.

output limiting *np*
The process of limiting the output sound pressure of a hearing aid (or other listening device) by means of peak clipping or compression.

output sound pressure level 90 (OSPL90) *np*
The maximum output of a hearing aid when an input signal of 90 dB SPL is presented. It is measured with the hearing aid volume full-on, with all controls set for maximum gain.

oval window *np*
The membrane-covered opening from the middle ear into the vestibule of the bony labyrinth. The stapes footplate is attached to the oval window by an annular ligament and transmits vibrations to the fluid in the cochlea.

overcompensation *n*
Covering up for a weakness or disability, e.g., hearing loss, by exaggerated concentration on some other aspect.

overmasking *n*
A term used when too much masking noise is applied to the nontest ear, such that the threshold is shifted in the test ear.

oversampling *n*
The process of generating additional samples (at a frequency higher than the Nyquist frequency) to create a more precise digital representation of an analog signal.

overtone *n*
Also: harmonic
A tone that is a component of a complex sound, where each frequency is a whole number (or integer) multiple of the fundamental frequency.

oxy- *prefix* [Gk *oxus* sharp]
1. Combining form denoting something sharp or acute. 2. Containing oxygen.

oxyacoia *n* [Gk *oxus* sharp + Gk *akoia* hearing]
Hypersensitivity to sound due to facial paralysis, especially involving the stapedius muscle.

pachyotia *n* păkē'ōshēa [Gk *pakhus* fat + Gk *ous* ear]
Pinnae that are abnormally coarse and thick.

Paget disease *np* 'păjĭt Named after Sir James Paget (1814–1899), an English surgeon, who described the clinical and pathologic features of this disease in 1877.
Also: osteitis deformans; Beethoven deafness
A skeletal condition in which there is excessive bone absorption followed by excessive poor abnormal bone formation, such that new bone is weak and bulky and liable to deformation and fracture. Bones affected can include the skull, and can lead to tinnitus, vertigo, and sensorineural hearing loss related to loss of bone mineral density in the cochlear capsule.

Paget disease, juvenile *np* Named after Sir James Paget (1814–1899), an English surgeon, who described the clinical and pathologic features of this disease in 1877.
Also: hereditary hyperphosphatasia
A rare recessive genetic disorder that affects bone growth throughout the skeleton. Characteristics include progressive bone deformity with pain and an enlarged thickened skull, which can result in sensorineural hearing loss.

paired comparison *np*
Options compared and tallied to find a winner.

palantype *n*
A British specialized shorthand typing machine (similar to the American stenograph) that can produce a simultaneous display of speech to text.

palatal *adj* 'pălatal [Lat *palatum* the palate]
Formed with the body of the tongue toward the hard palate, as in the production of the speech sound /y/.

palate *n* [Lat *palatum* the palate]
The upper part or roof of the mouth (part of the buccal cavity). Consists of two parts. The hard palate (bony structure) forms the main part of the upper mouth from behind the front teeth and reaches backward to the anterior faucial pillar, which separates the hard palate from the soft palate. The soft palate is the part at the back of the upper mouth that also forms the uvula at the posterior of the throat.

palate, cleft *np*
A palate in which some part has not fully formed (closed) before birth, resulting in swallowing and feeding difficulties and associated conductive hearing problems.

palatine tonsils *n* [Lat *palatum* the palate; Lat *tonsila* capstan or tonsil]
The two areas of lymphoid tissue on either side of the back of the throat.

palpebral reflex *np* 'pălpebral ('pălpēbral) [Lat *palpebra* eyelid]
Also: auropalpebral reflex; acoustopalpebral reflex; cochleo-orbicular reflex; cochleopalpebral reflex
A rapid eye blink caused by sudden loud sound.

palsy *n* 'pawlzē [medieval Fr *paralisie* (from Gk *paralusis* paralysis)]
Paralysis occurring due to damage or trauma of nerve fibers, which results in weakness or complete paralysis of the structures supplied by those nerves. It may also be accompanied by involuntary tremors.

pandemic *n* [Gk *pan* all + Gk *demos* people]
A disease prevalent across a wide geographic area involving a high proportion of the population, e.g., a rubella pandemic across Europe occurred in 1963–1965 causing many cases of permanent sensorineural deafness.

panic *n* [After the Greek god Pan who inspired terror in those who saw him]

A sudden unreasoning terror or fear; an anxiety disorder with a wide range of symptoms, e.g., palpitations, dizziness, hyperventilation.

panotitis *n* [Gk *pan* all + Gk *ous* ear + Gk *-ites* denoting disease of]
Inflammation of all parts of the ear.

paracentesis *n* [Gk *para* beside + Gk *kentesis* puncturing]
A procedure in which fluid is removed from a body cavity or from an outgrowth, e.g., middle ear paracentesis is a removal of fluid from the middle ear.

paracusia *n* păˈrakyūsēa [Gk *para* beyond + Gk *akousis* sense of hearing]
Also: auditory hallucinations
Sounds heard without auditory stimulus that appear real to the person hearing them; they are usually linked with mental or neurologic illness.

paracusis/paracousis *n*
Abnormal or disordered hearing.

paracusis loci *np* [Gk *para* beyond + Gk *akousis* sense of hearing; Lat *loci* of position]
An inability to determine the direction of sound.

paracusis Willisii *np* Named after Thomas Willis (1622–1675), an English physician, who first described the phenomenon. Hearing loss that is apparently improved in the presence of background noise. It is characteristic of conductive hearing loss and thought to be due to the tendency of others to raise their voice level in the presence of background noise.

paradigm *n* părˈadēm [Gk *paradeigma* example]
1. A universally recognized (or generally accepted in a field) model, example, perspective, solution, or achievement. 2. A particular experimental procedure.

parallel play *np*
The situation where young children play alongside each other, but do not join together in their play.

parallel processing *np*
Information processing in which more than one operation is carried out at the same time, usually without conscious thought, e.g., the process of reading requires parallel processing of written symbols, language rules, and meaning.

parallel vent *np*
The most usual type of vent, which runs through the earmold parallel to the sound bore.

paralysis *n* [Gk *paraluesthai* to be disabled at the side]
Loss of muscle function and/or sensation, e.g., facial muscle paralysis.

parameter *n* [Gk *para* beside + Gk *metron* measure]
1. A defining characteristic, factor, aspect, or element. 2. An independent variable in a set of parametric equations.

parametric *adj* [Gk *para* beside + Gk *metron* measure]
1. Relating to a parameter; having a measurable or quantifiable characteristic of a system. 2. Having a predictable distribution, e.g., interval and ratio data.

paranasal sinuses *np* [Gk *para* beside + Lat *nasus* nose; Lat *sinus* recess]
Also: accessory sinuses
Four pairs (maxillary, frontal, ethmoid, and sphenoid) of air-filled spaces in the skull that drain into the nasal cavity. The sinuses lighten the skull and resonate the voice.

parapharyngeal space *np* [Gk *para* beside + Gk *pharunx* throat]
A space beside the upper pharynx.

paraplegia *n* [Gk *paraplessein* to strike at the side]
Paralysis of the legs and part or all of the body due to damage to the spinal cord.

parasympathetic nervous system *np* [Gk *para* beside + Gk *sun-* with + Gk *pathos* feeling, suffering]
One of the main divisions of the autonomic (self-regulating) nervous system,

part of the peripheral nervous system that controls the internal environment of the body. Its effects include bronchiole and pupil constriction, alimentary canal and smooth muscle contraction, heart rate moderation, increases in saliva and mucus production, and some glandular secretion.

paresis *n* [Gk *parienai* to let go]
Weakness due to a nerve disorder that can cause loss of voluntary movement. A slight or incomplete paralysis.

parietal bone *np* pa'rīetal [Lat *paries* a wall]
The two parietal bones are posterior to the frontal bone and form the greater part of the sides and the roof of the cranial cavity.

Parkinson disease *np* Named after James Parkinson (1755–1824), an English physician, who gave a detailed description of the condition in 1817.
A progressive neurologic condition due to lack of dopamine in the brain caused by loss of nerve cells. It generally affects older individuals, over age 50, but early onset also exists. The main characteristics are tremors, slow movement and rigidity; speech may also be affected.

parosmia *n* [Gk *para* beside + Gk *osme* odor]
A disorder of the sense of smell, especially the subjective perception of smells that do not exist.

parotic/parotid *adj* [Gk *para* beside + Gk *ous* ear]
Near or beside the ear.

parotic/parotid gland *np* [Gk *para* beside + Gk *ous* ear]
A large salivary gland situated near the ear, below the jaw.

parotid tumor *np* [Gk *para* beside + Gk *ous* ear; Lat *tumor* a swelling]
A tumor in the parotid gland.

parotidectomy *np* [Gk *para* beside + Gk *ous* ear + Gk *ektome* cutting out]
Removal of the parotid gland.

parotitis/parotiditis *n* [Gk *para* beside + Gk *ous* ear + Gk *-ites* denoting disease of]
Inflammation of the parotid glands, e.g., in mumps.

paroxysm *n* [Gk *paroxunein* to exasperate]
1. A sudden increase or recurrence of a symptom or disease. 2. A sudden outburst of emotion.

pars flaccida *np* [Lat *pars* part; Lat *flaccidus* slack]
Also: Shrapnell membrane
The smaller upper portion of the tympanic membrane that has no fibrous layer and is therefore thin and slack or flaccid.

pars tensa *np* [Lat *pars* part; Lat *tensus* tight, rigid]
The lower and largest portion of the tympanic membrane, containing all three layers (cutaneous, fibrous, and mucous), it is fairly rigid, tightly stretched, elastic, and set into vibration by sound waves.

partial *n/adj* [Lat *pars* part]
-*n* Any one of the single-frequency components of a complex tone; not necessarily arithmetically related to the fundamental. -*adj* Involving a part.

partial recruitment *np*
Abnormal loudness growth where the loudness of a tone presented to the impaired ear is close to but always less than the perceived loudness in the normally hearing ear.

pascal (Pa) *n* Named after Blaise Pascal (1623–1662), a French mathematician, whose experiments increased our knowledge of atmospheric pressure.
The international unit of pressure. One pascal is equivalent to one newton per square meter.

passband *n*
The frequency range of an electronic filter that allows a preselected band of frequencies to pass through and be transmitted, without attenuation.

passive *adj*
Inactive.

passive filter *np*
An electronic filter that contains few components and does not require an external energy source, e.g., the simplest hearing aid tone controls are passive filters.

passive hearing protection *np*
Hearing protection, e.g., ear muffs, that provide an unchanging level of sound attenuation.

past-pointing *np*
The effect, due to vertigo, of objects moving away.

Patau syndrome *np* pahtū Named after Klaus Patau (1908–1975), a German-born American physician and geneticist, who described the condition in 1960.
Also: trisomy 13
A chromosomal abnormality in which there is an extra chromosome 13. The clinical features include structural defects of the brain, scalp lesions, small eyes, polydactyly (extra fingers or toes), and cardiac and renal malformations. The condition results in severe learning difficulty and physical impairments, which may include ear malformation and deafness.

patent *adj* [Lat *patere* to lie open]
1. Unobstructed, unoccluded, open, affording free passage, e.g., patent Eustachian tube. 2. A legal right that can be given to an inventor to make and use an invention.
Deriv: -n patency

pathogen *n* [Gk *pathos* suffering + Gk *-gen* giving rise to]
A microorganism or other agent that causes disease.
Deriv: -adj pathogenic

pathology *n* [Gk *pathos* suffering + Gk *-logia* study of]
The scientific study of the nature of disease and its causes, processes, development, and consequences.

patulous *adj* pătchūlus [Lat *patulus* lying open]
Abnormally open, widely spread apart or exposed.

patulous Eustachian tube *np*
A disorder of the Eustachian tube in which it remains intermittently open. This can cause the individual to hear echoes of body noise, e.g., heartbeat and respiratory noises.

PB word lists *np abbr*
Monosyllabic word lists that are phonetically balanced.

peak *n*
The maximum or highest level.

peak clipping *np*
Distortion of an output waveform caused by removing the extremes of alternating signal amplitudes at a predetermined level. This squares the waves and removes the extremes of the peaks and troughs.

peak clipping, soft *np*
A method of limiting the maximum output, e.g., of a hearing aid, by cutting off the peaks of the sound waves when the output reaches a predetermined level. The clipped peaks are rounded, but soft clipping still causes significant distortion of the output waveform.

peak clipping, symmetric *np*
A type of peak clipping in which the positive and negative extremes of the signal waveform are removed by an equal amount.

peak-equivalent peak sound-pressure level (dB peSPL) *np*
A measure of sound intensity where the maximum voltage of a transient stimulus (e.g., a click) is referenced to the voltage

of a tone stimulus of known intensity level in dB SPL.

peak sound-pressure level *np*
Also: LC peak
The instantaneous maximum value of sound pressure in any given period, e.g., measured in some noisy industries during the working day as the C-weighted peak.

peak-to-peak *adj*
The difference between maximum displacement in one direction and the maximum displacement in the other direction of a waveform.

pediatric (paediatric) *adj* [Gk *pais* child + Gk *iatros* doctor]
Concerning the branch of medical science that includes the study of childhood and the diseases of children.

peer *n* [Lat *par* equal]
One who has equal standing with another in what is being compared, e.g., age or intellect.

Pelizaeus-Merzbacher disease *np* pĕ-lēt'sāus-'mertsbăka Named after Fredrich Christoph Pelizaeus (1851–1942), a German psychiatrist and neurologist, who first reported the condition in 1885, and Ludwig Merzbacher (1875–1942), a German neuropathologist and psychiatrist, who further investigated the condition in one family in 1910.
A recessive dysmyelinating central nervous system disorder that is X-linked, i.e., it is passed by females but normally affects only males. Characteristics may include rotary nystagmus, tremor, and limited body control. It may include hearing loss.

Pendred syndrome *np* Named after Vaughan Pendred (1869–1946), an English physician, who first described the disorder in 1896.
An autosomal recessive genetic syndrome affecting the endocrine and central nervous system that begins in childhood. The characteristics include goiter

(thyroid swelling), profound deafness and occasionally some vestibular dysfunction.

penetrance *n* [Lat *penetrare* to penetrate]
The frequency of expression of inherited traits, i.e., the likelihood that a specific gene will result in disease.

pennate *adj* [Lat *pennatus* feathered, winged]
Ribbed, e.g., the stapedius muscle.

pentoxyfylline *n*
A vasodilator prescribed for circulation problems. Sometimes used to treat hearing loss that is due to reduced cochlear blood flow.

per- *prefix* [Lat *per* through]
A combining term meaning through, throughout, or all over.

perception *n* [Lat *perceptio* perception]
1. The process of becoming aware and acquiring knowledge through one of the senses, e.g., hearing. 2. The process of becoming aware of something through cognition.
Deriv: -*v* perceive; -*adv* perceptible

perceptive deafness *n obs*
Also: sensorineural hearing loss; nerve deafness
A hearing loss that involves the sensory and/or neural cells of the cochlea and their connections or occasionally cranial nerve VIII or brainstem lesions.

percutaneous *adj* perkyū'tānēus [Lat *per* through + Lat *cutis* skin]
Placed through the skin, e.g., percutaneous cochlear implantation; that is, implantation that uses a minimally invasive technique to reach the cochlea through a single drill port.

perforation *n* [Lat *perforare* to pierce through]
A hole or opening caused by disease or accident, e.g., a perforation of the eardrum.
Deriv: –*v* perforate

performance test *np*
1. A pediatric audiometric test in which the child responds to audible stimuli either via headphones or free-field presentation by performing an action, e.g., putting bricks in a box. 2. A test designed to measure nonverbal performance, used in intelligence tests, e.g., block design in which patterns are constructed from colored blocks.

perfusion *n* [Lat *perfundere* to pour through]
To cause or spread fluid through something.

peri- *prefix* [Gk *peri* around]
A combining form meaning around or about.

perichondritis *n* [Gk *peri* around + Gk *khondros* cartilage + Gk *-ites* denoting disease of]
A painful infection of the perichondrium of the external ear that can also occur in the perichondrium of cartilages of the larynx.

perichondrium *n* [Gk *peri* around + Gk *khondros* cartilage]
A dense membrane of fibrous connective tissue that covers all cartilage, except the joints.

perilymph *n* [Gk *peri* around + Lat *lumpha* water]
The extracellular fluid in the scala vestibuli and the scala tympani of the labyrinth, i.e., between the bony labyrinth and the membranous labyrinth. The fluid is high in sodium and low in potassium.

perilymph fistula *np* [Gk *peri* around + Lat *lumpha* water; Lat *fistula* pipe]
A tear in the membrane of either the oval window or the round window, releasing perilymph from the cochlea.

perinatal *adj* [Gk *peri* around + Lat *natalis* relating to birth]
During or around the time of birth. From the seventh month of pregnancy to the fourth week after birth.

period *n* [Gk *periodos* orbit, recurrence, course]
1. The time taken to complete one cycle of a repetitive sinusoidal waveform. 2. The period is the reciprocal of the frequency of a sinusoidal motion.

periodic *adj* [Gk *periodos* orbit, recurrence, course]
1. Appearing or occurring at intervals. 2. A sound that has a pressure/time waveform that is repetitive and consists of two or more pure tones.

perioperative *adj*
The time around surgery, i.e., the time from entry to a hospital or other place for an operation until discharge.

periosteum *n* pĕrē'ŏstīum [Gk *peri* around + Gk *osteon* bone]
Dense fibrous vascular connective tissue that overlays bone.

periotic *adj* [Gk *peri* around + Gk *ous* ear]
Enclosing the inner ear and formed by the fusion of the otic bones.

peripharyngeal *adj* [Gk *peri* around + Gk *pharunx* throat]
Encircling the pharynx.

peripheral *adj* [Gk *periphereia* circumference]
1. Outside or away from the center. 2. Situated or produced around the edge.

peripheral nervous system *np*
The part of the nervous system that is outside the brain and spinal cord.

peritympanic *adj* [Gk *peri* around + Gk *tumpanon* drum]
Deep in the bony portion of the ear canal, close to the eardrum, e.g., peritympanic hearing aid.

permanent threshold shift *np*
Permanent hearing loss due to excessive noise exposure.

Perrault syndrome *np* 'pĕrō Named after M. Perrault, a French physician, who reported the condition in 1951.

Also: XX gonadal dysgenesis with sensor-ineural hearing loss

An autosomal recessive disorder characterized by ovarian dysgenesis in females and associated with severe or profound sensorineural hearing loss.

personal amplification *np*
A device for increasing the sound level for the listener (e.g., a hearing aid) that is worn by an individual.

perstimulatory *adj*
Occuring during stimulation.

perstimulatory fatigue *np*
Auditory adaptation, i.e., reduction in hearing sensitivity in response to extended sound stimulation.

perturbation *n* [Lat *perturbare* to disturb]
A change from predicted or regular behavior.

petal *suffix* 'pĕtal [Lat *petere* to make for]
Toward, e.g., ampullopetal, utriculopetal.

petro- *prefix* [Gk *petros* stone]
Stone.

petrosa *n* [Lat *petrosus* stony]
The hard part of the petrous bone.

petrous *adj* [Gk *petros* stone]
Stone-like.

petrous bone *np*
A dense stone-like part of the temporal bone, of pyramidal shape, that contributes to the base of the skull and contains the middle and inner ear.

-pexy *suffix* [Gk *pegnumi* to fix]
Fixation.

Pfeiffer syndrome *np* 'fifer Named after Rudolph A. Pfeiffer (b 1931), a German geneticist, who described the condition in 1964.
An autosomal dominant congenital inherited condition; characteristics include short and broad big toes and thumbs, webbing of second and third digits, wide skull with high forehead, depressed cheeks, widely spaced prominent eyes,

and small nose. May have conductive hearing loss.

phagocytosis *n* [Gk *phagein* to eat + Gk *kutos* vessel, cell + Gk *-osis* denoting a diseased state]
The process by which cells engulf and digest other cells or debris.

phalangeal cells *np* [Gk *phalanx* a body of troops (with overlapping shields and spears)]
Supporting cells between the hair cells of the cochlea, e.g., cells of Deiter are the outer phalangeal cells.

phalangeal process *np*
A projection from the apical surface of the outer hair cells that flattens into a plate. The plates form the reticular membrane of the organ of Corti.

phalanges *n, pl* fa'lănjēz *sg* phalanx [Gk *phalanx* a body of troops (with overlapping shields and spears)]
The bones of the fingers and toes.
Deriv: -adj phalangeal

pharyngitis *n* [Gk *pharunx* throat + Gk *-ites* denoting disease of]
Inflammation of the pharynx.

pharyngoplasty *n* [Gk *pharunx* throat + Gk *plastos* molded, shaped]
Surgical reconstruction or alteration of the pharynx.

pharyngoplegia *n* [Gk *pharunx* throat + Gk *plessein* to strike]
Paralysis of the muscles of the pharynx.

pharyngotomy *n* [Gk *pharunx* throat + Gk *–tomia* cutting]
Incision into the pharynx.

pharynx *n* [Gk *pharunx* throat]
The upper part of the respiratory and digestive tracts, which forms the passageway between the mouth and nasal cavities and the larynx, i.e., the throat.
Deriv: -adj pharyngeal

phase *n* [Gk *phasis* appearance]
Any point in a cycle that can be described by its phase, e.g., the phases of the moon. One complete cycle can be likened to a

circle and therefore, like a circle, has 360°. The position or phase in the cycle can be described in terms of degrees.

phase, in *n*
The condition when two waves have the same direction of movement and the same speed. When two sound waves are exactly in phase, the amplitude is doubled and the sound will be heard much louder.

phase-locked *adj*
Maintaining a constant phase relative to a reference signal, e.g., the tendency of a neuron to respond to a particular phase of an acoustic signal.

phenotype *n* [Gk *phainein* to show + Gk *tupos* figure, shape, type]
The total in biochemical, physical, and physiologic nature of an individual that results from the expression of the genes (genotype) and interaction with environmental factors.

phlegm *n* [Gk *phlegma* inflammation]
Thick mucus secreted by glands in the respiratory system and sometimes coughed out of the mouth.

phobia *n* [Gk *phobos* fear]
An anxiety disorder in which an unreasonable fear is linked to a specific object or situation.

phon *n* [Gk *phone* sound]
A unit that equates to the dB SPL level of a 1 kHz tone to which the comparison tone sounds equally loud to someone with average normal hearing.

phonation *n* [Gk *phone* sound]
The production of voiced speech sounds.

phone *n* [Gk *phone* sound]
An individual speech sound.

phoneme *n* [Gk *phonema* sound]
The smallest meaningful unit of speech, e.g., the middle vowel of "cut" and "cat," which changes the meaning of the word.
Deriv: –*adj* phonemic

phonemic balance *np* fōˈnēmĭk
Word lists, used in speech tests, in which

each initial consonant, vowel, and final consonant appears with the same frequency of occurrence in every test list.

phonetic alphabet, International (IPA)
np fōˈnĕtĭk [Gk *phone* sound]
A set of standardized symbols used to represent the phonemes of speech.

phonetic balance (PB) *np*
The condition in which the relative frequency of occurrence of the phonemes in a test list approximates to that of a representative sample of everyday English.

phonetic reading *np*
Reading by decoding the phonetic significance of letter groups.

phonetics *np*
The study of speech sounds (phones), including study of the physiologic production of speech, acoustic properties, and auditory perception.

phonetics, acoustic *np*
A study of the transmission of speech from speaker to listener.

phonetics, articulatory *np*
The study of the production of speech.

phonetics, auditory *np*
The study of the reception of speech by the listener.

phonics *n, pl* [Gk *phone* sound]
A method of teaching reading that looks at the letter sounds rather than the whole words.
Deriv: –*adj* phonic

phonology *n* [Gk *phone* sound + Gk *-logia* study of]
The study of the sound system of a language.

phonometer *n* fōˈnŏmĭta [Gk *phone* sound + Gk *metron* measure]
An instrument with filters that correspond to equal loudness contours and measures loudness on the phon scale.

phonophobia *n* [Gk *phone* sound + Gk *phobos* fear]
An abnormal fear of sounds.

phonopsia *n* [Gk *phone* sound + Gk *opsis* seeing]
The condition in which an individual sees color in association with certain sounds.

physics *n* [Gk *phusis* nature]
The science concerned with the properties of matter and energy. It includes the study of mechanics, electricity, radioactivity, magnetism, heat, light, and sound.

physiology *n* [Gk *phusis* nature + Gk *-logia* study of]
The study of the functioning and activities of living organisms.
Deriv: –adj physiologic

pia mater *np* pēă 'maht*a*/pīă 'māt*a* [Lat *pia mater* soft matter]
The inner layer of the meninges, adjacent to the surface of the brain.

Pierre Robin syndrome/sequence *np*
Named after Pierre Robin (1867–1950), a French dental surgeon, who described the condition in 1923.
A congenital condition, characterized by small lower jaw (micrognathia), cleft palate, and a tongue that falls backward in the throat (glossoptosis). There may be difficulty in breathing and feeding. The jaw continues growing and the malformation is often corrected by adulthood. Hearing loss is common due to malformation and may be conductive and/or sensorineural.

piezoelectric *adj* pēāzōe'lĕktrĭk (pēātzōe 'lĕktrĭk) [Gk *piezein* to press + Gk *elektron* amber (from electrostatic effect of rubbing amber)]
Pertaining to crystals that produce voltages when they are deformed, e.g., a thin strip of piezoelectric material attached to a diaphragm is used in a crystal microphone; when the crystal is deflected by the diaphragm, the two sides of the crystal acquire opposite charges.

pili torti *np* pĭlī tawtī [Lat *pili torti* twisted hairs]
A condition in which hairs are twisted and brittle and which may be associated with congenital moderate to severe sensorineural hearing loss.

pillar cells *np*
Also: rods of Corti
The supporting cells that form the walls of the tunnel of Corti in the cochlea.

pilot study *np*
An initial trial with a few subjects prior to carrying out a full experiment or study.

pink noise *np* Named by analogy to light, which changes color according to its frequency distribution.
A random signal that falls off by 3 dB per octave, i.e., a signal that has equal energy per octave.

pinna *n pl* pinnae [Lat *pinna* wing]
Also: auricle; *colloq* the ear
The outer part of the ear that is readily viewed with the naked eye. It is a cartilagenous structure covered in skin and innervated with nerves and blood vessels.

pip *n*
1. A small ready-made ear insert. 2. A short duration tone burst.

pit *n*
A small hole or depression, e.g., a preauricular pit.

pitch *n*
The individual listener's subjective impression of frequency. High-frequency tones are heard as high pitch, and low-frequency tones are heard as low pitch.

pitch matching *np*
The process in which an individual matches the pitch of his/her tinnitus to the pitch of a tone.

pitch, periodicity *np*
Also: missing fundamental; virtual pitch
The phenomenon in which the brain interprets the pitch from the harmonics that are present even when the fundamental frequency is missing.

pitch, residue *np*
The perceived pitch of a complex tone

that corresponds to a missing fundamental.

pituitary gland *np* [Lat *pituitarius* secreting phlegm]
Major endocrine gland of vertebrates that produces several hormones that affect adrenal cortex activity, growth, thyroid activity, reproduction, and melanophore (containing melanin) cells.

placebo *n* plɑ′sēbō [Lat *placebo* I shall be pleasing]
A medical intervention that does not contain a drug, but which may cause an actual or perceived improvement due to the individual's expectation that it will.

place of articulation *np*
The point of contact of the articulators when forming consonant speech sounds. Places of articulation are part of a continuum along the upper surface of the vocal tract, e.g., bilabial, labiodental, alveolar, palatal, velar.

place theory *np*
A theory that states that different areas along the basilar membrane respond to different frequencies.

placode *n* [Gk *plax* flat + Gk *-oides* signifying likeness]
1. Any plate-like structure. 2. A thickening of primordial tissues of the human embryo that is a precursor to organs and body structures, e.g., the auditory/otic placode develops into the otic capsule and inner ear.

plagiocephaly *n* ′plājēosĕfɑlē [Gk *plagios* slanting + Gk *kephale* head]
An asymmetrical twisting condition of the head, usually seen in infants who sleep on their backs, which improves when the infant becomes mobile. It is also seen in infants with hypotonia, especially preterm babies who spend long periods lying on their sides in incubators.
Deriv: -adj plagiocephalism

plasma *n* [Gk *plasma* mold]
The straw-colored watery liquid in which blood cells are suspended.

plasma membrane *np* [Gk *plasma* mold; Lat *membrana* a partition]
A selectively permeable, lipid bilayer that surrounds cells, separating the intracellular and extracellular environments.

plasticity *n* [Gk *plastikos* moldable]
The capacity to be altered.

plasticity, neural *np*
The ability of the central nervous system to reorganize the neural pathways, e.g., for learning and memory and as an adaptive mechanism for recovery after brain injury.

-plasty *suffix* [Gk *plastos* molded, shaped]
Corrective surgery, e.g., otoplasty.

plateau *n*
A range of successive masking levels in the nontest ear at which the threshold of hearing in the test ear remains stable while the intensity of masking noise in the nontest ear is increased. This is an indication that accurate measurement of the threshold of the test ear has been obtained.

play audiometry *np*
A method of pediatric hearing in which the auditory stimuli are paired with an operant task, e.g., dropping a block in a bucket. This requires the active cooperation of the child.

plosive *n/adj*
–n A stop-consonant speech sound that is produced by creating an oral cavity closure, building air pressure behind the closure, and then releasing it (e.g., /p/, /b/, /t/, /d/, /k/, /g/). *–adj* Pertaining to a plosive sound.

pneumatic otoscopy *np* [Gk *pneuma* wind, air; Gk *ous* ear + Gk *skopein* to look at]
An otoscopic examination performed using an otoscope equipped with an air-filled bulb that releases pressure into the ear canal to visualize tympanic membrane movement.

pneumatization (pneumatisation) *n*
The formation of air cells, e.g., the mastoid air cells in the temporal bone.

polarity *n*
An electrical, magnetic, or ionic difference; the tendency of opposing physical properties to move in a certain direction because of attraction or repulsion.

polarization (polarisation) *n*
A sudden increase in the electrical potential of a membrane.

polar plot *np*
A graph showing the output of a microphone as a sound source rotates around the microphone. It is often used to illustrate the effect of a directional microphone system.

politzer inflation *np* Named after Adam Politzer (1835–1920), an Austrian physician, who developed this maneuver.
Inflation of the Eustachian tube and middle ear, by forcing air through the nose during swallowing. The olive-shaped nozzle of a Politzer bag is placed in the nostril corresponding to the ear into which the air is to be forced. The other nostril is closed while the cheeks are forcibly blown out. The bag is thus compressed and the raised intranasal pressure draws air up the Eustachian tube.

poly- *prefix* [Gk *polus* much, many]
Multiple or different.

polyarteritis nodosa *np* [Gk *polus* much, many + Gk *arteria* blood vessel, artery; Lat *nodosus* knotty]
An autoimmune disease causing spontaneous inflammation of the arteries, which can affect any organ of the body (e.g., heart, kidneys, muscles, nerves, skin) due to poor blood supply. It can be associated with sudden sensorineural hearing loss.

polychondritis *n* pŏlē'kŏndrītis [Gk *polus* much, many + Gk *khondros* cartilage + Gk -*ites* denoting disease of]
Inflammation of the cartilage.

polychondritis, relapsing *np*
A rare progressive condition in which the cartilage degenerates. All types of cartilage may be involved and usually the condition includes the cartilage of the ear. There may also be sensorineural or mixed hearing loss, secretory otitis media, and vestibular symptoms.

polyethylene *n/adj*
-*n* A semihard waxy material that can be used for earmolds where there are severe allergic reactions to other materials. -*adj* Made of polyethylene.

polymorphism *n* [Gk *polus* much, many + Gk *morphe* shape]
The occurrence of different forms (phenotypes) in organisms of the same species. To be considered as polymorphism, rather than due only to a new mutation, the form must be present in at least 1% of the population.
Deriv: -adj polymorphic

polyneuropathy *n* [Gk *polus* much, many + Gk *neuron* string, nerve + Gk *patheia* suffering, disease]
A neurologic disorder in which there is involvement of many peripheral nerves, leading to both sensory and motor problems. This can occur as part of a syndrome with hearing loss.

polyotia *n* pŏlē'ōsh(ē)a [Gk *polus* much, many + Gk *ous* ear]
A condition in which there is an additional pinna on one or both sides of the head.

polyp *n* 'pŏlĭp [Gk *polypous* cuttle fish (lit. many-footed)]
A small benign and usually insensitive growth from a mucous membrane. Polyps can have the appearance of tentacles or feet.

polysyllabic *adj* [Gk *polus* much, many + Gk *sullabe* syllable]
Consisting of two or more syllables.

polyvinyl chloride (PVC) *np*
A polymer of relatively strong soft plastic material used for earmolds that creates a

good seal but hardens, shrinks, and discolors over time.

pons *n* pŏnz [Lat *pons* bridge]
A portion of the brainstem just above the medulla and below the midbrain that connects the two halves of the brain at the level of the brainstem.

pontine *adj*
Of or relating to the pons.

pontobulbar palsy *np* [Lat *pons* bridge + Gk *bolbos* onion, bulb]
Also: Brown-Vialetto-Van Laere syndrome
A rare genetic type of muscular dystrophy, in which there is progressive sensorineural deafness accompanied by or followed by paralysis of a number of cranial nerves. It occurs mostly in females and characteristics include progressive deafness, clumsiness, weakness of the arms, shaking, slurred speech, and swallowing and respiratory difficulties.

population *n*
1. All the organisms belonging to a group that share one or more characteristics. 2. A group of people on whom a research study is focused, often represented by a sample selected from the full population.

positional nystagmus *np* [Gk *nustagmos* nodding, blinking, drowsiness]
1. Nystagmus that occurs in specific head positions. Positional nystagmus of short duration may be due to a benign lesion of the posterior semicircular canal. Positional nystagmus may also be found sometimes in serious brainstem and cerebellum lesions. 2. A test to identify the presence of nystagmus elicited by specific head positions.

positive middle ear pressure *np*
The condition in which the air pressure in the middle ear is greater than the atmospheric pressure, usually due to poor Eustachian tube functioning. Fluid may build up in the middle ear, which may cause bulging of the eardrum.

positive reinforcement *np*
The provision of some kind of reward to strengthen the behavior that preceded it, e.g., showing toys that light up when a child responds correctly to a tone presented during visual response audiometry (VRA).

positron emission tomography (PET) scan *np* 'pŏzĭtrŏn
Equipment that produces three-dimensional images that show where cells are particularly active. A radiotracer is used to build up small amounts of radioactivity, which is broken down into positrons (small particles) in the parts of the body to be examined. The scan detects gamma rays released by positrons as these are broken down.

post- *prefix* [Lat *post* behind, after]
Behind or after.

postaural *adj* [Lat *post* behind + Lat *auris* ear]
Behind the ear.

postauricular myogenic response (PAM) *np* [Lat *post* behind + Lat *auris* ear; Gk *mus* muscle + Gk –*genes* produced by]
A form of evoked response audiometry in which contraction of the muscle behind the pinna is evoked by sound.

postaxial acrofacial dysostosis (POADS) *np* [Lat *post* behind + Lat *axis* axle, axis; Gk *akron* tip + Lat *facies* face; Gk *dus-* bad + Gk *osteon* bone + Gk *-osis* denoting a diseased state]
Also: Miller syndrome
An autosomal recessive condition characterized by drooping lower eyelids, small jaws, cleft palate and lip, small cup-shaped pinnae, limb abnormalities, missing digits, external and middle ear anomalies, and possible conductive hearing loss.

posterior *adj* [Lat *posterior* behind]
Toward the back.

posterior incudal ligament *np* [Lat *posterior* behind; Lat *incus* an anvil; Lat *ligare* to tie]

The ligament from the short process of the incus to the posterior wall of the tympanic cavity of the middle ear; one of the ligaments that support the ossicular chain.

posterior semicircular canal *np*
One of the three semicircular canals of the vestibular system; a vertical canal that is parallel to the anterior semicircular canal. It joins the utricle at one end and combines with the anterior semicircular canal at the other before joining the utricle as a common canal and is involved in sensing movement in the vertical plane.

postlingual *adj* [Lat *post* after + Lat *lingua* language, tongue]
After the acquisition of speech and language.

postnatal *adj* [Lat *post* after + Lat *natalis* relating to birth]
Shortly after birth.

postoperative *adj*
Shortly after a surgical procedure.

postsynaptic receptor *np* [Lat *post* behind + Gk *sunhapsis* joining together]
A protein molecule in the postsynaptic membrane that contains a binding site for a neurotransmitter. Once binding occurs, the ion channel opens to permit the passage of specific ions into or out of the cell.

posturography *n*
A generic term for any technique that assesses balance.

posturography, computerized dynamic (CDP) *np*
A technique that involves standing on a moving platform while watching a visual target. Shifts in body weight are recorded to give information about the ability to maintain balance.

potassium (K+) *n*
An alkaline metal element that is important for maintaining the functioning of the body. Potassium and sodium are electrolytes, i.e., they have the capacity to conduct electricity, and intracellular fluid is high in positively charged potassium ions. An electrochemical gradient is maintained across all cell membranes such that the interior of the cell is negatively (less positively) charged in comparison to the outside of the cell. During action potentials, i.e., when nerve cells fire, chemically gated channels open to allow movement of potassium and sodium, which causes electrical signals that pass along the nerve fibers to the brain.

potential *n/adj* [Lat *potentia* power]
-n A difference in electrical charge that represents the work involved or energy released in the transfer of a quantity of electricity from one point to another, e.g., between two electrodes or across cell membranes. *-adj* Having power, capable of action.

potential, action (AP) *np*
Synchronous electrical response of numerous auditory nerve fibers that can be elicited in response to an acoustic event, e.g., the electrical activity of the inner hair cells of the cochlea.

potential, auditory evoked (AEP) *np*
The increase of combined electrical activity in the cochlea, auditory nerve, and auditory brainstem following presentation of an acoustic stimulus.

potential, membrane *np*
The electrical charge across a cell membrane, i.e., the difference in electrical potential inside and outside the cell.

potential, postsynaptic *np* [Lat *post* behind + Gk *sunhapsis* joining together]
A protein molecule in the postsynaptic membrane that contains a binding site for a neurotransmitter. Once binding occurs, the ion channel opens to permit the passage of specific ions into or out of the cell.

potential, resting *np*
The membrane potential of a neuron in its resting state, i.e., when it is not being altered by an action potential.

potential, summating *np*
A complex nonlinear response that occurs within the first two to three milliseconds following a sound stimulus. It arises from the hair cells and reflects the asymmetry of basilar membrane vibration. It is one of the main components of electrocochleography (together with the cochlear microphonic and the action potential) and usually appears as a hump on the first slope of the action potential wave.

potentiometer *n* poˈtĕnchēŏmˌĭter
Also: colloq abbr pot; variable resistor
A manually adjustable variable resistor, i.e., a screw or wheel that the user can turn to increase or decrease the resistance. This determines how much current flows through the circuit.

power *n/adj*
-*n* The rate at which energy is expended measured in watts. -*adj* Strong or forceful.

power contralateral routing of signals (CROS) *np*
A monaural power hearing aid fitting that has the microphone placed on the unaidable ear to provide high gain without feedback in the aided ear.

practice effect *np*
An improvement in performance due to learning having taken place, e.g., the retesting of 1 kHz in the first ear tested during a pure tone audiometric test is included to check for a practice effect.

practolol *n*
A beta-adrenergic antagonist (beta blocker) that may be used as an emergency treatment for cardiac arrhythmia. It can be ototoxic and may cause tinnitus and sensorineural hearing loss.

pragmatic *adj* [Gk *pragmatikos* relating to fact]
Realistic or practical and concerned with facts.

pragmatics *n* [Gk *pragmatikos* relating to fact]
Language in social contexts. The ways in which meaning is produced and understood, including contextual factors and the social rules of conversation.

pre- *prefix* [Lat *prae* before, in front of]
Before.

preamplifier *n*
An electronic device that increases the strength of the input signal prior to further amplification in subsequent stages.

preauricular *adj* [Lat *prae* before, in front of + Lat *auris* ear]
In front of the pinna.

preauricular cyst *np* [Lat *prae* before, in front of + Lat *auris* ear; Gk *kustos* box, container]
A capsule-like sac situated in front of the pinna.

preauricular pit/sinus *np*
A congenital malformation in the soft tissue in front of the pinna which may also lead to a sinus under the skin. It is thought to be due to defective development of the ear in the embryo.

preauricular tag *np*
A fleshy skin mound or appendage in front of the pinna.

precedence effect *np*
Also: Haas effect
When two brief sounds in close succession from different distances are perceived as coming from the nearest source rather than from both.

precentral gyrus *np*
The primary motor area in the brain, anterior to the central sulcus (fissure) in the frontal lobe.

precipitously falling audiogram *np* [Lat *praecipitare* to push over the edge]

Also: abruptly falling audiogram; *colloq* ski slope

An audiometric configuration in which the hearing loss is within normal limits in the low frequencies, but then falls dramatically in the mid/high frequencies.

predictor variable *np*
A variable that is used to predict the value of another variable. This may be an independent variable, but only if it is manipulated by the experimenter, as opposed to simply being measured.

prednisolone *n*
A corticosteroid used to treat inflammatory and allergic conditions, e.g., asthma.

preferred frequencies *np*
A series of recommended standard frequencies for audiometric testing.

prefrontal *adj* [Lat *prae-* in front of + Lat *frons* front]
1. Situated anterior to (in front of) a frontal structure. 2. Pertaining to the prefrontal bone, which is one of a pair of bones situated anterior to the frontal lobes of the brain, which forms the forehead and roof of the orbital and nasal cavities. 3. Pertaining to the prefrontal cortex, the part of the brain important for executive functioning, e.g., decision making and social control.

prejudice *n* [Lat *praeiudicare* to prejudge]
A biased judgment made because of a person's membership of a certain group. Prejudice usually involves a negative attitude, but may be positive, and may be associated with discriminatory behavior.

prelingual *adj* [Lat *prae-* before + Lat *lingua* tongue]
Before the acquisition of speech and language, generally taken to mean before the age of 2 years.

prenatal *adj* [Lat *prae-* before + Lat *natalis* relating to birth]
Before birth.

presby- *prefix* [Gk *presbus* old man]
Relating to old people.

presbycusis (presbyacusis) *n* prĕzbĕ′kyū-sĭs (prĕzbēā′kyūsĭs) [Gk *presbus* old man + Gk *akousis* sense of hearing]
A progressive bilateral sensorineural hearing loss that occurs as a cumulative effect of the aging experience.
Deriv: -adj presbycusic (presbyacusic)

presbytinnitus *n* [Gk *presbus* old man + Lat *tinnitus* ringing, tinkling]
The condition of tinnitus accompanying presbycusis.

presbyvertigo *n* [Gk *presbus* old man + Lat *vertigo* dizziness]
Age-related balance problems, e.g., due to aging of the otoconia and vestibular sensory cells.

prescription *n* [Lat *praescribere* to preset]
1. A plan of care written by a health professional. 2. A rule or guide, e.g., calculation of the gain and frequency response required for a particular hearing loss.
Deriv: -v prescribe

prescription of gain and output (POGO) *np*
A linear hearing aid prescriptive fitting method that gives target gain values for amplification.

preservation, hearing *np*
Prevention of hearing loss. This usually refers to a program of hearing conservation in industry that includes noise reduction, education, and use of hearing protection.

pressure *n/adj*
-n 1. Force per unit area. 2. The application of force. *-adj* Using force.

pressure method *np*
A method of measurement that uses a pressure-calibrated reference microphone to monitor and control the sound pressure level at a hearing aid microphone.

pressure vent *np*
A very small hole (of approximately 0.06 to 0.8 mm diameter) made through an earmold or a custom hearing aid to pro-

vide pressure equalization and that has little or no effect on the frequency response.

presynaptic *adj* [Lat *prae* before + Gk *sunapsis* joining together]
Situated before a synapse.

prevalence *n*
The number of individuals in a population, at a given time, affected by a condition. It may also be given as a ratio, calculated by the number of individuals with the condition divided by the number in the population or the sample examined, or as a percentage, i.e., the ratio multiplied by 100.
Deriv: -adj prevalent

primary auditory cortex *np pl* cortices
The superior portion of the temporal lobe of the brain responsible for auditory processing. The two auditory cortices (left and right) receive information from both ears.

primary auditory neurons *np*
The first sensory neuron in the afferent auditory pathway, which relays information from the hair cells in the organ of Corti to the cochlear nuclei of the central auditory system.

primary cell *np*
A nonrechargeable battery.

primary cortical area *np*
The area of the neocortex that receives direct information from ascending sensory pathways or gives rise to motor information from descending motor pathways.

probability *n*
The likelihood of something happening. In statistics, this is expressed as a number between 0 and 1, where 0 = certainty and 1 = impossibility. Conventionally, 0.05 is used as the point beyond which results are rejected as being likely to be due to chance.

probe *n* [Lat *probare* to test]
A long slim instrument which may be il-

luminated, e.g., an otoprobe used to place an otostop down the ear canal.

probe (tube) microphone *np*
A microphone apparatus that basically consists of a microphone attached to a small tube that can be placed in the ear canal. This facilitates measurement of sound pressure levels in the ear canal.

probe tip *np*
A disposable or reusable tip that is used to seal the ear, e.g., in tympanometry measurements.

probe tone *np*
The steady-state stimulus tone, e.g., used in tympanometry, typically 226 Hz (1 kHz for infants).

process *v/n* [Lat *procedere* to proceed]
–v To analyze information, e.g., the left and right hemispheres of the brain process information in different ways. The left tends to process information logically, while the right tends to integrate information based on insight and perception. *–n* A projection or prominence, e.g., the second ossicle, the incus, consists of a body and three processes: the short, long, and the lenticular process.

processing strategy *np* [Lat *procedere* to proceed; Gk *strategia* a plan of action]
1. A method of determining how an input signal shall be processed, e.g., the amount of amplification in the various frequency bands. 2. The method used in cochlear implants to transform the speech signal into a pattern of electrical stimulation.

profound deafness *np* [Lat *profundus* deep]
An average hearing level in excess of 90 dBHL (UK: > 95 dBHL; WHO: > 80 dBHL).

progeroid nanism *np* ˈprōjɛroid [Gk *pro* before + Gk *geras* old age + Gk *eidos* form, likeness; Gk *nanos* dwarf]
Also: Cockayne syndrome
A progressive disorder characterized by dwarfism, an abnormally small head (microcephaly), sensitivity to sunlight,

learning difficulty, impaired development of the nervous system, progressive
later-onset sensorineural hearing loss,
eye abnormalities, and bone abnormalities.

prognosis *n* prŏg'nōs*is* [Gk *pro* before +
Gk *gignoskein* to know]
A forecast of the probable course of a dis-
ease.

programmable hearing aid *np obs*
An analog hearing aid that can be digitally programmed.

**programmable increase at low levels
(PILL)** *np*
A type of programmable sound processing that increases low-level inputs for
specific frequencies.

progressive *adj* [Lat *progredi* to progress]
Increasing in extent or severity, e.g., of a
disease.

progressive diaphyseal dysplasia (PDD)
np [Gk *diaphusis* growing through; Gk
dus- bad + Gk *plasis* formation]
Also: Engelmann syndrome; Camurati-
Engelmann syndrome
A skeletal disorder, characterized by
muscle weakness, bone pain, and difficulty in walking due to progressively
thickening bones. Progressive sensorineural hearing loss may develop as the
skull bones may thicken and constrict
the passages carrying nerves and blood
vessels.

promontory *n* [Lat *promontorium* prom-
ontory]
A prominence of, or projection from, the
body, e.g., the cochlear promontory in
the middle ear, which is formed by the
first turn of the cochlea protruding between the oval window and the round
window.

propagate *v* [Lat *propagare* to multiply
from shoots]
To multiply or spread.
Deriv: –n propagation

prophylaxis *n* prōfĭlăktĭk [Lat *pro* for +
Gk *phulaxis* act of guarding]
Action to prevent disease.
Deriv: –adj prophylactic

proprioception *n* [Lat *proprius* own]
The ability to sense the weight, posture,
movement, and position of the body.
Deriv: –adj proprioceptive

prosody *n* [Gk *prosodia* song, tone of syl-
lable]
The suprasegmental aspects of speech,
e.g., stress, rhythm, pitch, and intonation.
Deriv: –adj prosodic

prospective study *np*
A study that follows a group of individuals over time.

prosthesis *n* *pl* prostheses [Gk *prosthesis*
(from Gk *prostithenai* to add)]
A device to replace or improve the function of a defective body part.

proximal *adj* [Lat *proximus* next to, near-
est]
Toward the center.

Prussak space *np* Named after Alexander
Prussak (1839–1897), a Russian otologist
and professor of otology at St. Petersburg
Academy, who investigated ear anatomy,
including the blood supply to the eardrum.
A small space in the middle ear, medial
to the eardrum and lateral to the neck of
the malleus, which is a possible site for
an attic retraction pocket.

pseudo- *prefix* [Gk *pseudes* false]
A combining term meaning false or spu-
rious.

pseudohypacusis/pseudohypoacusis *n*
[Gk *pseudes* false + Gk *hypo-* below + Gk
akousis sense of hearing]
Also: malingering; functional hearing
loss; nonorganic hearing loss
Feigned or exaggerated hearing loss with
no known organic cause.

psoriasis *n* soّriّasiّs [Gk *psoriasis* an itching]
A skin condition in which dead flaky skin builds up over red patches of immature skin cells due to an immune system error that causes skin cell production to speed up.

psychiatrist *n* [Gk *psukhe* soul + Gk *iatros* doctor]
A medically trained specialist in mental disorders.

psychoacoustics *n* [Gk *psukhe* soul + Gk *akoustikos* pertaining to hearing]
The study of the relationship between an acoustic stimulus and the behavioral response produced in the subject.
Deriv: -adj psychoacoustical

psychogenic *adj* [Gk *psukhe* soul + Gk *-genes* born of (from *gignomai* to be born)]
Originating from the mind.

psychogenic hearing loss *np*
Also: obs hysterical deafness
A rare form of deafness that has no organic basis but may be caused by shock or stress.

psychologist *n* [Gk *psukhe* soul + Gk *logia* study]
A person trained and qualified in the study of the mind and behavior.

psychologist, clinical *np*
A person trained and qualified in the assessment and treatment of mental illness.

psychologist, educational *np*
A person trained and qualified in the cognitive and emotional development of children.

psychologist, industrial/organizational *np*
A person trained and qualified in the study of workplace behavior.

psychology *n* [Gk *psukhe* soul + Gk *logia* study]
The study of the mind and behavior.

psychometric *adj* [Gk *psukhe* soul + Gk *metron* measure]
Concerned with the measurement of psychological factors, e.g., intelligence or personality.

psychophysical tuning curve *np* [Gk *psukhe* soul + Gk *phusis* nature]
A curve on a graph that plots masker level as a function of frequency and that is analogous to a neural threshold tuning curve for a single auditory nerve fiber. A psychophysical tuning curve is normally V-shaped with a sharp tip because the nerve fiber responds to a very small frequency range, i.e., it is finely tuned, at its threshold. It has a broader top because a wider area of the basilar membrane responds to louder sounds.

psychosis *n* [Gk *psukhe* soul + Gk *-osis* denoting a diseased state]
A condition in which the individual loses touch with reality. Symptoms include hallucinations, delusions, or disordered thoughts.

psychosomatic *adj* [Gk *psukhe* soul + Gk *soma* body]
Depending on mind and body. This generally relates to a physical disorder caused or heightened by psychological factors, but can relate to a mental disorder caused or heightened by physical factors.

psychotherapy *n* [Gk *psukhe* soul + Gk *therapeia* healing]
Therapeutic treatment for a mental disorder or problem, where the treatment involves talking about the problem and modifying behavior, e.g., cognitive-behavioral therapy.

psychotropic drugs *np* [Gk *psukhe* soul + Gk *trope* turn, turning]
Drugs that affect the brain, e.g., antidepressants and antipsychotic drugs.

pulsatile tinnitus *np* [Lat *pulsatilis* pulsating (from Lat *pulsare* to throb; Lat *tinnitus* ringing, tinkling)]

A pulsing sound heard in the ears or head that is usually related to the blood flow or to a vascular disorder in the head or neck, e.g., glomus tumor, carotid disease, high blood pressure, or a blood vessel malformation. This is an objective form of tinnitus that can be heard using a stethoscope.

pulse *n* [Lat *pulsare* to throb]
Short duration signal.

pulsed sound *np*
An acoustic stimulus, e.g., a pure tone, that is switched on and off at regular intervals.

pure tone *np*
Also: simple tone
A sound with a pressure/time waveform that exhibits sinusoidal wave motion and consists of only one frequency.

pure tone audiometry (PTA) *np*
A procedure in which tones of varying frequency and intensity are presented to establish an individual's hearing thresholds.

pure tone average *np*
The description of hearing level as an arithmetic average of hearing threshold levels across a number of specified frequencies, i.e., 250 Hz to 4 kHz (five frequency average), 500 Hz to 4 kHz (four frequency average), or 1 kHz to 4 kHz (three frequency average). The World Health Organisation (WHO) suggest classifying according to the hearing in the better ear using the four frequency average, but a diversity of methods continues to be used.

pursuit *adj*
Following or tracking.

pursuit tracking *np*
The smooth following of moving objects by the eyes.

pursuit tracking test *np*
A test used in electronystagmography for assessing the ability to keep an image focused on the fovea of the eye.

purulent *adj* ˈpyur(y)ulent [Lat *purulentus* producing pus]
Producing pus.

push-pull amplifier *np*
A balanced amplifier that uses two transistors to supply more power in an alternating manner to the load than is possible with a single output transistor. One transistor delivers current to the load while the other rests, and vice versa.

Pyle disease *np* ˈpīel Named after Edwin Pyle (1891–1961), an American orthopedic surgeon, who reported the first known case in 1931.
Also: craniometaphyseal dysplasia
A condition in which tubular bones widen and there is overgrowth of the facial and skull bones. Characteristics may include a large broad head and frontal bossing. Cranial nerves may be affected due to stenosis and narrowing of the foramina, resulting in facial nerve paralysis, atrophy of the optic nerve, and sensorineural deafness.

pyramid *n* [Gk *puramis* pyramid]
A small bony projection or conical structure, e.g., the pyramid of the middle ear, a hollow prominence that contains the stapedius muscle.
Deriv: -adj pyramidal

pyramidal tract *np* ˈpīramidal [Gk *puramis* pyramid; Lat *tractus* drawn out]
A large bundle of motor axons in the brain carrying voluntary impulses from areas of the cerebral cortex.

Q factors (quality factors) *np* [Lat *quantus* how much]
1. A measure of the strength of the damping in a resonator, e.g., a bell. A low Q factor indicates a highly damped resonator, a high Q factor indicates a resonator that will ring for longer. 2. A convention used in quantifying the sharpness of tuning of auditory hair cells and neurons, e.g., Q 10 dB is the characteristic frequency divided by the bandwidth of the frequency tuning curve at 10 dB above threshold.

qualitative research *np*
A research-based approach to social science that seeks to investigate perceptions and behaviors and that can include observation, case study, interviews, questionnaires, etc.

quality *n* [Lat *qualis* of what sort]
1. Capacity, characteristic, ability, or skill. 2. The degree to which a sample of reproduced sound resembles a sample of the original sound. 3. A general description of freedom from various types of acoustic distortion in sound-reproducing systems. 4. The timbre or quality of a note that depends upon the number and magnitude of harmonics of the fundamental.

quality of life (QoL) *np*
A subjective rating of the quality and functionality of a person's life when living with a particular disease or condition. It is usually determined by a psychological questionnaire, e.g., the Tinnitus Handicap Inventory (THI).

quantum *n/adj pl* quanta [Lat *quantus* how much]
-*n* 1. A minimum amount of a physical quantity that can exist; quantity changes are measured as multiples of this discrete value. 2. A small, discrete amount of neurotransmitter released by a presynaptic cell (including a hair cell) onto a neuron at a synaptic junction. -*adj* Relating to the theory of matter at the atomic level.

quantization *n/adj* kwŏntĭ'zāshon [Lat *quantus* how much]
-*n* The act of converting data to a digital form, i.e., subdividing data into small, measurable parts, e.g., the process of assigning a sequence of discrete values to represent the continuous variation in amplitude and frequency of an analog signal. -*adj* Pertaining to the conversion of data to digital form.

quantization noise *np* [Lat *quantus* how much]
A signal distortion that results when too few quantization levels are used when digitizing a signal.

quarter-wave resonator *np*
The wavelength of the resonant frequency of a tube that is closed at one end and open at the other, e.g., the ear canal. The wavelength is equal to four times the length of the tube.

quasi-free field *np* 'kwāzī- [Lat *quasi* as if]
A sound field that approximates a free field.

quench *v/n/adj*
-*v* To extinguish. -*n* Loss of superconductivity. -*adj* Pertaining to quenching.

questionnaire *n*
A list of questions seeking information from a particular sample or population, often used in statistical studies.

quick phase *np*
The fast eye movement in nystagmus toward one direction, followed by a slow adjusting eye movement.

quinine *n*
A drug used to treat malaria. It can be ototoxic and cause temporary or, less commonly, permanent hearing loss.

quinsy *n* 'kwĭnzē
Acute suppurative tonsillitis or peritonsillar abcess. Acute inflammation of the tonsil with formation of pus around it.

quotient *n* [Lat *quotiens* how many times]
The number that results from the division of one number into another.

radial *adj* [Lat *radialis* ray, radius]
Characterized by divergence or moving out from the center.

radical *adj* [Lat *radicalis* pertaining to the root of a plant]
Complete removal or rooting out of diseased tissue.

radical mastoidectomy *np* [Lat *radicalis* pertaining to the root of a plant; Gk *mastoeides* breast-shaped + Gk *ektome* excision]
The surgical removal of mastoid bone and middle ear structures to completely remove diseased tissue.

radio *n* [Lat *radiare* to emit rays]
The wireless transmission and reception of radio frequency electromagnetic waves.

radiography *n* [Lat *radiare* to emit rays + Gk *graphia* writing]
The process of producing an image using x-ray or gamma radiation.

radio hearing aid *np*
A wireless system where the signal is sent from a transmitter (microphone) by means of frequency modulated (FM) radio waves to a receiver worn by a listener. It is used to overcome the effects of noise, distance, and reverberation and is widely used in education, where the teacher wears the microphone and the pupil wears the receiver.

radiology *n* [Lat *radiare* to emit rays + Gk *-logia* study of]
The study of body structures using x-rays, high-energy radiations and radioactive substances. It includes computed tomography (CT) scans used to determine the state of ear structures prior to surgery, e.g., the cochlea prior to implant surgery.
Deriv: –adj radiologic

radio receiver *np*
The receiving part of a radio (FM) hearing aid. It receives incoming radio waves and converts them to acoustic signals and delivers them to the user's hearing aid.

radiotherapy *n* [Lat *radiare* to emit rays + Gk *therapeia* healing]
Treatment of disease, usually of cancer, using radiation.

radio transmitter *n*
The transmitting part of a radio (FM) hearing aid. It transmits an acoustic signal in the form of modulated radio waves.

Rainville test *np obs* Named after Maurice J. Rainville, a French audiologist, who published his test in 1959.
An early test that sought to assess the degree of conductive hearing loss by comparing the intensity of masking, by air and bone conduction, needed to mask an air-conducted pulsed signal.

Rainville test, modified *np obs* Named after Maurice J. Rainville, a French audiologist, who published his test in 1959.
A test in which the bone conductor, placed on the forehead, was used to mask a pulsed air conduction signal presented to the test ear. The amount of masking noise, above that required with normal hearing, to mask the air-conduction signal indicated the degree of sensorineural hearing loss.

raised threshold *np*
A threshold of hearing that is elevated, i.e., worse than an average normal hearing threshold. A raised hearing threshold level for air and bone conduction indicates a sensorineural hearing loss. A raised hearing threshold level for air conduction and a normal threshold for bone conduction indicates a conductive hearing loss.

Ramsay-Hunt syndrome *np* Named after James Ramsay-Hunt (1872–1937), an American neurologist, who described the syndrome in 1921.
Also: herpes zoster oticus
A painful rash around the pinna caused by the varicella zoster virus, which also

causes chickenpox and shingles. It may be preceded or followed by painful neuralgia. Other characteristics may include unilateral hearing loss, vertigo, and weakness or paralysis of one side of the face.

random *adj*
A stream or flow having no regular pattern, e.g., random noise.

range *n*
The distance between the least and greatest values of a frequency distribution of variables or attributes, i.e., the difference between the two most extreme values.

Ranvier, node of *np* ˈrŏnvēā Named after Louis-Antoine Ranvier (1835–1922), a French histologist and pathologist, who discovered these nodes in 1878.
A constriction in the myelin sheath of a nerve where there is a high concentration of ion channels. The action potential is able to jump from one node of Ranvier to the next.

rapid deafness *np*
1. Hearing loss that occurs rapidly, e.g., within 90 days. 2. Hearing loss that occurs within 90 days.

Rapp-Hodgkin syndrome *np* Named after R.S. Rapp and W.E. Hodgkin, who published a description of the syndrome in a family with an affected mother, son, and daughter in 1968.
Also: Hay-Wells syndrome; ankyloblepharon ectodermal dysplasia cleft lip/palate syndrome (AEC)
An autosomal dominant genetic syndrome that is characterized by ectodermal dysplasia, cleft palate and lip, sparse hair, and abnormal or missing teeth and nails. Conductive hearing loss due to chronic otitis media is common

rapport *n*
A harmonious relationship.

rarefaction *n* [Lat *rareficio* to rarefy]
1. Reduction in air density. 2. The negative part of a sine wave, i.e., the part in which there is a reduction in air density.

rarefaction click *np*
A click produced by a negative polarity electric pulse.

Rassmusen, bundle of *np* ˈrăsmusen Named after Grant Litster Rasmussen (1905–1989), an American anatomist, who first described the olivocochlear bundle.
Also: olivocochlear bundle
An efferent bundle of fibers that originates in the superior olivary complex and exits the brainstem on the vestibular nerve before joining the cochlear nerve and running to the outer hair cells.

rate *n*
1. The computed quantity. 2. The number of repetitions of a stimulus per unit of time (normally in one second).

rating scale *np*
A classification in which the rated object is assigned a number giving the order or grade.

ratio *n* [Lat *ratio* account, reckoning]
A relationship between two numbers, determined by the number of times one contains the other.

ratio, compression *np*
The ratio of change in the output level that occurs when there is a change in input level.

ratio, data *np*
Quantitative items that can be measured on a scale in which the numbers are multiples of each other and where zero has a meaning, e.g., age.

ratio, signal-to-noise (S/N) *np*
The difference between the signal level and the ambient sound level at the listener's ear. This is given as a number +/-, e.g., a speech signal of 60 dB and a noise level of 55 dB results in a signal-to-noise ratio of +5 dB.

rationale *n*
A statement of reasons.

Raynaud phenomenon *np* ˈrānō Named after A.G. Maurice Raynaud (1834–1881), a French physician, who discovered the condition.
A disorder in which the blood vessels in the extremities contract causing discoloration of the fingers and toes. It is usually triggered by cold or emotional stress and may be associated with hearing loss due to vasoconstriction.

reactance *n*
1. The nonresistive component of impedance. 2. The opposition to the flow of acoustic energy usually due to stiffness.

reaction time *np*
The time taken between a stimulus and a response, e.g., hearing a pure tone and pressing the response button. Reaction time increases when sounds are near threshold.

real ear *adj*
Pertaining to measurements made in the ear canal using a probe tube microphone.

real ear-aided response (REAR) *np*
A graph that shows the value in decibels of the sound-pressure level of a specified soundfield, across the frequency range, measured in the ear canal with a hearing aid in place and switched on.

real ear gain *np*
Also: insertion gain; etymotic gain; transmission gain
The mathematical difference in dB between the sound-pressure level in the ear canal without and with a hearing aid.

real ear insertion gain (REIG) *np*
The value in decibels of the real ear insertion response at a given frequency.

real ear insertion response (REIR) *np*
The difference in decibels across frequency between the unaided response (REUR) and the aided response (REAR) obtained at the same measurement point

in the same soundfield. The electroacoustic equivalent of functional gain.

real ear occluded response *np*
The SPL or the gain when the ear is occluded with a turned-off hearing aid, measured in decibels across the frequency range at a specified point in the ear canal in a specified sound field.

real ear to coupler difference (RECD) *np*
The difference in sound pressure level (measured across the frequency range) between the output of a hearing aid in the real ear and measured in a 2-cc coupler.

real ear unaided response (REUR) *np*
The sound pressure level (measured across the frequency range) in the open ear canal, i.e., without a hearing aid, at a specified point in the ear canal in a specified sound field. It is used as the reference value for calculating the insertion or real ear gain.

real time *adj*
Having virtually instantaneous processing and display.

real-time clock *np*
Also: complementary metal oxide semiconductor (CMOS)
An integrated circuit employing miniature chip capacitors that set and track the current time.

receiver *n*
The output transducer of a hearing aid that converts electrical to acoustic energy.

receiver-in-the-ear (RITE) *np*
A type of hearing aid in which the receiver is located in the ear canal with the remaining assemblies contained in a behind the ear case.

receptive aphasia *np* [Lat *recipere* to receive; Gk *aphatos* speechless]
An inability or difficulty in understanding spoken and written language which may be due to adventitious brain injury, e.g., a stroke.

receptor cells *np*
Cells that respond to stimuli in the environment, e.g., the hair cells in the cochlea, which respond to sound.

recess *n* [Lat *recedere* to recede, go back]
An indentation, dip, or depression, e.g., a sinus.

recessive *adj* [Lat *recedere* to recede, go back]
Pertaining to a hereditary trait whose effect is often hidden. A recessive gene is one that is not expressed unless passed to the offspring by both parents.

recognition *n* [Lat *recognoscere* to recognize]
The action of acknowledging or identifying.

recovery time *np*
Also: release time
1. The period during which a nerve cannot be activated. It is the period that immediately follows the firing (depolarization) of the nerve impulse. 2. In compression, the time taken for the compressor to react to a decrease in input level and return to its steady state.

recruitment *n* [Lat *recrescere* to grow again, increase (from Fr *recrute*)]
An abnormally rapid increase in the rate of loudness growth, associated with cochlear hearing loss.

recurrent *adj*
1. Repeated. 2. A disease or condition repeated more than three times in a 6-month period.

redundant *adj* [Lat *redundare* to surge, to be surplus]
Exceeding what is necessary or normal; able to be eliminated without loss of information.

reference *n/adj/v*
-*n* 1. A measure that forms the standard for comparison. 2. A source of information, e.g., a book or article, that has been mentioned. 3. A letter (written by someone other than the individual in ques-

tion) that provides information about an individual, e.g., for a prospective employer. -*adj* Constituting the standard for measuring, constructing, or comparing to. -*v* To mention or to provide with references.

reference coupler *np*
Also: 2 cc coupler; standard coupler
A device that joins the receiver of a hearing aid to the microphone of a sound level meter. Designed with a standard volume of 2cc. Used for measuring the acoustic output of hearing aids.

reference electrode *np*
Also: common electrode
The evoked potential electrode that is taken as zero.

reference equivalent threshold force level (RETFL) *np*
The equivalent force level that is required to produce audiometric zero for bone conduction testing.

reference equivalent threshold sound pressure level (RETSPL) *np*
The equivalent sound pressure level that is required to produce audiometric zero in a 6-cc coupler.

reference level *np*
The zero point on a scale.

reference microphone *np*
A monitoring microphone.

reference pressure, audiologic *np*
The minimum sound pressure required to cause the sensation of hearing in the mid-frequency region, i.e., 0.00002 pascals (Pa).

reference test frequency *np*
In testing hearing aid performance, the reference frequency is based on the high frequency average of 1 kHz, 1.6 kHz, and 2.5 kHz (ANSI S3.22: 2003 and IEC 60118-7: 2005).

reference test gain (RTG) *np*
The amount of gain when the hearing aid is at the reference test setting, e.g., (ANSI S3.22: 2003 and IEC 60118-7: 2005) the

volume control position when the high-frequency average gain is 77 dB below OSPL 90. Reference test gain is a standardized setting that is intended to approximate a "user" volume setting.

reflection *n*
1. The return of sound waves that have impinged upon a resistant surface, i.e., when sound is reflected or thrown back by a barrier. 2. The act of considering.

reflective practice *np*
Reviewing and evaluating professional experiences to lead to greater understanding and improved outcomes.

reflex *n/adj* [Lat *reflexus* a bending back] -*n* An involuntary action. -*adj* Involuntary.

reflex, acoustic *np*
An involuntary activation of one or both of the middle ear muscles (tensor tympani and/or stapedius muscle) to high intensity acoustic stimulation.

reflex, auropalpebral *np* awrō'pălpebrǎl
An involuntary eye blink on being startled by a loud sound.

reflex arc *np*
The neural pathway involved in a reflex action. The pathway consists of a sensory receptor, a sensory neuron, an integrating center (the spinal cord or brainstem), a motor neuron, and an effector (e.g., a muscle).

reflex decay *np*
A reduction in a reflex action in response to constant stimulation, e.g., the stapedial reflex decay.

reflex, light *np*
Also: cone of light
The triangular-shaped light that is reflected back from the eardrum during otoscopic examination.

reflex, Moro *np* 'mawrō
A startle response to sound, characterized by extending and moving the arms, hands, and fingers; and normally seen in infants in the first 3 months of life.

reflex, vestibulooccular (VOR) *np*
Compensatory eye movements in response to signals from the semicircular canals.

reflux *n/v* [Lat *refluere* to flow backward] -*n* A flowing back. -*v* To boil a liquid in a vessel attached to a condenser so that the vapor returns into the vessel after condensing.

refraction *n* [Lat *refringere* to bend]
The bending of a sound wave as it passes from one medium to another.

refractory period *np*
The recovery time following the firing of a nerve or the excitation of a muscle fiber. The refractory period can be subdivided into the absolute refractory period and the relative refractory period. During the absolute refractory period, no impulse can be initiated but during the relative refractory period, although a normal stimulus will not initiate an action potential, a larger stimulus will initiate an impulse.

Refsum syndrome *np* Named after Sigvald Bernjard Refsum (1907–1991), a Norwegian physician and professor of neurology at Oslo University, who described this syndrome in his doctoral thesis in 1946.
A rare autosomal recessive disorder of lipid metabolism in which phytanic acid cannot be broken down and accumulates in the blood and tissues. Characteristics include night blindness, progressive sensorineural deafness, progressive tunnel vision, retinitis pigmentosa, peripheral sensory and motor neuropathy, unsteadiness, nystagmus, loss of smell, and bone and skin abnormalities.

regression *n* [Lat *regredi* to step backward]
1. The action of returning to a former or less developed state. 2. A statistical analysis to assess the strength of the relationship between one dependent variable (usually denoted by Y) and a series of independent or changing variables.

rehabilitation *n*
The reestablishment (fully or partially) of normal capacity.

Reichert canal *np* ˈrīkert Named after Karl Bogislaus Reichert (1811–1883), a German anatomist, who is remembered for his work on the anatomy of the inner ear.
Also: reuniens canal/duct; Hensen canal
The small channel that joins the cochlea to the saccule of the vestibular system.

reinforcement *n*
The process by which a behavior is learned or strengthened. Positive reinforcement is used when testing children's hearing, e.g., by praising the child for giving correct responses.

Reissner membrane *np* ˈrīsnez Named after Ernst Reissner (1824–1878), a Latvian anatomist and professor of anatomy at the University of Dorpat (now known as the University of Tartu in Estonia), who studied the formation of the inner ear and described this membrane of the scala media in 1851.
Also: vestibular membrane
The membrane that separates the scala media from the scala vestibule in the cochlea. One end of the Reissner membrane is attached to the spiral ligament, the other to the inner part of the spiral limbus.

relaxation therapy *np*
A therapeutic method to train the individual to recognize the difference between tension and relaxation and to use this knowledge to consciously relax.

release from masking *np*
Also: masking level difference (MLD)
A measure of the improvement in detection of a masked signal under dichotic listening conditions.

release time *np*
Also: recovery time
1. The period during which a nerve cannot be activated. It is the period that immediately follows the firing (depolari-

zation) of the nerve impulse. 2. In compression, the time taken for the compressor to react to a decrease in input level.

reliability *n*
The degree to which something is repeatable under the same conditions.

reliability, internal *np*
A method of assessing the consistency of something, e.g., a questionnaire written in such a way that it can be seen if some of the answers are contradictory.

remote *adj*
Situated at a distance, e.g., remote control; remote microphone.

renal *adj* ˈrēnəl [Lat *renes* kidneys]
Pertaining to the kidneys.

renal disease *np*
Kidney dysfunction, sometimes associated with hearing loss.

renal-genital syndrome *np*
A rare genetic disorder in which the main characteristics are kidney, genital, and middle ear malformations. There may also be a small jaw.

renal tubular acidosis *np*
Also: Fanconi pancytopenia syndrome; Fanconi anemia syndrome
A rare condition that may be genetic or acquired. Characteristics include patchy brown pigmentation, short stature, microcephaly (small head), kidney problems, delayed puberty, learning difficulty and extra or fewer digits. The external ear may also be malformed, and there may be conductive and sensorineural hearing loss.

repair strategy *np*
Tactics intended to rectify a breakdown in communication.

repetition rate *np*
1. The rate at which repeated signals are produced. 2. The rate per minute at which words are repeated.

representative sample *np*
A group of subjects that is representative of the population under test.

resect *v* [Lat *resecare* to cut back]
To cut away.
Deriv: -*n* resection

reserve gain *np*
The additional or residual amplification that is available for use by the hearing-aid wearer. The difference in gain between the volume setting of the user and the maximum volume setting possible without feedback.

residual *adj*
Remaining.

residual hearing *np*
The degree of hearing that remains when a hearing loss is present.

residual inhibition *np*
Also: postmasking effect
A temporary reduction or complete removal of tinnitus after tinnitus masking noise has ceased.

residue pitch *np*
Also: virtual pitch; pitch periodicity
The perceived pitch of a complex tone that corresponds to a missing fundamental.

resistance *n*
Opposition, e.g., the opposition of a body to the pressure of another.

resistor *n*
A passive electronic device that limits current flow.

resonance *n* [Lat *resonare* to ring out]
The continuation of sound due to reflection.

resonance, concha *np*
The constructive enhancement of sound, by about 5 to 10 dB at frequencies between 5.5 and 7 kHz. that occurs in the concha.

resonance, ear canal *np*
The constructive enhancement of sound, by about 10 dB at frequencies between 2.5 and 3.5 KHz., that occurs in the ear canal.

resolution *n* [Lat *resolvere* to divide up into its constituent parts]
The separation into component parts.

resonant frequency *np*
Also: natural frequency
The object's natural frequency of vibration, i.e., it will vibrate with the greatest amplitude and with the least effort at a certain frequency. The specific frequency depends upon the physical properties of the vibrating body.

response *n*
1. A measure of the output. 2. An observable behavior, e.g., one that indicates that a sound has been heard during a pure tone audiometric test.

response, frequency *np*
A graph showing the output of a hearing aid as a function of frequency.

response time *np*
The amount of time it takes for an individual to respond to a stimulus, e.g., a pure tone.

resting potential *np*
The membrane potential of a neuron in its resting state, i.e., when it is not being altered by an action potential.

reticular *adj* ˈrĕtĭkyūlə [Lat *reticulum* small net]
Pertaining to a network.

reticular lamina/membrane *np*
The stiff membranous network that is formed by the phalangeal processes of the supporting cells and the cuticular plates of the hair cells. The reticular lamina isolates the stereocilia of the hair cells from their cell bodies.

retinitis pigmentosa *np* ˈrĕtĭnītĭs ˈpĭgmĕntōza [Lat *rete* net + Gk -*ites* denoting disease of; Lat *pigmentosus* colored]
Progressive blindness due to retinal atrophy. Symptoms appear first in childhood and develop gradually into adulthood. The condition starts with night blindness, later tunnel vision, and finally loss

of central vision and may be associated with sensorineural deafness.

retraction *n* [Lat *retrahere* to draw back]
Drawing back.

retraction pocket *np*
A condition in which a part of the eardrum is sucked inward due to negative pressure in the middle ear, and adheres to the medial wall of the middle ear.

retro- *prefix* [Lat *retro-* backward]
Behind.

retrocochlear *adj* [Lat *retro-* backward + Lat *cochlea* snail shell, spiral]
Pertaining to the part of the auditory system that is beyond the cochlea, i.e., the auditory nerve and the auditory centers of the brain.

retrognathia *n* rĕtro'nãthēa [Lat *retro-* backward + Gk *gnathos* jaw]
A jutting-out lower jaw, which is the most common jaw deformity.

retrosigmoid *adj* [Lat *retro-* backward + Gk *sigmoides* S-shaped]
From behind the sigmoid sinus, an approach that may be taken in surgery for an acoustic neuroma.

retrospective study *np*
A study in which information is taken from previous records for analysis.

reuptake *n*
A rapid reabsorption of neurotransmitter from the synaptic cleft.

reuniens, canal/duct *np* [Lat *reuniens* joining, reuniting]
Also: Hensen canal; Reichert canal
The small channel that joins the cochlea to the saccule of the vestibular system.

reverberation *n*
The persistence of sound in a space due to multiple simultaneously occurring incident and reflected sound waves.
Deriv: -adj reverberant

reverberation time *np*
The time required for the intensity of a sound to decrease by 60 dB from the original level after the source has ceased.

reverse horn *np*
An earmold tubing modification in which the tubing coming from the earhook decreases from a large diameter to a small diameter, providing a poor impedance match to the ear that results in reduction of the transmission of high frequencies and an increase in low-frequency gain.

reverse slope *np*
An audiometric configuration in which the greatest hearing loss is in the low frequencies, which is opposite to the common configuration.

rhesus (Rh) incompatibility *np* 'rēsus
Probably named after Rhesus, Prince of Thrace.
A condition that occurs when a rhesus-negative mother carries a rhesus-positive fetus. Antibodies from the mother may attack red blood cells in the fetus, resulting in severe jaundice, which is a high-risk factor for hearing loss.

rhinitis *n* [Gk *rhis* nose + Gk *-ites* denoting disease of]
Inflammation of the nose.

rhino- *prefix* [Gk *rhis* nose]
Pertaining to the nose.

rhinolaryngology *n* [Gk *rhis* nose + Gk *larunx* throat + Gk *-logia* study of]
Study of the diseases of the nose and throat, usually also including study of the ear.

rhinosinusitis *n* [Gk *rhis* nose + Lat *sinus* recess, bend + Gk *-ites* denoting disease of]
Inflammation of the nose and sinuses.

rhombencephalon *n* 'rŏmbĕnsĕfalŏn [Gk *rhombos* square + Gk *enkephalon* brain]
Also: hindbrain
The rear area of the brain that contains the pons, cerebellum, and medulla oblongata.

rhythm *n* [Gk *rhuthmos* a flowing, rhythm]
An ordered recurrent pattern of strong and weak elements, e.g., the stress, tim-

ing, etc., in the flow of speech production.

Deriv: -adj rhythmic

ribonucleic acid (RNA) *np*
A molecule that carries the genetic sequence or code that determines the precise protein produced.

ribosome *n* ˈrībōsōm
A small protein structure in the cytoplasm that is involved in protein synthesis.

Richards-Rundle syndrome *np* Named after Barry Wyndham Richards and A.T. Rundle, British physicians, who described five siblings with the syndrome in 1959.
Also: ataxia-hypogonadism syndrome
A genetic hormonal disorder that progresses in childhood before becoming static. Characteristics include ketoaciduria (excess keto acids in the urine), learning difficulties, underdeveloped secondary sex characteristics, deafness, ataxia (poor muscle coordination), and peripheral muscle wasting.

Rinne test *np* ˈrīne Named after Heinrich Adolf Rinne (1819–1868), a German otologist, who developed the test.
A monaural tuning fork test that compares sensitivity by air conduction with sensitivity by bone conduction.

ripple *n*
The degree to which a filter, e.g., in a hearing aid, is flat. Filtering is not perfect and the degree of ripple is usually below 3 dB and may be below 1 dB.

rise time *np*
1. In compression, the time taken for the signal to rise from -60 dB to within 1 dB of its steady state. 2. The time taken for a stimulus to reach its maximum.

Rivinus notch/incisure *np* Named after August Quirinus Bachmann (1652–1723), a German anatomist and botanist and professor of pathology at the University of Leipzig, who published widely in medicine and anatomy. August's father had changed his surname from Bachmann to Rivinus, and August was more commonly known as August Quirinus Rivinus.
Also: tympanic notch; incisura tympanica
A gap in the tympanic sulcus (the groove in the temporal bone that holds the tympanic membrane) that is bridged by the pars flaccida.

Roberts syndrome *np* Named after John B. Roberts, who published a description in 1919, of the syndrome in three siblings. The earliest description of the syndrome is thought to be that of Francois Bouchard in 1672, who carried out an autopsy on an individual with the condition.
Also: pseudothalidomide
A rare autosomal recessive disorder characterized by phocomelia (shortening or absence of limbs) and craniofacial abnormalities, including cleft lip and palate that may be associated with hearing loss.

rodent ulcer *np* [Lat *rodere* to gnaw; Lat *ulcus* an ulcer]
Also: basal cell carcinoma
A skin cancer that grows slowly and rarely spreads to other parts of the body.

rods of Corti *np*
Also: pillar cells
The supporting cells that form the walls of the tunnel of Corti in the cochlea.

roll-off *np*
A smooth downward slope in the response of a hearing aid at either the upper or lower ends of the frequency range.

rollover *n*
1. A turning upside down. 2. The area in the plot of a performance-intensity function for speech recognition where further increases in sound intensity produce a reduction (fall off) in performance.

Romberg sign *np* Named after Moritz H. Romberg (1795–1873), a German neurologist, who wrote the first systemic book on neurology.
An inability to stand with the feet togeth-

er and the eyes shut, indicating loss of a sense of position.

root mean square (rms) *np*
The square-root of the mean of the squares of several samples of a signal over a specified period, i.e., the long-term overall power level of a signal.

Rosenberg-Chutorian syndrome *np*
Named after Roger N. Rosenberg and Abe Milton Chutorian (b 1929), American physicians, who reported two brothers with the syndrome in 1967.
Also: optic atrophy; Charcot-Marie-Tooh neuropathy X type 5
A rare X-linked genetic syndrome. Characteristics include progressive visual deterioration, progressive severe high-frequency sensorineural hearing loss and polyneuropathy, especially affecting the arms and legs.

Rosenthal canal *np* ˈrōzentahl Named after Friedrich-Christian Rosenthal (1780–1829), a German surgeon and anatomist, who described this canal in his late work.
The spiral channel in the bony core of the cochlea that contains the spiral ganglion.

rostral *adj* [Lat *rostrum* a beak]
1. Beak-like. 2. Situated near the front of the body, especially in the mouth and nose area.
Deriv: -*adv* rostrally

rostrum *n* [Lat *rostrum* a beak]
An anatomic term, referring to a beak-like projection, e.g., from the sphenoid bone.

rotary nystagmus *np*
Also: torsional nystagmus
Nystagmus with a rotary movement. (Most nystagmus resulting from vestibular dysfunction has a rotary component).

round window *np*
The membrane-covered opening that separates the middle ear from the scala tympani of the cochlea and that is found behind and below the oval window in the cochlea.

round-window membrane *np*
The membrane that covers the round window.

round-window niche *np*
The depression in the temporal bone in the middle ear cavity that holds the round-window membrane.

rubella *n* [Lat *rubellus* reddish]
Also: rubeola; *colloq* German measles
A congenital viral infection passed from the mother to the fetus, which can result in sensorineural deafness that is often severe to profound. Other characteristics may include conductive hearing loss, heart disease, learning difficulties, cataracts or glaucoma, and "salt and pepper" retinal pigmentation.

running speech *np*
Continuous speech.

sabin/Sabine *n* ˈsābĭn/ˈsābīn Named after Wallace C. Sabine (1868–1919), an American acoustician and professor at Harvard University, who developed a formula for calculating the reverberation time in a room.
The unit of Sabine absorption that is used in calculating the sound absorbency in a room, where 0 is completely reflective and 1 is completely absorbent.

Sabine (reverberation) formula *np* Named after Wallace C. Sabine (1868–1919), an American acoustician and professor at Harvard University, who developed a formula for calculating the reverberation time in a room.
A formula used to calculate the reverberation time of an enclosure based on the volume of the enclosure and the absorption coefficient in Sabines.

sac *n* [Lat *saccus* sack]
A pouch, e.g., the endolymphatic sac.

saccade *n* să'kād (să'kahd) [Fr *saccade* violent pull]
A rapid jumping movement of the eye from one position to another.

saccadic eye movement *np* să'kădĭk
Movements used both voluntarily and reflexively to initiate the eye quickly toward an object of interest and to stop and fix to the target accurately. This allows the viewer to refix their gaze with minimal duration of retinal slip.

saccule *n* [Lat *sacculus* a small sack]
1. A small sac. 2. The smaller of the two sacs in the membranous labyrinth of the vestibule.

saddle nose and myopia *np*
Also: Marshall syndrome; ectodermal dysplasia; lobster-claw syndrome
A rare genetic pigmentary disorder characterized by distinctive facial features that include a flattened nasal bridge, upturned nose and widely spaced eyes, also lobster-claw deformity of hands and feet, nearsightedness, cataracts, and congenital progressive moderate-to-severe sensorineural, conductive, or mixed hearing loss and poor vestibular function.

saggital *adj* ˈsăjĭtal [Lat *saggita* arrow]
Vertical.

sagittal plane *np*
The plane that runs through the length of the body parallel to the spinal column.

sagittal section *np*
A vertical slice through the brain parallel to the spinal column.

salicylate *n* săˈlĭsĭlāt (săˈlĭsĭlat)
A pain-relieving drug derived from salicylic acid, e.g., aspirin, which is ototoxic in large doses and can cause tinnitus and/or mild-to-moderate sensorineural hearing loss.

saliva *n* [Lat *saliva* saliva]
A watery secretion containing amylase, invertase, lipase, and protease, produced by the salivary glands. Its function is to lubricate the passage of food and carry out part of its digestion.

salivary glands *np*
Glands found in many animals, the ducts of which open in or near the mouth.

salping- *prefix* ˈsălpĭnj- [Gk *salpinx* trumpet]
Trumpet.

salpingemphraxis *n* [Gk *salpinx* trumpet + Gk *emphraxis* blocking, fencing]
Obstruction of the Eustachian tube (which is trumpet-shaped).

salpingian *adj*
Relating to the Eustachian tube.

salpingitis *n*
Inflammation of the Eustachian tube.

saltatory conduction *np* ˈsăltătawrī [Lat *saltare* to dance, jump; Lat *conducere* to conduct]
The conduction of action potentials by myelinated axons. The axon potential jumps from one node of Ranvier to the next, increasing the speed of transmission.

sample *v/n*
-v To measure a signal at discrete and regular times. *–n* 1.The measurement of a signal at discrete and regular times. 2. A representative part of a larger whole, e.g., a sample taken from a population for study.

Sanfilippo syndrome *adj* Named after Sylvester Sanfilippo (b 1926), an American pediatrician, who described the condition in 1963.
A genetic metabolic condition in which glycosaminoglycans (long sugar molecules previously known as mucopolysaccharides) cannot be properly broken down. It results from an enzyme deficiency and characteristics include deafness and loss of vision, cardiovascular problems, and severely decreased intellectual functioning. The condition is progressive and death usually occurs before age 20.

sanguinous *adj* săng'wĭnŭs [Lat *sanguineus* bloody (from *sanguis* blood)]
Bloody.

sarcoidosis *n* [Gk *sarx* flesh + Gk *eidos* shape + Gk *-osis* denoting a disease]
Also: sarcoid; Bessnier-Boeck disease; Bessnier-Boeck-Schaumann disease
A disorder, thought to be due to an abnormal immune response, in which granulomas appear on the body, most commonly affecting the lungs, skin, eyes, and lymph glands, but which can affect any organ, e.g., the auditory nerve causing hearing loss, which can be unilateral and may be fluctuating.

sarcoma, soft tissue *np* [Gk *sarx* flesh + Gk *–oma* denoting tumor, swelling]
A cancer that begins in connective tissue, e.g., bone, muscle, fat, blood vessels, etc.

saturating nonlinearity *np*
The nonlinear response of the basilar membrane to incoming sounds, i.e., the gain decreases with increasing stimulus intensity.

saturation *n* [Lat *saturare* to be saturated]
1. The state where an increase in input signal, e.g., to a hearing aid, cannot produce any further increase in the output signal. 2. The condition in which an auditory nerve fiber reaches its maximum firing rate.

saturation sound pressure level (SSPL) *np*
Also: saturation sound pressure level with 90 dBSL input (SSPL 90); output sound pressure level with 90 dBSL input (OSPL 90); *colloq* maximum power output (MPO)
The highest possible sound pressure level obtainable from an amplifier, e.g., in a hearing aid.

sawtooth wave *np*
A wave that has the appearance of a jagged saw edge and contains all the integer harmonics of the fundamental frequency.

scala *n/adj* 'skahla [Lat *scala* ladder]
-n A stair-like structure. *-adj* Stair-like.

scala media *np* [Lat *scala* ladder; Lat *medius* middle]
Also: endolymphatic space; cochlear duct
The middle chamber of the cochlea that is filled with endolymph and contains the organ of Corti.

scala tympani *np* [Lat *scala* ladder; Gk *tumpanon* drum]
The chamber of the cochlea that is filled with perilymph and extends from the round window to the helicotrema and is separated from the scala media by the basilar membrane.

scala vestibuli *np* [Lat *scala* ladder; Lat *vestibulum* entrance]
The chamber of the cochlea that is filled with perilymph and extends from the oval window to the helicotrema and is separated from the scala media by the basilar membrane.

scanning electron microscopy *np*
The use of a focused beam of high-energy

electrons to analyze the structure of a specimen.

scaphoid fossa *np* ˈskǎfoid [Lat *scapha* boat + Gk *eidos* shape; Lat *fossa* ditch, depression]
A boat-shaped depression between the helix and the antihelix of the pinna.

scarlet fever/scarlatina *np*
A contagious bacterial infection that causes a rough red rash that spreads to many parts of the body, e.g., the ears, neck, and chest including the face, and which may cause conductive and/or sensorineural hearing loss.

Scarpa ganglion *np* [Gk *ganglion* nerve center] Named after Antonio Scarpa (1752–1832), an Italian surgeon and professor of anatomy at the University of Modena, who described the structure of the round window.
The ganglion (a mass of nerve cell bodies) of the vestibular nerve located in the internal auditory canal.

Scarpa membrane *np* [Lat *membrana* a covering] Named after Antonio Scarpa (1752–1832), an Italian surgeon and professor of anatomy at the University of Modena, who described the structure of the round window.
The membrane that covers the round window.

scar tissue *np*
Dense fibrous connective tissue that forms externally or internally over a healing wound.

scattergram *n*
A graph that shows two sets of measurement as dots and where a strong correlation is indicated by clusters of the dots in a particular pattern.

Scheibe dysplasia *np* ˈshībe [Gk *dus-* bad + Gk *plasis* formation] Named after A. Scheibe, a German pathologist, who first described the condition in 1892.
Also: cochleosaccular dysplasia
Gross malformation of the cochlea and saccule in which the organ of Corti may

be fully or partially missing and the cochlear duct collapsed or distended. It is often present in congenital profound deafness of autosomal recessive inheritance.

schema *n* ˈskēma [Gk *schema* figure, form]
A store of information about previous experiences that is used to make future decisions.

Schwabach test *np* ˈshvahbahk (ˈshvahbǎk) Named after Dagobert Schwabach (1846–1920), a German otologist, who published widely on hearing tests.
A tuning fork test that compares a patient's hearing by bone conduction to that of a normal-hearing person (the examiner).

Schwann cells *np* shwǒn (shvǎn) Named after Theodor Ambrose Hubert Schwann (1810–1882), a German anatomist and physiologist, who discovered the myelin sheath of the nerves.
The myelin sheath that forms a continuous envelope around each nerve fiber of a peripheral nerve.

schwannoma, vestibular *np*
Also: acoustic neuroma
A benign tumor that grows from the vestibular branch of the eighth nerve, caused by an overgrowth of the Schwann cells of the myelin sheath. Unilateral hearing loss is often the first sign of the condition. Bilateral tumors are very rare, but may be associated with neurofibromatosis.

Schwartze sign *np* shvahtze Named after Hermann Schwartze (1837–1919), a German physician, who described the condition in 1873.
A reddish color sometimes seen behind the eardrum in otosclerosis due to an excessive accumulation of blood in the mucous membrane around the promontory.

scientific method *np*
A systematic pursuit of knowledge involving recognition, definition, and for-

mulation of a problem, the collection of data through observation and experiment, and the formulation and testing of hypotheses.

sclerectomy *n* [Gk *skleros* hard + Gk *ektome* cutting out]
Removal of fibrous adhesions following chronic otitis media.

sclerosis *n* [Gk *skleros* hard + Gk *-osis* denoting a diseased state]
Hardening of the tissues.
Deriv: -adj sclerotic

sclerosteosis *n* [Gk *skleros* hard + Gk *osteon* bone + Gk *-osis* denoting a diseased state]
An autosomal recessive condition characterized by progressive osteosclerosis. Thickening of the skull can narrow the cranial nerve canals causing facial palsy, sensorineural hearing loss, and visual problems.

scoop, ear *np*
A spoon-shaped instrument that is used for removing wax from the ear.

screening *n*
The use of quick tests to identify individuals who require further diagnostic testing.

screening, hearing *np*
Testing hearing using a limited range of frequencies and intensities (and without masking), which is used to identify individuals who need further investigation.

scroll ear *np*
An ear in which the pinna is rolled forward.

sebaceous cyst *np* se'bāshus (si'bāshus) [Lat *sebum* wax; Gk *kustos* container]
Named sebaceous cysts because it was thought they arose from the sebaceous glands; however, this is incorrect.
A small closed sac under the skin filled with semifluid keratin material.

secondary *adj*
Caused by or following another condition.

secondary cell *np*
A battery in which the electrochemical reaction is reversible, i.e., a rechargeable battery.

secondary tumor *np*
An additional tumor arising from cells carried around the body from the original or primary tumor.

second-order neuron (neurone) *np*
A neuron that relays information from the spinal cord to the thalamus.

secretory *adj* se'krētorē
Concerning the secretion of fluid, e.g., secretory otitis media.

section *v/n*
-v To cut. *-n* Part of a whole; a subdivision or a part cut off.

segment *n*
1. Each part into which a thing is or can be divided. 2. Part of a circle or sphere cut off by an intersecting line or plane.

segmental *adj*
Pertaining to divisions or segments, e.g., the phonemes in a word are segmental.

select-a-vents *n, pl*
A selection of inserts that can be installed within the aperture of a vent in an earmold or custom aid to reduce vent size.

selective listening *np*
Attending to a particular sound source, in the presence of other sounds that are ignored.

self-curling electrode *np*
A cochlear implant electrode array that is curved during manufacture so that, after insertion, it will curl closely to the modiolus and therefore to the auditory nerve.

self-recording *adj*
Making an automatic record, e.g., a self-recording audiometer.

self-recording audiometry *np*
A type of audiometry, often used in industrial hearing screening, in which the signal is automatically introduced by the audiometer and the individual under test records their response by pressing a but-

ton when they first hear the sound and releasing it when they no longer hear it. This is repeated a number of times for each frequency. The results are recorded graphically.

semantics *n* [Gk *semantikos* significant]
The study of meanings of words and combinations of words.

semicircular canal *np*
One of the three fluid-filled ducts in the vestibular (balance) system that are concerned with angular acceleration (turning the head) in certain directions.

semipermeable/semi-permeable membrane *np*
A membrane that is not permeable to all molecules. Although many ions may pass through it, they may do so to different degrees, and large molecules are unable to pass through.

semivowel *n*
A sound that is formed like a vowel but functions as a consonant, e.g., /w/ and /y/.

senile *adj* [Lat *senilis* old]
Pertaining to old age.

sensation level (SL) *np*
The level of a stimulus in dB presented above a person's pure tone or speech threshold.

sense organ *np*
A bodily organ, e.g., the ear, that conveys external stimuli to the sensory system.

sensitive *adj*
1. Acutely susceptible to external stimuli or impressions. 2. Capable of receiving a stimulus. 3. (Instrumentation) Able to respond to or record slight changes. 4. Easily offended or hurt and requiring tactful treatment or secrecy.

sensitivity *n*
1. A statistical measure of the proportion of people who have a disease or disorder who are correctly identified by a given test. The inverse of specificity. 2. The ability to respond to a stimulus. 3. The sound pressure level required for a cochlear im-

plant speech processor to behave in a certain way, e.g., to generate a T-level stimulus.

sensitize *v*
To make sensitive.
Deriv: -n sensitization

sensor *n*
A device for detecting or measuring a physical property.

sensorineural *adj*
Involving the sensory and/or neural cells of the cochlea and their connections, e.g., the cause of a sensorineural hearing loss may be due to eighth nerve or brainstem lesion (damage).

sensorineural acuity level test (SAL) *np obs*
A modification of the Rainville test, in which the air-conduction threshold is obtained both in quiet and in the presence of a fixed level of bone-conducted narrow band noise. The sensorineural element of a hearing loss is determined by comparing the degree of threshold shift in the presence of the noise with the degree of shift for a normally hearing listener with the same level of noise.

sensory *adj*
Stimulated by the senses (e.g., auditory, visual, tactile).

sensory adaptation *np*
An increase or decrease in the intensity or strength of a response. A decrease due to changes in the state of a receptor organ after repetitive or lengthy stimulation or a corresponding increase due to recovery of a receptor from such stimulation.

sensory deprivation *np*
The reduction or removal of stimulation of one or more of the senses.

sensory input *np*
Input consisting of different sensory modalities (e.g., auditory, visual, tactile) that is provided to a person or other living organism.

sensory radicular neuropathy *np*
A nervous system disorder characterized by pains in the arms and legs, foot ulcers, and progressive sensorineural hearing loss.

sentence tests *np*
Speech tests that present sentences rather than single words, which are intended to provide a more natural representation of normal speech than single nonconnected words. They may be used in clinical audiometry and in hearing aid fitting and certain sentence tests are intended to assess central auditory function, e.g., the dichotic sentence test (competing sentences presented to each ear at different sensation levels above threshold).

Senter syndrome *np* Named after Thomas P. Senter (b 1946), an American dermatologist, who described the syndrome in the *Journal of Pediatrics* in 1978.
Also: ichthyosiform erythroderma deafness keratitis; Desmond syndrome; keratitis ichthyosiform/ichthyosis deafness (KID) syndrome; *colloq* fish-skin disease
A rare genetic syndrome in which there is congenital deafness, noninflammatory scaling of the skin, thin or absent hair, and gradual destruction of the cornea, which can lead to blindness. The condition is due to glycogen deposited in the skin and liver, which can also result in the need for a liver transplant.

sepsis *n* [Gk *sepsis* rotting]
A dangerous condition of bacterial infection in the bloodstream.
Deriv: -adj septic

septum *n* *pl* septa [Lat *septum* enclosure]
A dividing wall or membrane, e.g., the cartilage in the nose, which divides the nostrils.

sequela *n* sĭˈkwēla *pl* sequelae [Lat *sequela* consequence]
A condition that occurs after a disease and as a result of it.

sequential *adj* [Lat *sequi* to follow]
Following or resulting from.

sequential implant *np*
A second cochlear implant added after unilateral implantation to create a binaural system.

serial *adj* [Lat *series* row, chain]
Forming a series, e.g., serial pure tone audiograms.

series *n*
1. A number of similar or related things.
2. A set of electrical circuits or components arranged so that the same current passes through each successively.

seroma *n* seˈrōma [Lat *serum* whey + Gk *–oma* denoting tumor, swelling]
A localized collection of serous fluid in the tissue.

serous membrane *np* [Lat *serum* whey; Lat *membrana* a partition]
One of the delicate membranes of connective tissue that line the internal cavities of the body.

serum *n* ˈsĭrŭm (ˈsĭerŭm) *pl* sera [Lat *serum* whey]
A thin, watery sterile liquid.

service life *np*
The expected or acceptable working life of a device.

sessile *adj* [Lat *sedeo* I sit]
1. Attached; fixed in one place and having no connecting neck or stalk. 2. Immotile (of cells).

seventh cranial nerve *np*
Also: facial nerve
Cranial nerve VII, which provides innervation to the facial muscles and from the tongue and soft palate.

severe hearing loss *np*
1. A subjective description of a severe to profound level of hearing loss. 2. Average hearing level between 71 dBHL to 90 dBHL (UK: 71–95 dBHL; WHO: 61–80 dBHL)

sex-linked *adj*
Of genes, characters or diseases carried on the X chromosome.

sex-linked inheritance *np*
The phenotypic expression of an allele that is dependent upon the sex of the individual and directly tied to the sex chromosome.

sex-linked trait *np*
A genetic characteristic that occurs completely or mostly in one sex.

shadow curve *np*
A configuration of thresholds in the test ear that mirrors the threshold configuration of the nontest ear. It is usually due to crossover from the signal in the test ear and lack of masking in the nontest ear, i. e., the signal introduced to the poor ear is loud enough to be heard by the nontest (good) ear on the opposite side via bone conduction.

shadow point *np*
A false hearing threshold due to cross hearing.

sharply falling audiogram *np*
A hearing loss that falls by 15 dB or more per octave.

shear *v*
To cut or thrust through.
Deriv: –adj shearing

shearing action/motion *np*
Deflection with a cutting or shaving movement, e.g., the movement between the tectorial membrane and the basilar membrane in the cochlea causes a shearing motion that bends the stereocilia of the hair cells back and forth.

sheath *n*
The surrounding layer.

sheath, myelin *np* [Gk *muelos* marrow]
The fatty layer that covers the axons of nerve cells.

shelf life *np*
The length of time over which something remains fit for use, e.g., a battery.

shell *n*
1. A hard protective covering. 2. An earmold that fills the concha.

shell, carved *np*
A silicone shell earmold where the interior has been carved out to make it lightweight and flexible.

shift *n*
A movement.

shift, temporary threshold *np*
A change in hearing threshold due to excessive noise exposure that returns to previous levels after a short time out of the noise.

shift, threshold *np*
A change in a hearing threshold.

shingles *n*
Also: herpes zoster
An infection caused by the same virus that causes chickenpox. Usually affects a single area causing pain and a rash. May be due to a dormant chickenpox virus that becomes active again. If the auditory nerve is affected, there is sensorineural hearing loss with pain.

shoe *n*
Also: boot
A coupling device attached to behind-the-ear hearing aids that allows wired or FM signals to be input to the hearing aid.

shore value *np*
The hardness of a material after curing (hardening due to polymerization) is complete. The higher the shore value the harder and more rigid the material.

short circuit *np*
1. A situation where current is accidentally or intentionally allowed to flow between points of low resistance that normally have high resistance. 2. An electrode anomaly in a cochlear implant.

short-duration signal *np*
A signal of less than 200 ms duration.

short increment sensitivity index test (SISI) *np*
A test of the patient's ability to detect small intensity changes (1dB) at near threshold levels. The ability to do so is indicative of cochlear damage.

short latency response *np*
An evoked auditory potential that occurs within the first 12–15 ms following the stimulus onset.

short process of malleus *np*
The small white knob of bone that extends from the upper end of the malleus that can be visualized during otoscopic examination.

Shrapnell membrane *np* Named after Henry Jones Shrapnell (1792–1834), an English surgeon, who described the anatomy of the eardrum, dividing it into the pars tensa and pars flaccida in 1830.
Also: pars flaccida
The smaller upper portion of the tympanic membrane that has no fibrous layer and is therefore thin and slack or flaccid.

shunt *n*
A passage or tube that allows fluid drainage.

SI (Systeme International) *n abbrev*
A system of coherent metric units used internationally.

sibilant *n* [Lat *sibilare* to hiss]
A hissing consonant sound made by forcing air through a restricted passage, e.g., /s/.

sigmoid sinus *np* [Gk *sigmoides* S-shaped; Lat *sinus* recess, bend]
A pair of sinuses that arise below the temporal bones and that drain blood into the internal jugular vein.

sign *n* [Lat *signum* a sign]
1. A visible medical finding, e.g., swelling, discharge, etc. 2. A visually transmitted word or message.

signal *n*
An object, gesture, act, or event that conveys information.

signal averaging *np*
Also: computer averaging
A method of averaging successive samples to remove unrelated signals or noise.

signal-to-noise ratio (SNR or S/N) *np*
The signal level compared to the level of background noise. It is expressed as the signal level plus or minus the competing noise level, e.g., a signal of 60 dB(A) with background noise of 70 dB(A) results in a signal-to-noise ratio of -10 dB SNR. A signal of 70 dB(A) in noise of 60 dB(A) is expressed as +10 SNR.

sign language *np*
A manual system of communication.

sign-supported English (SSE) *np*
Speech that is accompanied by simultaneous signing.

signed English *np*
A sign language that follows the rules of English grammar. A system of signing that may be used in education, but which is not the natural sign language of the deaf community.

significance *n* [Lat *significare* to signify]
A statistical conclusion that is unlikely to have occurred by chance, normally expressed as the probability (*p*-value) that a result is due to chance, e.g., a *p*-value of 0.05 indicates a 5% probability that the result is due to chance.

silicone *n/adj* [Lat *silex* flint, stone]
-n A soft rubber-like polymeric compound used to make ear impressions and soft earmolds. *-adj* Made from silicone.

simple harmonic motion *np*
A repetitive pendulum or spring-like motion back and forth across its resting position, e.g., the movement of air molecules due to the passage of a sound wave. The acceleration that causes simple harmonic motion is proportional to and op-

posite to the displacement from the equilibrium (resting position).

simple tone *np*
Also: pure tone
A sound with a pressure/time waveform that exhibits sinusoidal wave motion and consists of only one frequency.

simulate *v* [Lat *simulare* to copy]
1. To pretend to be, have, or feel. 2. To imitate or copy. 3. To reproduce the conditions of something. 4. To produce a computer model of a process.

simulated *adj*
Imitating particular conditions, e.g., simulated real ear measurements.

sine wave *np*
Also: sinusoid
A waveform that moves with simple harmonic motion.

sinistral *adj* ˈsĭnĭstrəl [Lat *sinister* left]
Situated on the left side.

sinus *n* ˈsīnus [Lat *sinus* recess, bend]
A cavity, recess, or channel.

sinus, ethmoid *np* [Lat *sinus* recess, bend; Gk *ethmos* sieve + Gk *eidos* form]
A collection of many small spaces situated beside the bridge of the nose.

sinus, frontal *np* [Lat *sinus* recess, bend; Lat *frons* forehead]
A pair of sinuses situated in the frontal bone above the eyes.

sinus, maxillary *np* [Lat *sinus* recess, bend; Lat *maxilla* jaw]
Relatively large sinuses situated within the cheekbones.

sinus, paranasal *np* [Lat *sinus* recess, bend; Gk *para* beside + Lat *nasus* nose]
Four pairs (maxillary, frontal, ethmoid, and sphenoid) of air-filled spaces in the skull that drain into the nasal cavity. The sinuses lighten the skull and resonate the voice.

sinus, sigmoid *np* [Lat *sinus* recess, bend; Gk *sigmoides* S-shaped]
A pair of sinuses that arise below the temporal bones and that drain blood into the internal jugular vein.

sinus, sphenoid *np* [Lat *sinus* recess, bend; Gk *sphen* wedge + Gk *eidos* form]
A sinus, with the appearance of a bat with wings extended, that is situated at the base of the skull in the sphenoid bone.

sinusitis *n*
Inflammation of the mucous membrane of the paranasal sinuses.

sinusoid *n*
Also: sine wave
A waveform, e.g., of a pure tone, that moves with simple harmonic motion, i.e., a smooth repetitive oscillation.

SISI (short increment sensitivity) test *np*
A test of the ability to detect small (1 dB) increases in intensity close to threshold, which may be indicative of cochlear pathology.

sisomicin (sisomycin) *n* sĭsōˈmĭsĭn
An ototoxic antibiotic related to gentamycin.

six cc coupler *np*
An artificial ear used for the calibration of audiometer headphones.

skeleton earmold (earmould) *np*
An earmold in which the central concha portion has been cut away.

skewed *adj*
Varying from the normal. A statistical term that is applicable where the majority of scores from a test, when plotted graphically, are clumped toward one end or the other.

skewed, negatively *np*
A distribution where the majority of scores or events are located below the mean.

skewed, positively *np*
A distribution where the majority of scores or events are located above the mean.

ski-slope *adj*
Having normal hearing in the low frequencies followed by a rapid increase in thresholds in the higher frequencies, equal to or greater than 25 dB per octave.

skirt, filter *np*
The range of frequencies either side of the center frequency.

slit leak *np*
A pathway for the escape of sound from around the circumference of an earmold, which may be undesirable.

slope *n*
The steepness of the ascent or descent, e.g., the steepness of a filter.

slow phase *np*
A slow adjusting eye movement that occurs in nystagmus following the quick phase, i.e., when there is a rapid eye movement in one direction.

slow vertex response (SVR) *np*
Also: cortical evoked response audiometry
A cortical evoked response to sound recorded at 50-500 ms latency.

socioacusis *n* sōsēōakʹyūsĭs [Lat *socius* companion + Gk *akousis* sense of hearing]
Hearing loss due to aging, diseases, and the noises encountered in normal everyday living (but excluding hearing loss due to occupational noise exposure).

sodium (Na+) *n*
An alkaline metal element that is important for maintaining the functioning of the body. Potassium and sodium are electrolytes, i.e., they have the capacity to conduct electricity, and intracellular fluid is high in positively charged potassium ions. An electrochemical gradient is maintained across all cell membranes, such that the interior of the cell is negatively (less positively) charged in comparison to the outside of the cell. During action potentials, i.e., when nerve cells fire, chemically gated channels open to allow movement of potassium and sodium, which causes electrical signals that pass along the nerve fibers to the brain.

sodium potassium pump *np*
A protein found in the membrane of all cells that transports sodium and potassium across the cell membranes. It corrects the overshoot that occurs after an action potential and returns the membrane to its resting value by pumping out sodium ions and moving potassium ions in.

soft failure *np*
A problem with a cochlear implant, in which the implant does not sound as it should, but upon investigation, no error can be found with the device.

soft palate *np*
Also: velum
A fold of tissue at the back of the roof of the mouth that separates the mouth from the pharynx. It is used during swallowing and in producing velar speech sounds, e.g., /k/ and /g/.

soft surgery *np*
Surgery that specifically sets out to minimize damage, e.g., in cochlear implantation when the surgeon uses a range of measures to prevent damage, such as making a minimal entry hole to the cochlea, ensuring no debris falls into the cochlea and using chemicals or steroids to reduce inflammation.

solid earmold (earmould) *np*
A custom-made earmold that fills the whole concha and which is used mainly with high-powered hearing aids.

solvent, wax *np*
A product used to soften ear wax.

soma *n* sōmᴀ [Gk *soma* body]
The cell body of a neuron containing the nucleus.

somat- *adj*
Pertaining to the body.

somatic cells *np*
Cells of an organism, other than germ cells.

somatic nervous system *np*
The part of the peripheral nervous system that controls the movement of skeletal muscles or transmits somatosensory information to the central nervous system.

somatosensory *adj*
Pertaining to sensory information from the skin (touch) and internal organs. The information is relayed from the peripheral receptors of the body via unipolar sensory neurons that have their cell bodies in the dorsal root ganglia, and enters the spinal cord through the dorsal nerve root before being transferred to the brain. Conscious awareness and localization of sensory stimuli is a function of the somatosensory cortex in the post central gyrus of the parietal lobe.

sone *n* [Lat *sonus* sound]
A unit of loudness. Loudness does not grow equally across the frequency range, but grows more rapidly with increasing intensity for low-frequency tones. One sone is equal to the loudness of a 1 kHz tone presented at 40 phons. Two sones is equal to a sound that is judged to be twice as loud, etc.

sonic *adj*
Pertaining to sound within the range of human hearing.

sonics *n*
A general term for the study of mechanical vibrations in matter.

sonorant/sonant *adj* [Lat *sonare* to sound]
Pertaining to a voiced sound produced with relatively unobstructed air flow, e.g., /w/, /n/, /m/, etc. and vowels.

sonotubometry *n* [Lat *sonus* sound + tube + Gk *metron* a measure]
An assessment of the Eustachian tube in which sound is introduced through the nose and measured in the ear canal.

sound *n*
Vibrations in a transmitting medium that are capable of producing the sensation perceived by the hearing mechanism.

sound absorption *np*
The reduction of sound energy through the use of certain materials; generally the energy is converted to heat.

sound absorption coefficient *np*
Also: acoustic absorption coefficient; acoustic absorbency
A single number rating that indicates how much sound is absorbed by a material or medium. It is the ratio of absorbed sound energy to the energy in the incident sound. An ideal absorber, i.e., where no sound is reflected, has a coefficient of 1.00.

sound attenuation *np*
A decrease in the magnitude, amplitude, or intensity of sound by absorption or the use of electrical resistors and capacitors (an attenuator).

sound bore *np*
The channel through the earmold along which amplified sound is directed into the ear canal.

sound exposure *np*
The amount of sound received by the ear over a given period.

sound field *np*
1. Any environment that contains sound. 2. A region through which sound waves, standing or progressive, propagate from a sound source. 3. An enclosed space in which the diffused sound waves are random in magnitude, phase, and direction, constituting reverberant sound.

sound generator *np*
1. A device that creates sound. 2. A device that emits sound intended to mask tinnitus (fully or partially); *colloq* a tinnitus masker.

sound intensity *np*
Also: sound power
The absolute power (in watts [W]) of a sound source, measured as the average rate at which sound energy passes through a unit area, normal to the direction of propagation.

sound intensity level (SIL) *np*
The intensity of a sound, expressed in decibel (dB SIL) above the reference level, 10–12 W/m2. Sound pressure is the result of sound power and because sound intensity level is difficult to measure, it is common to measure the sound-pressure level instead.

sound-level meter (SLM) *np*
A device, consisting of a microphone, an amplifier and a meter, that is used to measure sound pressure.

sound pressure *np*
The deviations in pressure (away from atmospheric pressure) caused by a sound wave.

sound-pressure level (SPL) *np*
A ratio between the sound pressure and the standard audiologic reference pressure, which is 0.00002 pascals (20 micropascals). This sound pressure corresponds to 0 dB SPL and is based on the minimum pressure required to cause hearing in the mid frequency region. The dB SPL scale takes no account of the way hearing varies with frequency.

sound processor *np*
Also: speech processor
A device that encodes the speech signal and transmits it to a receiver, e.g., in a cochlear implant.

soundproof *adj*
Pertaining to preventing sound from entering a space.

sound shadow *np*
A region in which a sound field is reduced in magnitude in relation to the free field value as a result of its incidence on an obstacle.

sound-treated *adj*
Pertaining to the reduction of sound from outside, e.g., having sound absorbent material used in the construction.

space of Nuel *np* Named after Jeanne-Pierre Nuel (1847–1920), a Luxembourgian physician and professor of ophthalmology and physiology of sensory organs, who published a description of this space in addition to many other observations of the anatomy of the cochlea.
A fluid-filled cleft between the inner and outer tunnels of the organ of Corti through which nerve fibers pass.

spasm *n* [Gk *spasmos* violent pull]
A sudden muscular contraction.

spasmodic dysphonia *np* [Gk *spasmos* violent pull; Gk *dus-* bad + Gk *phone* sound]
An involuntary movement of the muscles in the larynx that causes brief disruption of the voice.

spatial processing disorder (SPD) *np*
An inability to separate a speech or other desired signal from competing environmental sounds, a form of central auditory processing disorder.

spatial unmasking *np* ˈspāshᵁl
An improvement in the identification of sounds that occurs when they arrive from a different location to simultaneous masking sounds.

speaking tube *np obs*
A type of ear trumpet with a voice pipe for conveying speech over a short distance.

specific *adj*
Clearly defined or relating to a particular subject.

specification sheet *np*
A document that provides a variety of performance characteristics, e.g., gain, frequency response, and maximum output, for a specified hearing aid.

specific language disorder *np*
A language impairment in the absence of any intellectual disorder or hearing loss, etc.

specificity *n* ˈspěsĭˈfĭsĭtē
1. A statistical measure of the proportion of people who do not have a disease who are correctly identified by a given test. The inverse of sensitivity. 2. The narrowness of a range, e.g., where a substance will be effective.

spectacle aid *np*
A hearing aid attached to or part of a pair of glasses. This may be an air-conduction or bone-conduction hearing aid.

spectral *adj* [Lat *spectrum* image, appearance]
Pertaining to frequency or a specific frequency range.

spectral analysis *np*
The analysis of the individual frequency components of an acoustic signal.

spectral cues *np*
Monaural sound cues due to spectral amplification (i.e., pinna echoes interact with the various frequencies received at the ear), which assist in determining localization of sound in the vertical direction.

spectral peak (SPEAK) *np*
A sound-coding strategy used in cochlear implants.

spectrogram *n* [Lat *spectrum* image, appearance + Gk *gramma* thing written]
The graph produced by a spectrograph that plots the way frequency and intensity vary over time. Frequency is plotted against time with intensity indicated by the darkness of the trace.

spectrograph *n* [Lat *spectrum* image, appearance + Gk *graphos* writing]
A device that splits a sound wave into its component frequencies and produces a spectrogram.

spectrum *n* [Lat *spectrum* image, appearance]
1. The pure tones that make up a wave envelope (the spectral envelope). 2. A distribution of components arranged according to certain characteristics, e.g., component colors, component electromagnetic wavelengths, component frequency sounds, etc. 3. A wide range.

speculum *n* *pl* specula [Lat *speculum* mirror]
The small funnel that affixes to an otoscope for examining the ear canal.

speech *n*
Oral language.

speech and language therapist (SLT) *np*
A professional who is qualified to assess and treat speech, language, and communication problems.

speech audiogram *np*
A graph that shows how an individual's ability to discriminate speech varies with intensity.

speech audiometry *np*
A method of assessing an individual's hearing for speech.

speech banana *np colloq*
Also: long-term average speech spectrum (LTASS)
The long-term average speech spectrum superimposed on the audiogram.

speech coding *np*
A signal processing strategy to compress audio data, e.g., used in cochlear implants.

speech detection *np*
The ability to recognize the presence of speech sounds.

speech detection level *np*
The point at which speech sounds are just audible (but not generally comprehended).

speech discrimination *np*
The ability to perceive the difference between speech sounds.

speech frequencies *np*
1. The frequencies that are considered most important for the perception of speech. 2. The frequencies within which speech occurs.

speech intelligibility *np*
The amount of speech, expressed as a percentage, that is understood by a listener.

speech intelligibility index *np*
Also: articulation index
A means of quantifying the amount of the speech signal available to the listener.

speech mapping *np*
Also: visible speech mapping
A version of real ear measurement in which live or recorded speech is used as an input signal. The individual's auditory residual area and the processed speech signal from a hearing aid or cochlear implant are visually displayed simultaneously.

speech processor *np*
Also: sound processor
A device that encodes the speech signal and transmits it to a receiver, e.g., in a cochlear implant. Used in fitting and verification.

speech-reading *n*
The use of lip-reading, facial expression, and body language to aid speech understanding.

speech-reception threshold (SRT) *np*
The lowest level at which a person can just (i.e., 50% of the time) understand speech.

speech tracking *np*
A method of evaluating speech reception in which the individual has to repeat segments of a text over a given period. The number of words repeated correctly is given as a percentage of the total number of words presented.

speech trainer *np*
A device consisting of a microphone, amplifier, and a set of headphones, which may be used to provide a high quality sound signal in individual speech teaching sessions for deaf children.

speech-weighted noise *np*
Noise that has a sound pressure level that is constant from 125 Hz to 1 kHz and falls by 12 dB per octave from 1 kHz to 6 kHz. This corresponds to the long-term average speech spectrum.

speed of sound *np*
A measure of how fast sound travels through a given medium and at a given pressure and temperature. Standard values that are often used for sound in air are approximate values, i.e., speed of sound in air = 350 m/s.

sphenoid bone *np* sfēnoid [Gk *sphen* wedge + Gk *eidos* shape]
An irregularly shaped bone that lies in the middle of the floor of the cranial cavity and holds the other cranial bones tightly together. Its shape resembles a butterfly with outstretched wings.

sphenoid sinus *np* [Gk *sphen* wedge + Gk *eidos* form; Lat *sinus* recess, bend]
A sinus that has the appearance of a bat with wings extended that is situated at the base of the skull in the sphenoid bone.

spherical wave *np* [Gk *sphaira* ball]
A propagated wave in which the wave fronts are ever-expanding concentric spheres.

spike *n*
A rapid increase in voltage followed by a rapid decrease.

spiral *adj*
A winding around a center or pole that gradually recedes from or approaches it, thus forming a succession of turns or curves, e.g., the cochlea and the spiral organs within it.

spiral ganglia *np* [Gk *ganglion* nerve center]
A mass of nerve tissue containing the cell nuclei, that spirals through the cochlea.

spiral lamina *np* [Lat *lamina* thin layer]
The thin bony shelf in the cochlea that juts out from the modiolus in the cochlea and to which the inner edge of the basilar membrane is attached.

spiral ligament *np* [Lat *ligare* to bind]
The connective tissue that joins the outer edge of the basilar membrane to the wall of the cochlea.

spiral limbus *np* [Lat *limbus* edge, border]
Also: inner spiral sulcus
The thickened periosteum border of the spiral lamina that forms a curved lip to which the tectorial membrane is attached.

SPL-ogram *n*
A graph that shows all measurements converted into real ear sound-pressure level (SPL) to facilitate direct comparison and that can be used in hearing aid fitting with targets typically shown for soft, medium, and loud sounds.

spondee *n* [Gk *spondeios* spondeic (the kind of meter used in songs to accompany wine offerings) from Gk *sponde* a wine offering]
A word of two syllables, each having equal stress, e.g., mushroom.
Deriv: –*adj* spondaic

spongy bone *np*
Also: trabecular bone; cancellous bone
Bone composed of a network of branching bony spicules that has the appearance of a sponge with bone marrow contained in the spaces, e.g., the type of bone that develops around the stapes footplate in otosclerosis.

spontaneous *adj* [Lat *sponte* of one's own accord]
Occuring without an evoking stimulus, e.g., spontaneous nystagmus.

sporadic trait *np* [Gk *sporas* scattered]
A characteristic that appears in an individual without any evident genetic basis.

squamous *adj* ˈskwāmus [Lat *squamosus* scaly]
Having scales.

squamous cell carcinoma *np*
Skin cancer that occasionally spreads to nearby lymph nodes and other organs.

square wave *np*
A wave form that contains only odd harmonics of the fundamental frequency, which gives it a repetitive square appearance with equal high periods and low periods. It is used in digital switching circuits.

squelch *n*
Also: expansion; noise-gating
The ability to listen selectively, e.g., to pick speech out of background noise. This is possible when listening binaurally and it is attributed to suppression by the central auditory system.

staggered spondaic word test (SSW) *np*
A test in which the first syllable of a spondee is presented to one ear and the second syllable is presented simultaneously to the other ear.

standard *np*
A recognized exemplar that prescribes rules for judging quality and accuracy, e.g., European or American hearing aid standards.

standard coupler *np*
Also: 2 cc coupler; reference coupler
A device that joins the receiver of a hearing aid to the microphone of a sound level meter. It is designed with a standard volume of 2 cc and used for measuring the acoustic output of hearing aids.

standard deviation *np*
A statistical measurement of the dispersion of a frequency distribution away from the mean.

standing wave *np*
Also: stationary wave
A wave that appears to be stationary that is caused by two identical trains of simple harmonic waves following the same

path in a medium, but going in the opposite direction. It occurs when a reflected wave and an incident wave interact, such that there are points of increased intensity and other points where there are dead spots or areas of decreased intensity.

stapedectomy *n* [Lat *stapes* stirrup + Gk *ektome* excision]
Surgery to remove the stapes and insert a prosthesis.

stapedius/stapedial *adj*
Of the stapes.

stapedius muscle *np*
The muscle attached to the neck of the stapes that pulls the stapes away from the oval window and stiffens the ossicular chain.

stapedial reflex *np*
The contraction of the stapedius muscle in response to a loud sound.

stapedotomy *n* [Lat *stapes* stirrup + Gk –*tomia* cutting]
A modified stapedectomy in which the stapes footplate is left in the oval window. A hole is drilled in the footplate to receive the prosthesis.

stapes *n* ˈstāpīz [Lat *stapes* stirrup]
Also: colloq stirrup
The innermost bone of the ossicular chain that transmits sound vibrations to the oval window of the cochlea. It is the smallest bone in the human body.

stapes crura *np* [Lat *stapes* stirrup; Lat *crura* legs]
The two sides of the arch of bone that joins the footplate to the head and neck of the stapes.

stapes fixation *np*
Also: stapes ankylosis
Progressive hardening of abnormal bone growth around the stapes fixing it in the oval window, as occurs in otosclerosis. Causes conductive hearing loss.

stapes footplate *np*
The base of the stapes that transmits sound vibrations to the oval window.

staphylococcus *n* stăfˈīlōˈkŏkus *pl* staphylococci [Gk *staphule* bunch of grapes + Gk *kokkos* berry]
Clusters of bacteria (most commonly staphylococcal aureus) that cause staphylococcal infections, such as skin infections, e.g., furuncles, and invasive infections, e.g., blood poisoning.

startle reflex *np*
A reflex to loud sounds present in normal babies between newborn and about 3 months of age. The reflex involves a sudden stretching out of the arms with fanned fingers and flexing of the legs.

-stasis *suffix* [Gk *stasis* stoppage]
Slowing or stopping.

static *adj* [Gk *statikos* causing to stand]
At rest.

static pressure *np*
Constant unchanging pressure.

stationary wave *np*
Also: standing wave
A wave that appears to be stationary that is caused by two identical trains of simple harmonic waves following the same path in a medium, but going in the opposite direction. It occurs when a reflected wave and an incident wave interact, such that there are points of increased intensity and other points where there are dead spots or areas of decreased intensity.

statoconia *n, pl* stătoˈkōnēa *sg* statoconium [Gk *statos* standing + Gk *konia* dust]
Also: otoconia
Minute granules of calcium carbonate in the gelatinous otolithic membrane of the vestibular system. Cilia are embedded in the membrane and movement of these stimulates sensory cells to pass positional information to the brain, which is important in the maintenance of the body's upright position in respect to gravity.

steady-state *adj*
In an unvarying state.

stellate *adj* [Lat *stellatus* star-shaped]
Star-shaped, e.g., stellate ganglion.

Stenger test *np* Named after E. Stenger, who described the test in 1900.
A test of nonorganic unilateral hearing loss that is based on the principle that when two simultaneous tones of the same frequency are played to the ears only the most intense can be heard.

stenograph *n* [Gk *stenos* narrow + Gk *graphia* writing]
An American specialized shorthand typing machine (similar to British palantype) that can record speech by means of phonograms.

stenosis *n* stĕnōsĭs *pl* stenoses [Gk *stenosis* narrowing]
Abnormal narrowing of a passage, e.g., stenosis of the ear canal.
Deriv: -adj stenotic

stereocilia/stereovilli *n, pl sg* stereocilium/stereovillus [Gk *stereos* solid, stiff + Lat *cilium* hair, eyelash; Lat *villi* shaggy hair]
The stiff hairlike nonmotile projections from the hair cells in the inner ear that play a vital role in the transduction of electrical impulses to the auditory nerve fibers.

steroid *n*
A chemical of low molecular weight derived from cholesterol. Steroid hormones affect their target cells by attaching to receptors and initiating chemical changes within the cell.

Stewart Bergstrom syndrome *np*
Named after Janet M. Stewart and LaVonne Bernadene Bergstrom (1928–2008), American pediatric otolaryngologists, who reported the condition in the *Journal of Pediatrics* in 1971.
An autosomal dominant syndrome characterized by hand malformation, including curved fingers, and mild to severe sensorineural hearing loss.

Stickler syndrome *np* Named after Gunnar B. Stickler (1925–2010), a German-American pediatrician, who defined the condition in 1965.
Also: hereditary progressive arthroophthalmopathy
A progressive genetic disorder that affects the connective tissues. Characterized by a flattened facial appearance, caused by underdeveloped bones in the middle of the face, eye abnormalities including retinal detachment, joint problems, and progressive hearing loss that is usually conductive. Cleft palate, a large tongue, and small lower jaw are also common.

stigma *n pl* stigmata; stigmas [Gk *stigma* a mark]
1. A mark of negative discrimination, shame, or discredit. 2. A sign of some specific disease or disorder.

stimulus *n* [Lat *stimulare* to stimulate]
Something that increases activity or produces a reaction.

stimulus rate *np*
The number of stimuli per unit of time.

stock hearing aid *np*
A hearing aid in the possession of the provider, usually intended for temporary use or trial.

stone deaf *np colloq* Possibly named from noise-induced hearing loss caused by working in stone quarries.
Profoundly deaf or having the appearance to a layman of being completely deaf.

stop *n*
A brief silence that occurs within a word, between two consonants.

stop consonant *np*
A consonant formed by stopping the airflow briefly followed by its sudden release.

stop, glottal *np* [Gk *glotta* tongue]
Closure of the glottis causing a brief stoppage of the airstream. It is used in some

dialects, often as a replacement for /t/, e.g., "bo(tt)le."

stored equalization *np*
Used in real ear measurement systems to record the leveling (equalizing) data at the reference microphone before a measurement is made.

strepto- *prefix* [Gk *streptos* twisted]
Occurring in chains, e.g., *Streptococcus* bacteria.

streptomycin *n*
A powerful aminoglycoside antibiotic that is ototoxic.

stressor *n*
A psychological, social, or physical factor that causes stress to an individual, e.g., bereavement, illness, debt, etc.

stria *n* ˈstrīə *pl* striae [Lat *stria* a furrow or a stripe]
1. A small groove. 2. A stripe.

stria vascularis *np* [Lat *stria* a stripe; Lat *vascularis* pertaining to a vessel]
The vascular upper portion of the spiral ligament located on the lateral wall of the cochlea. Produces endolymph and helps to maintain the endocochlear potential, i.e., the ionic concentrations in the endolymph.

striate *adj* [Lat *striatus* striped]
Striped.

stroke *n*
1. Lack of oxygen to the brain due to an interruption in the blood supply that causes brain damage which may produce permanent difficulties, e.g., paralysis, aphasia. 2. A blow given or received. 3. *obs* The mark or bruise left by a blow. 4. *obs* An electric shock.

stylo- *prefix* [Gk *stulos* a pillar]
A pointed pillar or process.

stylomastoid *adj* [Gk *stulos* a pillar + Gk *mastos* breast + Gk *eidos* shape]
Pertaining to the styloid.

stylomastoid foramen *np* [Gk *stulos* a pillar + Gk *mastos* breast + Gk *eidos* shape; Lat *foramen* hole, opening]

A passage into the bone between the styloid and mastoid processes where the facial nerve canal ends.

styrene *n* Named after the resin obtained from the storax tree from which it was first isolated.
Also: vinylbenzene; phenylethane
An ototoxic hydrocarbon liquid that is a by-product of petrol, used in the production of polystyrene and other materials. Styrene is toxic to many parts of the body, e.g., kidney, lungs, etc., and high exposures may cause hearing loss.

sub- *prefix* [Lat *sub* below]
Below.

subacute *adj*
1. Between acute and chronic. 2. Having a specific duration between acute and chronic, e.g., of 3 weeks to 3 months in otitis media.

subarachnoid space *np* sŭbarˈăknoid [Lat *sub* below + Gk *arakhne* spider's web + Gk *eidos* shape]
A cerebrospinal fluid-filled space that cushions the brain. It is situated between the pia mater and the arachnoid membrane.

subcortical *adj* [Lat *sub* below + Lat *cortex* bark, outer layer]
Below the cerebral cortex.

subdural *adj*
Situated below the dura mater.

subjective *adj*
1. Having its source in the mind. 2. Not objective, but relying on the cooperation of the individual, e.g., pure-tone audiometry is subjective as it relies on the individual pressing a button, etc.

subsonic *adj* [Lat *sub* below + Lat *sonus* sound]
Below the range of human hearing.

substitution *n* [Lat *substituere* to put in place of]
Replacement, e.g., 1. Consonant substitution, which is common in the speech of young children and profoundly deaf indi-

viduals. 2. Substitution therapy, which is used in retraining patients with no vestibular-ocular reflex (VOR) function (i.e., eye movements that normally compensate for head movement), to strengthen the use of other senses to improve balance.

subthreshold *adj*
A sensory stimulus that is below threshold, i.e., too weak to be perceived.

subtotal *adj*
1. Partial or less than total, e.g., subtotal hearing loss. 2. Removal of a part, not the whole, e.g., part of an organ.

sudden deafness *np*
A hearing loss that occurs suddenly, e.g., within one week, such as with perilymph fistula.

sulcus *n* 'sŭlkus *pl* sulci [Lat *sulcus* furrow, wrinkle]
A groove, furrow, or fissure.

sulcus, inner spiral *np*
Also: spiral limbus
The thickened periosteum border of the spiral lamina that forms a curved lip to which the tectorial membrane is attached.

summating potential *np* [Lat *summa* total]
A complex nonlinear response that occurs within the first 2–3 ms following a sound stimulus that arises from the hair cells and reflects the asymmetry of basilar membrane vibration. It is one of the main components of electrocochleography (together with the cochlear microphonic and the action potential) and usually appears as a hump on the first slope of the action potential wave.

summation *n*
A cumulative effect.

summation, binaural *np*
The enhancement of hearing that occurs when listening with both ears, i.e., approximately 3 dB–6 dB increase in loudness in comparison with monaural listening.

superficial *adj*
Pertaining to the surface.

superior *adj* [Lat *superior* upper]
Above.

superior canal dehiscence syndrome (SCDS) *np* [Lat *superior* upper; Lat *dehiscere* to gape open]
A condition in which the part of the temporal bone over the superior semicircular canal is thin or absent. Characteristics may include low-frequency conductive hearing loss, a feeling of fullness in the ear, hearing own body noises as loud, pulsatile tinnitus, headache, hyperacusis, and sound-induced vestibular symptoms.

superior cerebellar artery syndrome *np* [Lat *superior* upper; Lat *cerebellum* small brain; Gk *arteria* artery]
A syndrome caused by obstruction of the superior cerebellar artery, characterized by vertigo, partial hearing loss, slurred speech, cerebellar hemiataxia (palsy of one side), loss of sensation of pain and temperature on the opposite side, hypotonia (low muscle tone), and tremor.

superior colliculus *np* colliculi [Lat *superior* upper; Lat *colliculus* little hill]
One of a pair bumps, situated on the roof of the midbrain, concerned with integrating sensory information, including that concerned with hearing.

superior olive *np*
The collection of nuclei in the lower brainstem where binaural stimulation first occurs.

superior semicircular canal *np*
The uppermost canal in the vestibular system that responds to angular motion.

supersonic *adj obs* [Lat *super* above + Lat *sonus* sound]
Also: ultrasonic
Pertaining to frequencies above the limit of audible hearing.

suppression *n*
1. Stopping or lowering. 2. Prevention of electrical interference. 3. The conscious act of subduing a thought or feeling. 4. Nondevelopment of a body part.

suppurative *adj* 'sūpyu(e)rətĭv [Lat *sub* below + Lat *pus* pus]
Producing pus.

supra- *prefix* [Lat *supra* above]
Above.

supraaural *adj* [Lat *supra* above + Lat *auris* ear]
Over the ear, e.g., supraaural headphones.

suprasegmental *adj* [Lat *supra* above + Lat *segmentum* portion]
The prosodic features of speech, e.g., pitch, loudness, stress, rhythm, and intonation.

suprathreshold *adj*
Above threshold level, e.g., speech discrimination tests.

surfer's ear *np colloq*
Also: exostosis
The growth of bone from another bone or cartilage, which occurs frequently found in the bony portion of the ear canal, which occurs frequently in people participating in water-related sports like swimming or surfing, due to prolonged exposure to cold water.

surgery *n* [Gk *kheirourgia* handwork, surgery]
The practice of treating medical conditions by operating.

susceptance *n*
The ease with which an alternating current can pass through a capacitance or inductance.

sustentacular cells *np*
Also: supporting cells; border cells of Held
Supporting cells of the epithelium found in the organ of Corti.

suture *n* 'sūcher ('sūtyuer) [Lat *sutura* sewing]
A stitch or a row of stitches holding together two parts of a wound.

sweep *n*
1. A swift and smooth movement. 2. A continuous increase over a given range, e.g., in frequency or pressure.

sweep frequency *np*
A continuous increase in frequency through a wide frequency range, maintaining a constant output level for each frequency.

swimmer's ear *np colloq* Named this because one possible cause of the condition is water remaining in the ear canal after swimming, resulting in a moist environment in which bacteria can thrive.
Also: otitis externa
Inflammation of the external ear.

swim plug *np*
A molded solid earplug that prevents water from entering the ear canal.

switch on *v/np*
-v To activate. *-np* The point at which a cochlear implant processor is fitted and activated for the first time.

syllabic compression *np*
Compression with a low threshold of activation, low compression ratio, and a short attack and release time (shorter than a typical speech syllable), which is intended to reduce the differences between vowels and consonants to make soft sounds louder without causing vowels to be too loud.

syllable *n* [Gk *sullabe* (from Gk *sun-* together + Gk *lambanein* to take)]
A unit of speech that can be spoken as a single element and that is composed of a vowel, with or without an accompanying consonant or consonants.
Deriv: -adj syllabic

symmetric *adj* [Gk *sun-* together + Gk *metron* measure]
1. Equal distribution about a dividing line. 2. Having a balanced arrangement, e.g., a symmetric hearing loss is one that is very similar in each ear.

sympathetic nervous system *np* [Gk *sun* with + Gk *pathos* feeling]
Part of the autonomic nervous system that originates in the spinal cord and brainstem. Increases blood pressure and heartbeat and slows digestion, important in the "fight or flight" response.

symphalangism *n* ˈsĭmfălănjĭzm [Gk *sun-* together + Gk *phalanges* finger/toe bones]
Fusion of the finger and/or toe joints.

symptom *n* [Gk *sumptoma* chance, symptom]
Subjective evidence of disease or physical disturbance, i.e., a feature noticed by the individual suffering from it, e.g., pain, throbbing, etc.

synapse *n* ˈsĭnăps (ˈsīnăps) [Gk *sun-* together + Gk *hapsis* a joining]
The junction between two neurons.
Deriv: –adj synaptic

synaptic cleft/gap *np*
The space at the synapse that separates the pre- and postsynaptic membranes. Nerve impulses pass through the extracellular fluid in the synaptic cleft by means of a chemical neurotransmitter.

syndactyly *n* sĭnˈdăktĭlē [Gk *sun-* together + Gk *daktulos* finger]
Also: webbing
The joining of digits by soft tissue.

syndrome *n* [Gk *sundrome* syndrome]
A condition characterized by a set of associated symptoms.

synesthesia (synaesthesia) *n* [Gk *sun-* together + Gk *aesthesis* sensation]
A phenomenon due to crosstalk in the brain, in which sound (or other stimulus) evokes a combined sensory experience, e.g., sound and color, or sound and taste.

syntax *n* [Gk *suntaxis* arrangement]
The way linguistic elements are put together, i.e., word order.

synthetic speech *np* [Gk *suntithenai* to place together]
Computer-generated speech.

syphilis *n* [From *Syphilus*, the fictional name for the supposed first sufferer of the disease in a poem of 1530]
Syphilis is a sexually transmitted bacterial disease that can be treated with antibiotics. In its early stages, there may be few symptoms, e.g., painless sores and swollen lymph nodes. Later fever, fatigue, rashes, aches, and pains develop and eventually it leads to heart, brain, and nervous system problems, including hearing loss.

syphilis, congenital *np*
A disease that may be passed from the pregnant mother to the infant who may be born deaf.

systemic *adj* [Gk *sustema* arrangement]
1. Pertaining to the whole system. 2. Freely transported within the body.

systemic disease *np*
A disease that affects many organs or the body as a whole, e.g., autoimmune disease, which may include ear, nose, and throat problems.

T

tacrolimus *n* ˈtăkrolĭmŭs
An immunosuppressant medication used to prevent organ rejection after transplantation, which may be a rare cause of sudden hearing loss with tinnitus.

tactile *adj* [Lat *tactilis* pertaining to touch]
Relating to touch.

tactile aid *np*
An aid that delivers speech signals as a sensation of touch to provide limited acoustic information.

tag *n*
A rudimentary appendage of tissue that is sometimes seen on the face in front of the pinna.

talk-forward *n*
The facility to speak through a microphone to someone wearing headphones, e.g., during a hearing test.

target *n*
A fixed objective, e.g., the target gain for a hearing aid.

target cell *np*
A type of cell directly affected, e.g., by a hormone.

Tartini tone *np* ˈtahtēnē Named after Giuseppe Tartini (1692–1770), an Italian violinist and composer, who is credited with the discovery of this phenomenon.
A third tone that may be noticeable when two tones are played simultaneously and that causes a low-pitch buzzing sound that has a frequency equal to the difference between the frequencies of the two tones.

tectorial membrane *np* [Lat *tectorium* a covering; Lat *membrana* partition]
The gelatinous structure that is attached along one edge to the spiral limbus and the other edge to the outer border of the organ of Corti and that lies over the stereocilia of the hair cells in the organ of Corti.

tegmental wall *np* [Lat *tegumentum* a covering]
The thin wall of bone, part of the temporal bone, that forms the roof of the middle ear.

telecoil (T) *n*
A small coil of wire around a core that picks up a magnetic signal, i.e., an analogous electric current is induced in the presence of an alternating magnetic field. It is part of an inductive loop system used as the input source on a hearing aid instead of (or as well as) the microphone.

telencephalon *n* [Gk *tele-* far off + Gk *enkephalon* brain]
The most highly developed part of the forebrain, i.e., the anterior part that contains the cerebral hemispheres.

telephone theory *np obs* [Gk *tele-* far off + Gk *phone* sound]
A theory put forward in 1866 by William Rutherford (1839–1899), a British physician, that suggested any hair cell may be stimulated anywhere along the basilar membrane, and that the basilar membrane vibrates as a whole in the same way as the diaphragm of a telephone and that the analysis of sound occurs in the brain.

temporal *adj* [Lat *tempora* temples (sides of forehead)]
1. Pertaining to the temples and the skull behind the eye sockets. 2. Pertaining to time.

temporal bones *np*
The two bones of the skull that contain the middle and inner ears and articulate with the two parietal bones. Each temporal bone is divided into four portions: squamous, mastoid, petrous, and tympanic.

temporal coding *np* [Lat *tempus* time]
The way in which timing information is carried in the pattern of firing in the auditory nerve, believed to be primarily a result of neural phase locking to the stimulus waveform.

temporal integration *np*
The ability to hear longer duration sounds as louder or stronger.

temporal resolution *np*
The ability to detect brief changes in an acoustic waveform.

temporary threshold shift (TTS) *np*
Hearing loss of short duration following exposure to loud noise.

temporomandibular joint (TMJ) *np* těm-pawrō'măndĭbyulα [Lat *tempora* temples (sides of forehead) + Lat *mandibula* jaw bone]
The joint between the head of the lower jawbone and the temporal bone.

temporomandibular joint dysfunction *np* těmpawrō'măndĭbyulα
A disorder of the temporomandibular joint and associated structures that may cause pain, limited mouth opening and joint noises, e.g., clicking or crackling.

TEN (threshold equalizing noise) test *np*
A test to indicate dead regions in the cochlea, developed by Brian Moore (b 1946), professor of auditory perception, and colleagues at the University of Cambridge (2000). The test involves finding the hearing threshold for a tone presented in a masking noise known as threshold equalizing noise, using a similar method to that used in traditional pure tone audiometry. A threshold for the tone that is 10 dB higher than the normal value is taken as indicating a dead region. There are also modified versions of the test, e.g., the TEN (HL) test and the TEN (ER3).

tendon *n* [Gk *tenon* sinew]
A band of tough fibrous tissue that connects a muscle to the bone.

tensor *adj* 'těnsaw [Lat *tendere* to stretch]
A muscle that tightens part of the body.

tensor tympani *np* 'těnsaw 'tǐmpǎnī [Lat *tendere* to stretch; Gk *tumpanon* drum]
A muscle of the middle ear attached by a tendon to the manubrium of the malleus.

The tensor tympani and stapedius muscles contract to stiffen the ossicles in response to loud sound or tactile stimulation to parts of the face, which helps to protect the inner ear from noise damage, especially from low-frequency noise.

tensor palati/tensor veli palati *np* 'těnsaw pα'lahtī/'těnsaw 'vēlī pα'lahtī [Lat *tendere* to stretch; Lat *velum* covering, veil; Lat *palatum* palate]
The muscle that arises from the scaphoid fossa of the sphenoid bone and is attached to the cartilage of the Eustachian tube. It assists in opening the Eustachian tube during yawning and swallowing to allow air pressure in the tympanic cavity to equalize with that in the ear canal.

teratogen *n* te'rătajen [Gk *teras* monster + Gk *-genes* produced by]
Any drug, chemical, disease, or process that causes malformation in the fetus.
Deriv: –adj teratogenic

teratoma *n* těrα'tōmα *pl* teratomata [Gk *teras* monster + Gk *-oma* denoting tumor, swelling]
A germ cell tumor formed from tissue foreign to the site of the growth. Some tumors may contain teeth, jawbone or fingers, etc. Teratoma may occur (rarely) in the head and neck.

terminal button/bouton *np*
The expanded knob at the end of an axon branch that forms the synapse with another neuron.

test *v/n*
–v To examine. *–n* A process to determine or evaluate something.

test battery *np*
Any variety of tests being used for testing, e.g., pure tone audiometry, tympanometry, and speech audiometry could form a battery of tests.

test box *np*
A box or device used to provide a quiet environment for testing the performance of hearing aids.

test ear *np*
The ear to be evaluated and into which a test signal is directed.

test-retest reliability *np*
The extent to which a test will provide the same results when repeated on the same subject and under the same conditions.

tetanus antitoxin *np* [Gk *tetanus* muscular spasm; Gk *anti* against + Gk *toxikon* poison]
A vaccine given to provide immunization against tetanus that can be a rare cause of hearing loss.

tetracycline *n*
An antibiotic used to treat bacterial infections such as acne, gonorrhea, and chlamydia, which may be ototoxic (rare).

text telephone *np*
A keyboard and modem that allows a person to communicate by telephone without speaking.

thalamus *n* [Gk *thalamos* chamber]
A dual-lobed mass of gray matter, situated in the posterior part of the forebrain, below the cerebral cortex, that relays auditory and other sensory impulses to the cerebral cortex.

theory *n* [Gk *theoria* contemplation, speculation]
An explanation that is supported by observable data.

therapy *n* [Gk *therapeia* healing]
A process to help someone overcome psychological difficulties.

third octave *adj*
Having a bandwidth of one third of an octave.

third-octave filter *np*
A bandpass filter with a bandwidth of one third of an octave.

third-order neurons (neurones) *np*
Neurons that transmit information from the thalamus to the primary cortex.

three neuron (neurone) arc *np*
Also: vestibuloocular reflex (VOR)
The reflex arc between the vestibular system and the muscles of the eyes, which maintains gaze stability by causing compensatory eye movements when the head is rotated.

threshold *n*
Also: limen
The limit below which a stimulus cannot be detected.

threshold, absolute *np*
Also: absolute sensitivity
The lowest intensity of a stimulus that is just detectable (50% of the time).

threshold, aided *np*
The level at which an acoustic signal, e.g., a pure tone, first becomes audible for an individual using a hearing aid.

threshold difference *np*
Also: just noticeable difference (JND) in intensity; difference limen for intensity (DLI); differential threshold
The least difference in intensity that can be detected between two stimuli (50% of the time), e.g., the smallest detectable change in intensity of a pure tone.

threshold of discomfort *np*
Also: uncomfortable loudness level
The level at which sound becomes uncomfortably loud for an individual.

threshold of excitation *np*
The value of the membrane potential that must be reached to produce an action potential.

threshold of hearing *np*
The minimum level of sound that is just audible for an individual. In audiometry, usually taken to be the lowest level heard 50% of the time in a series of ascending trials.

threshold kneepoint/knee point (TK) *np*
The point at which a hearing aid circuit changes from linear to nonlinear amplification, i.e., the point at which the intensity of the input (or output) signal acti-

vates the compression circuit and begins to reduce the gain. On a graph, the change in angle looks like a knee joint.

threshold level (T-level) *np*
The lowest stimulation level at which a train of electrical pulses is consistently detected and identified as sound by a cochlear implant recipient.

threshold of overload *np*
Also: threshold of aural overload
The minimum intensity level at which nonlinear distortion, evidenced by the presence of harmonics, starts to occur in the cochlea.

threshold of pain *np*
The point at which sound becomes painfully loud for an individual.

threshold shift *np*
A change in a hearing threshold due to masking, or over time.

thrombosis *n* [Gk *thrombos* blood clot + Gk *-osis* denoting a diseased state]
The formation or presence of a thrombus.

thrombus *n* [Gk *thrombos* blood clot]
A blood clot.

thyroplasty *n* [Gk *thureoeides* shield-shaped + Gk *plasis* formation]
Surgical alteration of the cartilage in the larynx to improve the voice.

Tietz syndrome *np* tētz Named after W. Alexander Tietz (1864–1927), a German surgeon, who published a description of the condition in a large three-generation family in 1963.
Also: oculocutaneous albinism
An autosomal dominant genetic syndrome of hypopigmentation and deafness, which is characterized by a white forelock; white spots on the arms, legs, and abdomen; blue eyes; and bilateral profound congenital sensorineural deafness.

timbre *n* ˈtămbₐ (ˈtămbrₐ) [Gk *tumpanon* drum]
The quality of a sound that allows an individual to distinguish between complex sounds with the same loudness and pitch, mainly due to the harmonic content.

tinnitus *n* tĭnˈītus (ˈtĭnĭtus) [Lat *tinnitus* ringing, tinkling]
Also: aural murmurs; acuphen
A sensation of sound in the head or ears without external origin.

tinnitus aurium *np* tĭnˈītus (ˈtĭnĭtus) ˈowrēum [Lat *tinnitus* ringing, tinkling; Lat *aurium* of the ears]
A sensation of sound in the ears without external origin.

tinnitus cerebri *np* tĭnˈītus (ˈtĭnĭtus) sĕˈrēbrē [Lat *tinnitus* ringing, tinkling; Lat *cerebri* of the brain]
A sensation of sound in the head without external origin.

tinnitus, objective *np*
1. Tinnitus that can be heard externally by others. 2. Tinnitus that can be linked to causes such as vascular anomalies.

tinnitus masker *np colloq*
Also: sound generator
A device that emits sound intended to mask tinnitus (fully or partially).

tinnitus matching *np*
The process in which an individual matches the pitch of his/her tinnitus to the pitch of a tone.

tinnitus, muscular *np*
Also: Leudet tinnitus
A type of objective tinnitus, e.g., clicking, snapping, or fluttering sounds caused by muscle spasm (myoclonus) of the soft palate or middle ear muscles.

tinnitus, pulsatile *np* [Lat *tinnitus* ringing, tinkling; Lat *pulsare* to throb]
Also: vibratory tinnitus
A type of objective tinnitus due to turbulent blood flow. Possible causes include vascular anomalies, vascular tumors, valvular heart disease (e.g., aortic stenosis), high blood pressure, etc.

tinnitus retraining therapy (TRT) *np*
A form of habituation therapy using

counseling, retraining, and sound enrichment to reduce the individual's perception of their tinnitus.

tip-link *n*
A fiber strand from the tip of one stereocilium to the next. Each tip link works as a gated spring for opening and closing the ion channels in the organ of Corti.

tissue expander *np*
A device similar to a balloon for stretching the skin and encouraging it to grow, e.g., for reconstruction of a pinna.

titanium *n/adj* 'tītānēum ('tītānēum)
Named after the mythical Titan metal forgers who made Zeus' thunderbolt.
-*n* A light strong metal that is biocompatible and highly resistant to corrosion. It is used in surgical devices and implants, e.g., bone-anchored hearing aids. -*adj* Formed of titanium.

tobramicin (tobramycin) *n* tōbra'mīsĭn
An aminoglycoside antibiotic that can be used against bacterial ear infections. Tobramycin ear drops may be ototoxic if they enter the middle ear via a perforation.

tolerance *n*
1. The permissible deviation from specified values given in a standard, e.g., the deviation allowed during calibration of an audiometer. 2. Resistance to a substance, e.g., a drug, after repeated exposure. 3. The acceptance of differences.

tomography *n* [Gk *tomos* slice, section + Gk *graphia* writing]
A technique used in radiology to produce images of sections of the body.

-tomy *suffix* [Gk –*tomia* cutting]
Involving a surgical operation.

tone *n* [Gk *tonos* tone]
An ongoing sound of one or more frequencies that has pitch, loudness, and timbre.

tone burst *np*
A short-duration tone.

tone, complex *np*
A sound consisting of more than one frequency.

tone control *np*
A control that alters the frequency response of a hearing aid.

tone decay *np*
Also: auditory fatigue; Albrecht effect; auditory adaptation
A reduction in the perception of loudness of a continuous tone.

tone pip *np*
Also: brief tone
A sinusoidal signal of less than 200 ms duration.

tone, pure *np*
A tone consisting of one frequency only. A sound with a pressure/time waveform that exhibits sinusoidal wave motion and exhibits pressure fluctuations of only one frequency.

tonotopic *adj* tōno'tŏpĭk [Gk *tonos* tone + Gk *topos* place]
In a fixed positional arrangement, such that separate frequency information is carried along separate tracts, e.g., as occurs along the auditory nerve.

tonsillectomy *np* [Lat *tonsilla* a capstan or mooring post + Gk *ektome* excission]
The surgical removal of the tonsils.

tonsils, palatine *np* [Lat *tonsilla* capstan or mooring post; Lat *palatum* palate]
The two areas of lymphoid tissue on either side of the back of the throat.

topical *adj* [Gk *topos* place]
Also: local
Applied to a localized area of the skin.

topography *n* [Gk *topos* place + Gk *graphia* writing]
The study of regions or parts.

topography, anatomic *np*
The study of a region of the body, the systems within it, and how they are related to each other.
Deriv: -adj topographic

torsional nystagmus *np* [Lat *torquere* to twist; Gk *nustagmos* blinking, nodding, drowsiness]
Nystagmus with a rotary movement. Most nystagmus resulting from vestibular dysfunction that has a rotary component.

total communication *np*
A communication philosophy that utilizes together both signed and spoken language.

total deafness *np*
The condition of having no measurable hearing.

total harmonic distortion (THD) *np*
Frequencies that are whole number multiples of the input signal that appear in the output signal and are not present in the input signal. They are due to nonlinearity in the amplifying system, e.g., an input frequency of 350 Hz may result in additional harmonics in the output signal at 700, 1050, 1400 Hz, etc.

toxin *n* [Gk *toxikon* poison]
A poison.

toxoplasmosis *n* [Gk *toxikon* poison + Gk *plasma* a shaping or forming + Gk *-osis* denoting a diseased state]
A disease caused by microorganisms in the blood, which is very serious for a fetus.

toy test *np*
A type of speech test for children in which the required response is usually pointing to a toy.

Toynbee maneuver (manoeuvre) *np*
Named after Joseph Toynbee (1815–1866), an English oral surgeon, who observed that swallowing with the nose and mouth closed caused air to enter the middle ear to relieve the pressure sensation after Valsalva maneuver.
Swallowing with the mouth and nose closed to force air out of the middle ear.

trabecular bone *np* [Lat *trabecula* little beam]
Also: cancellous bone; spongy bone
Bone composed of a network of branching bony spicules that has the appearance of a sponge, with bone marrow contained in the spaces.

traceability *n*
The ability to verify that the measurements stated on a calibration certificate are properly referenced back to an agreed (e.g., national or international) standard.

trachea *n* ˈtrākēa (traˈkēa) [Gk *trakheia (arteria)* rough (vessel or artery)]
Also: colloq windpipe
The tube that connects the pharynx or throat to the lungs.

tracking, connected discourse *np*
A speech test of hearing instrument benefit in which a passage is read in sections to the hearing-impaired listener, who must repeat it back. It is scored as words tracked per minute. It is also used as a rehabilitative strategy, especially in cochlear implant rehabilitation.

tract *n* [Lat *tractus* a drawing out]
A pathway or a system that is assembled longitudinally. May consist of organs, nerves, glands, or other tissues, e.g., the vocal tract.

tragion *n* ˈtrăjēon [Gk *tragion* little tragus]
A notch just above the tragus of the ear.

tragus *n* ˈtrăgus *pl* tragi [Gk *tragos* a goat, referring to a tuft of hair resembling a goat's beard]
Also: antilobium
A small cartilagenous prominence in front of the external opening to the ear canal.

trait *n* trāt
An enduring personal characteristic.

trans- *prefix* [Lat *trans* across]
Across or through.

transcranial *adj* [Lat *trans* across + Lat *cranium* skull]
Across the skull.

transcranial transmission loss *np*
The attenuation that occurs when a signal is applied to a test ear that crosses through the head so that it is heard in the nontest ear.

transducer *n* [Lat *trans* across + Lat *ducere* to lead]
A device that converts energy from one form to another, e.g., acoustic energy to electrical energy.
Deriv: -*v* transduce

transduction *n* [Lat *trans* across + Lat *ducere* to lead]
The means by which sound energy is converted to electrical impulses in the auditory nerve fibers.

transfer function *np* [Lat *transferre* to carry across]
Also: network function; system function
A mathematical relationship between the output of a control system and the input, e.g., Fourier transform is a transfer function that separates the output wave into its component frequencies.

transient *adj* [Lat *transire* to pass by]
Fleeting, of nearly instantaneous onset and lasting less than 0.1 ms.

transient distortion *np*
Inexact reproduction of an amplified waveform due to sudden changes in load or voltage.

transient evoked otoacoustic emission (TOAE) *np*
Emissions evoked by very brief sounds, usually clicks, but that can be tone bursts.

transistor *n*
A solid-state silicon device that regulates or amplifies current flow.

transition *n*
A rapid change.

transmission *n* [Lat *trans* across + Lat *mittere* to send]
The act of traveling from one medium in-to another.

transmitting coil *np* [Lat *transmitere* to send across]
The external coil of a cochlear implant, which is used to transmit radio signals to the implanted part of the device.

transparency, acoustic *np*
The ability to pass sound waves without change or distortion.

transposition *n* [Lat *transponere* to trans-pose]
The moving of something from one place to another.

transposition, frequency *np*
The shifting of high-frequency inputs to lower frequencies, e.g., as in a frequency transposition hearing aid.

transtympanic *adj* [Lat *trans* across + Gk *tumpanon* drum]
Across the tympanic cavity, usually through the tympanic membrane, e.g., transtympanic electrodes.

transudate *n* 'trăns(y)ūdāt ('trănz(y)ūdāt) [Lat *trans* across + Lat *sudare* to sweat]
A thin watery fluid exuded from a tissue.

transverse *adj*
Lying across.

transverse fracture *np*
A fracture in the horizontal plane.

transverse wave *np*
A wave in which the direction of particle displacement is parallel to the wavefront.

trapezoid body *np* 'trăpezoid [Gk *trapezoides* table-shaped]
A bundle of transverse nerve fibers that carry auditory impulses to the opposite superior olivary complex in the brain-stem.

trauma *n* [Gk *trauma* a wound]
An accident or injury.

traveling wave *np*
A longitudinal or radial wave that pro-gresses from its vibratory source through a medium over time.

Treacher-Collins syndrome *np* Named after Edward Treacher-Collins (1862–1932), an English ophthalmologist, who first reported the condition.
Also: mandibular dysostosis; first arch syndrome
A syndrome characterized by craniofacial deformities including downward sloping eyelid fissures, depressed cheek bones, receding chin, large fishlike mouth, and abnormalities of the external and middle ear, e.g., pinna abnormalities, atresia, and middle ear deformities. Hearing loss is usually severe conductive, but may be mixed if there is also inner ear deformity.

treble increase at low levels (TILL) *np*
A type of sound processing that achieves a higher frequency emphasis at low-input levels than at high-input levels by providing most compression in the high-frequency region.

triangular fossa *np* [Lat *fossa* ditch, depression]
The triangular-shaped dip in the upper part of the pinna where the antihelix splits into two.

triangular wave *np*
A periodic waveform that consists of odd integral multiples of the fundamental frequency and has the appearance of a series of triangular pulses.

trigeminal nerve *np* [Lat *trigeminus* three-fold; Gk *neuron* string, nerve]
One of the pair of cranial nerve V, a sensory and motor nerve that divides into three branches, ophthalmic, maxillary, and mandibular. The mandibular branch innervates the teeth, muscles of mastication, part of the tongue, the external ear, and the tensor tympani muscle.

trimester *n* [Lat *tri-* three + Lat *mensis* month]
A 3-month period.

trimethoprim-sulpamethoxazole *n* ˈtrīmĕthōˌprĭm sŭlpaˌmĕˈthŏksaˌzŏl
An antibiotic used for various bacterial infections, e.g., ear infections. Side effects of this antibiotic can include tinnitus and hearing loss, which may occur after large doses.

trimmer *n*
A device on a hearing aid to adjust the frequency response performance of the instrument. It may be operated by a screwdriver or electronically via programming software.

trisomy *n* trīˈsōmē (ˈtrīsomē) [Lat *tri-* three + Gk *soma* body]
Malformation due to chromosome irregularities that may include malformed ears.

trisomy 21 *np*
Also: Down syndrome; *obs* mongolism
A congenital genetic disorder. Characteristics include some physical and cognitive impairments, together with distinctive facial features (such as slanting eyes, square-shaped face, and macroglossia) and a high incidence of conductive and sensorineural hearing loss.

trisomy 18 *np*
Also: Edwards syndrome
A congenital genetic disorder caused by the presence of three copies of chromosome 18. Characteristics include microcephaly (small head) with the triangular shape due to a prominent chin, an undernourished appearance, heart disease, renal abnormalities, cleft lip, malformed ears, and learning difficulty.

trisomy 13-15 *np*
A congenital chromosomal disorder. Characteristics may include abnormally small eyes; cleft lip; extra fingers; learning disabilities; deafness; low set, malformed ears; and middle and inner ear deformities.

trochee *n* ˈtrōkē [Gk *trokhaion (pous)* running (foot)]
A two-syllable word in which the first syllable is stressed, e.g., finger.
Deriv: –*adj* trochaic

trochleariform process *np* 'trŏklēărē-fawm [Lat *trochlea* pulley + Lat *forma* shape, form]
Also: cochleariform process
A thin bony plate in the mesotympanum above the oval window. The tensor tympani muscle makes a right angle at this process before it runs laterally to attach at the neck of the malleus.

trough-shaped audiogram *np*
Also: colloq cookie bite
An audiogram that shows relatively good hearing in the high and low frequencies, but poor mid-frequency (1 to 2 kHz) hearing, which falls by 20 dB or more in comparison with the loss at 500 Hz and 4 kHz.

T-tube *n*
A long-term grommet or ventilation tube.

tube lock *np*
A small device that affixes to the tubing of the earmold with a flange that secures the tube in position.

tubercle *n* [Lat *tuberculum* a small swelling]
A small projection.

tuberculosis (TB) *n* [Lat *tuberculum* a small swelling + Gk *-osis* denoting a diseased state]
A contagious slow-developing bacterial infection that can be fatal if untreated and which is passed by droplet infection. It usually affects the lungs, but can spread to other organs, e.g., the central nervous system. Hearing loss may develop due to the disease or as a side effect of antibiotic (e.g., aminoglycoside) treatment.

tuberculosis luposa *np* [Lat *tuberculum* a small swelling + Gk *-osis* denoting a diseased state; Lat *lupus* a wolf]
Also: lupus vulgaris
A progressive form of skin tuberculosis in which there are raised brownish lesions on the skin, especially of the face.

tuberculum auriculae *np* [Lat *tuberculum* a small swelling; Lat *auriculae* of the ear]
Also: helix
The rolled edge of the pinna.

tubing expander *np*
A device for stretching the tubing of an earmold to make it easier to fit onto the earhook of a hearing aid.

tubotympanic *adj* [Lat *tubus* a tube + Gk *tumpanon* drum]
Pertaining to the Eustachian tube and the tympanic cavity.

Tullio phenomenon *np* 'tūlēō Named after Pietro Tullio (1881–1941), an Italian biologist, who discovered the effect when experimenting on pigeons.
Vertigo and nystagmus induced by sound, which may occur in Ménière syndrome and superior semicircular canal dehiscence syndrome (SCDS).

Tumarkin otolith crises *np* [Gk *ous* ear + Gk *lithos* stone] Named after Alexis Tumarkin (1900–1990), an honorary aurist at Bootle General Hospital in the UK, who described the condition in the *British Medical Journal* in 1936.
Also: otolithic catastrophe
Drop attacks without warning. The sudden falls may be due to inappropriate stimulation of the saccule, causing the interpretation of gravity having changed, before visual and proprioceptive input can be asssessed for accuracy of the situation.

tumor *n* [Lat *tumor* a swelling]
A growth (benign or malignant).

tune *v*
To program, e.g., each electrode of a cochlear implant speech processor is tuned for the electrical threshold and most comfortable level.

tuning curve, psychophysical *np*
A curve on a graph that plots masker level as a function of frequency and that is analogous to a neural threshold tuning curve for a single auditory nerve fiber. A

psychophysical tuning curve is normally V-shaped with a sharp tip because the nerve fiber responds to a very small frequency range, i.e., it is finely tuned, at its threshold. It has a broader top because a wider area of the basilar membrane responds to louder sounds.

tuning fork *np*
A mechanical device designed to produce a pure tone when struck.

tunnel of Corti *np*
Also: cuniculum internum; inner tunnel; canal of Corti
The triangular channel formed by the inner and outer pillars of the organ of Corti.

turbinate *n* [Lat *turbo* spinning top]
One of the curved ridges of spongy bone that are shaped like long sea shells and extend along the length of the nasal cavity. Their functions are to warm and moisten the incoming air.

Turner syndrome *np* Named after Henry Hubert Turner (1892–1970), an American endocrinologist, who described the syndrome in 1938.
Also: gonadal dysgenesis; XO syndrome
A chromosomal disorder in which there is not the usual pair of X chromosomes that affects only females. It is characterized by small stature, broad flat chest, absent or incomplete puberty, infertility, webbing of the neck, kidney and heart defects, and hearing loss, which may be conductive and/or sensorineural.

tweeter *n*
A small loudspeaker designed to operate in the high-frequency part of the audible range.

twenty two q/22q 11.2 deletion syndrome *np*
Also: DiGeorge syndrome; velocardiofacial syndrome; conotruncal anomaly face syndrome
A rare (1 in 4000 live births) syndrome that is genetic in only about 10% of cases. The signs and symptoms are very varia-

ble and may include congenital heart defects, cleft palate, kidney problems, autism, learning difficulty, an asymmetric crying face, poor growth, autism, skeletal abnormalities, e.g., spinal problems and extra fingers and toes, and external ear abnormalities. The syndrome is due to the deletion of a small amount of genetic material on the short or q arm of chromosome 22.

two-cc/2 cc coupler *np*
Also: reference coupler; standard coupler
A device that joins the receiver of a hearing aid to the microphone of a sound level meter and is designed with a standard volume of 2 cc. It is used for measuring the acoustic output of hearing aids.

two–tailed test *np*
A statistical test used when experimental results may be greater or lesser than a given value.

tympanic *adj* [Gk *tumpanon* drum]
Pertaining to the middle ear cavity.

tympanic cavity *np*
Also: middle ear
The portion of the ear between the eardrum and the cochlea. An irregular air-filled space in the temporal bone that contains the ossicles and is ventilated by the Eustachian tube. The ossicles connect the lateral and medial walls of the tympanic cavity and convey sound vibrations to the oval window of the cochlea.

tympanic membrane *np* [Gk *tumpanon* drum; Lat *membrana* partition]
Also: eardrum; myrinx
The elastic membrane between the external auditory canal and the middle ear. Its normal color is pearly gray with a cone-shaped light visible during otoscopic examination.

tympanic notch/incisure/incisura *np*
Also: Rivinus' notch/incisure
The indentation in the tympanic sulcus at the top of the tympanic membrane.

tympanic sulcus *np* [Gk *tumpanon* drum; Lat *sulcus* furrow, wrinkle]
The groove in the temporal bone that holds the tympanic membrane.

tympanocentesis *n* [Gk *tumpanon* drum + Gk *kentesis* a puncturing]
The removal of fluid from the middle ear.

tympanogram *n* [Gk *tumpanon* drum + Gk *gramma* thing written]
A graph of the results from tympanometry. These may be classified according to the shape of the tympanogram peak, as "A" (normal), "As" (shallow), "Ad" (deep), "B" (flat), and "C" (peak occurs at negative pressure).

tympanometry *n* [Gk *tumpanon* drum + Gk *metron* measure]
The procedure for measuring the acoustic impedance or admittance of the middle ear, which is used in the identification of middle ear conditions.

tympanometry, compensated *np*
Immittance measurements that are adjusted by the removal of the contribution of the ear canal.

tympanoplasty *n* [Gk *tumpanon* drum + Gk *plassein* to form, shape]
Surgery to repair the eardrum and the ossicular chain.

tympanosclerosis *n* [Gk *tumpanon* drum + Gk *skleroun* to harden]
A deposit of chalky patches on the tympanic membrane following disease or other injury.

tympanostomy tube *np* [Gk *tumpanon* drum + Gk *stoma* mouth]
Also: grommet
A ventilation tube that is inserted into the eardrum to resolve otitis media.

tympanum *n* *pl* tympana [Gk *tumpanon* drum]
1. The eardrum. 2. The middle ear and eardrum.

U

ulcer *n* [Lat *ulcus* ulcer]
An external or internal open sore that sometimes secretes pus, e.g., sensory radicular neuropathy includes ulcers on the feet (as well as sensorineural hearing loss) among its characteristics.
Deriv: -adj ulcerated

ultra- *prefix* [Lat *ultra* beyond]
Above.

ultrasonic *adj* [Lat *ultra* beyond + Lat *sonus* sound]
Pertaining to frequencies above the limit of audible hearing.

umbo *n* [Lat *umbo* shield boss, protuberance]
The central point where the handle of the malleus is attached to the tympanic membrane.

uncertainty of measurement *np*
Inaccuracies associated with all measurement, e.g., due to inherent inaccuracies of equipment. A general rule of thumb often used is that the equipment used to calibrate should be 10 times more accurate than the equipment being calibrated.

uncomfortable loudness level (ULL) *np*
Also: discomfort level; uncomfortable level (UCL); loudness discomfort level (LDL); threshold of discomfort
The sound level at which the listener begins to experience discomfort.

unidirectional *adj* [Lat *unus* one]
Responsive in one direction.

unilateral *adj* [Lat *unus* one + Lat *latus* side]
On one side.

unimodal *adj* [Lat *unus* one + Lat *modus* type]
Also: unisensory
Using only one sense.

unipolar *adj* [Lat *unus* one + Gk *polos* axis, pole]
1. Produced by a single electric or magnetic pole. 2. Having a single fibrous process (applied to nerve cells). 3. Pertaining to a depressive mood disorder.

unipolar lead *adj*
An asymmetrical system of electrodes in which there is a single positive recording electrode and an indifferent electrode.

unit *n*
1. A group of children (e.g., deaf children) partially integrated into a mainstream school. 2. A standard amount.

unity gain *np*
No gain or loss.

unmasked *adj*
A psychoacoustic term for a reduction in the effectiveness of masking when an additional sound is introduced.

unoccluded *adj* [un- + Lat *occludere* to block, shut up]
Also: open
Not blocked.

unvoiced *adj*
A speech sound produced without vocal cord vibration, e.g., /s/, /k/, /p/.

upward spread of masking *np*
The tendency for low frequency sounds to mask higher frequency sounds.

uranoschisis *n* 'yūrănŏskǐsǐs [Gk *ouranos* sky, palate + Gk *schisis* a split]
Also: cleft palate
A congenital fissure in the median line of the palate.

use (user) gain *np*
The amount of gain when a hearing aid is set at the wearer's normal volume position.

Usher syndrome *np* Named after Charles Howard Usher (1865–1942), a Scottish ophthalmologist, who published a description of the syndrome in 1914.
A recessive genetic disorder in which there is congenital profound deafness and late-onset retinitis pigmentosa,

which leads to progressive loss of vision. The visual problems start with night blindness, usually in the teenage years, progressing to tunnel vision and eventually total blindness. There may also be additional problems, e.g., vestibular dysfunction, epilepsy, and psychosis. Usher syndrome is relatively common (up to 10%) among profoundly deaf children.

utricle   *n*   [Lat *utriculum* a little leather sack, bag]
Also: utriculus
The largest of the two sacs in the vestibule of the vestibular system into which the semicircular canals open.

uvula   *n*   ˈyūvyūl*a* [Lat *uvula* a little (bunch of) grape(s)]
The fleshy pendant that hangs from the posterior border of the soft palate.

V

vagus nerve *np* ˈvāgus [Lat *vagus* wandering; Gk *neuron* string, nerve]
Also: pneumogastric nerve; cranial nerve X
A motor and sensory nerve that originates in the brainstem and wanders down the body supplying nerve fibers to many organs, e.g., external ear, pharynx, larynx, lungs, heart, intestines, etc. A small branch of the vagus nerve in the ear canal may be stimulated during impression-taking and can cause a cough reflex.

valacyclovir *n*
An oral antiviral drug used in the treatment of herpes viruses, e.g., herpes zoster oticus (shingles affecting the auditory nerve). Possible side effects include dizziness and tinnitus.

validity *n* [Lat *validus* strong]
The strength of the conclusions reached in a study or experiment, i.e., the degree to which a measurement actually reflects what it is supposed to measure.

validity, face *np*
The degree to which test items represent what they claim to test.

Valsalva maneuver (manoeuvre) *np*
Named after Antonio Maria Valsalva (1666–1723), an Italian physician and professor of anatomy in Bologna, who discovered this method of inflating the middle ear.
A method of opening the Eustachian tube by increasing pressure in the nasopharynx, achieved by taking a breath, holding the nose and forcibly trying to blow down the nose. The eardrum should be able to be seen to move outwards and a click may also be heard.

Van Buchem syndrome *np* văn ˈbūkem
Named after Francis van Buchem (b 1922), a Dutch physician, who described the syndrome in 1955.

Also: endosteal hyperostosis; hyperostosis corticalis generalisata; hyperphosphatasemia tarda
A genetic bone disorder characterized by overgrowth of the mandible and thickening of the long bones and the forehead and brow area. The bone growth may trap cranial nerves, causing facial palsy, sight, and hearing problems.

Van der Hoeve syndrome *np* văn der ˈhūve Named after Jan Van der Hoeve (1878–1952), a Dutch ophthalmologist, who emphasized the syndromic relationship of blue sclera, brittle bones, and deafness in osteogenesis imperfecta tarda in 1918.
Also: osteogenesis imperfecta tarda; osteogenesis imperfect type 1
A less-severe form of osteogenesis imperfecta. Characteristics may include frequent fractures, often starting when the child begins to walk, normal or near normal height, blue sclera, and progressive conductive hearing loss similar to that in otosclerosis.

variable *adj* [Lat *variare* to change]
Having a value that is subject to change, i.e., a quantity that may assume any one of a set of values.

variable, continuous *np*
A value measured on a continuous scale that can be subdivided such that the difference between items can be calculated.

variable, discrete *np*
A value measured on a fixed scale, which may be arbitrary, e.g., a rating scale of hearing aid benefit.

variable resistor *np*
Also: potentiometer
A potentiometer, i.e., a screw or wheel that the user can turn to increase or decrease the resistance. This determines how much current flows through the circuit.

variance *n*
A measure of the dispersion or variation in a set of scores. The larger the variance, the more scattered are the scores.

varicella *n* văriˈsĕla [Lat *varicella* a little pustule]
Also: chickenpox
One of the herpes viruses that causes chickenpox, and in adults, shingles.

vascular *adj* [Lat *vas* vessel]
Relating to blood vessels. The cochlea is rapidly affected by any disruption of the blood supply. Circulatory disorders may result in sensorineural hearing loss and vestibular symptoms. Low-frequency areas of the cochlea are affected first as these areas are the most distal.

vascular compression *np*
Pulsatile compression or irritation of a nerve, usually at the brainstem, by a blood vessel. If cranial nerve VIII is involved, there may be severe tinnitus and/or vertigo.

vascular dementia (VaD) *np* [Lat *vas* vessel; Lat *dementia* madness]
A form of dementia caused by cerebrovascular disease.

vaso- *prefix* ˈvāzō- [Lat *vas* vessel]
Channel.

vasoconstrictor *n* [Lat *vas* vessel + Lat *constringere* to constrict, narrow]
An agent or drug that causes narrowing of the blood vessels.

vasodilation *n* [Lat *vas* vessel + Lat *dilatare* to spread out, widen]
An agent or drug that causes the blood vessels to widen.

vasospasm *n* [Lat *vas* vessel + Gk *spasma* convulsion]
An involuntary contraction of a blood vessel.

vas spirale *np* [Lat *vas* vessel; Lat *spiralis* spiral (from Gk *speira* a coil)]
The largest blood vessel that runs the length of the basilar membrane. It is found below the tunnel of Corti in the vascular covering (mesothelium) of the basilar membrane.

vein *n* [Lat *vena* vein]
A blood vessel that carries deoxygenated blood back toward the heart.

velar *adj* ˈvēla [Lat *velum* sail, curtain, covering]
Formed with the point of contact at the back of the mouth, as in the production of the speech sounds /k/ and /g/.

velocardiofacial syndrome (VCFS) *np* [Lat *velum* sail, curtain, covering + Gk *kardia* heart + Lat *facies* face]
Also: DiGeorge syndrome; conotruncal anomaly face syndrome; 22q 11.2 deletion syndrome
A chromosomal disorder, in which a small part of chromosome 22 is usually missing, that causes a wide range of developmental defects. Characteristics may include congenital heart defects, cleft palate, mild learning difficulties, hearing loss, and minor malformation of the pinna.

velocity *n* [Lat *velocitas* swiftness]
Also: colloq speed
The measurement of rate of change of position along a straight line with respect to time, i.e., speed in a given direction.

venous sinus *np* [Lat *vena* vein; Lat *sinus* recess, bend]
A large vein or passage for deoxygenated blood.

vent *n* [Lat *ventus* wind]
A hole drilled through the earmold of a hearing aid to reduce the response of the lower frequencies and to assist in the reduction of the occlusion effect, but which can cause acoustic feedback.

vent, diagonal *np*
A vent where there is insufficient room for a parallel vent due to a small ear canal; the vent is therefore joined into the sound bore when the canal becomes too narrow. This type of vent causes an adverse effect on the high-frequency region.

vent, external *np*
A vent where there is insufficient room for the entire vent to be within the earmold due to a small ear canal.

vent, parallel *np*
The most usual type of vent, which runs through the earmold parallel to the sound bore.

vent, select-a- *n*
A selection of inserts that can be installed within the aperture of a vent in an earmold or custom aid to reduce vent size.

ventilation tube *np*
Also: grommet; tympanostomy tube
A small tube, similar in shape to a cotton reel, that is inserted into the eardrum to resolve otitis media by allowing air to enter the middle ear.

ventral *adj* [Lat *venter* belly]
Pertaining to the front part of the body.

ventricle *n* [Lat *ventriculus* a little belly]
A cavity, e.g., the four connected cavities in the central portion of the brain that are continuous with the central canal of the spinal cord and filled with cerebrospinal fluid. Enlarged ventricles may be associated with deterioration in dementia.

vernix *n* [Lat *veronix* fragrant resin]
A fatty substance that covers the skin of the fetus, which is sometimes found in a neonate's ear canal.

vertex *n* *pl* vertices [Lat *vertex* crown of head]
The top of the head. In evoked response audiometry, the forehead may be used as the vertex placement for the reference electrode.

vertical semicircular canal *np*
A vertical canal, one of the three semicircular canals, which is parallel to the posterior semicircular canal. It joins the utricle at one end and combines with the posterior semicircular canal at the other before rejoining the utricle as a common

canal. It is involved in sensing movement in the vertical plane.

vertigo *n* ˈvertĭgō [Lat *vertigo* whirling or dizziness]
An illusion of movement.
Deriv: -*adj* vertiginous

vertigo, rotational *np*
Also: torsional nystagmus
A feeling of spinning when neither the environment or the body is moving.

vesicle *n* ˈvĕsĭkel [Lat *vesicula* a little bladder]
A small membranous sac, cyst, or blister that is usually filled with fluid.

vestibular *adj* [Lat *vestibulum* entrance hall]
Pertaining to balance.

vestibular labyrinth *np* [Lat *vestibulum* entrance hall; Gk *laburinthos* labyrinth or maze]
The vestibular pathways in the petrous part of the temporal bone. It consists of the semicircular canals, the saccule, and the utricle.

vestibular membrane *np* [Lat *vestibulum* entrance hall; Lat *membrana* covering]
Also: Reissner membrane
The membrane that separates the scala media from the scala vestibule in the cochlea. One end of the vestibular membrane is attached to the spiral ligament, the other to the inner part of the spiral limbus.

vestibular nerve *np* [Lat *vestibulum* entrance hall; Gk *neuron* a string, nerve]
The branch of cranial nerve VIII that serves the vestibular system.

vestibular neuronitis/neuritis *np* [Lat *vestibulum* entrance hall + Gk *neuron* a string, nerve]
Inflammation of the vestibular nerve that is usually of abrupt onset and causing acute rotational vertigo and may be due to a reactivation of the herpes simplex virus. Spontaneous horizontal nystagmus with the fast phase toward the healthy

ear is characteristic, but hearing is not affected.

vestibular schwannoma *np*
Also: acoustic neuroma/neurinoma/neurilemoma; cerebellopontine angle tumor
A benign tumor that grows from the vestibular branch of the eighth nerve, caused by an overgrowth of the Schwann cells of the myelin sheath. Unilateral hearing loss is often the first sign of the condition. Bilateral tumors are very rare, but may be associated with neurofibromatosis.

vestibular system *np*
The sensory mechanism of the inner ear that detects movement and controls balance.

vestibule *n* [Lat *vestibulum* entrance hall]
1. A body cavity that opens into another cavity. 2. A cavity in the central part of the bony labyrinth of the inner ear into which the semicircular canals open.

vestibulocochlear nerve *np* [Lat *vestibulum* entrance hall + Lat *cochlea* snail shell, spiral]
Cranial nerve VIII that supplies the cochlea and the vestibule of the inner ear.

vestibulometry *n* [Lat *vestibulum* entrance hall + Gk *metron* measure]
The testing of vestibular function.

vestibuloocular reflex (VOR) *np* [Lat *vestibulum* entrance hall + Lat *oculus* eye]
Also: three-neuron arc
The reflex arc between the vestibular system and muscles of the eyes, which maintains gaze stability by causing compensatory eye movements when the head is rotated.

vibration *n* [Lat *vibrare* to vibrate]
Oscillating movement.

vibrator *n*
A device that causes an object to vibrate, e.g., a bone conduction vibrator.

vibrotactile *adj* [Lat *vibrare* to vibrate + Lat *tactilis* touchable]
The sensation of touch or feeling induced

by vibration, e.g., the responses by a profoundly deaf individual, when given high sound levels during a hearing test, may be vibrotactile.

videootoscopy *np* [Lat *videre* to see + Gk *ous* ear + Gk *skopein* to look at]
A form of otoscopy in which the image from the ear canal is projected onto an external monitor.

virtual pitch *np*
Also: pitch periodicity; missing fundamental
The perceived pitch of a complex tone that corresponds to a missing fundamental.

virus *n* [Lat *virus* slime, venom, poison]
A microscopic infectious agent that can only grow and replicate itself once inside the cells of a living host.
Deriv: -adj viral

viscosity *n* [Lat *viscosus* sticky (from *viscum* bird lime)]
The resistance of a substance to flow. A measurement of the consistency of a material, e.g., ear impression material, before curing (hardening due to polymerization) occurs. A low-viscosity material has a soft consistency, a high viscosity material is relatively dense and firm.

viseme *n* ˈvīzēm [Lat *videre* to see]
One of a group of speech sounds that appears identical by lipreading alone, e.g., /m/, /p/, /b/.

visispeech *n*
Computer software used by speech and language therapists to deliver a real-time display of aspects of voice, e.g., pitch, energy, and voicing, which can assist in the recognition and production of speech sounds.

visual reinforcement audiometry (VRA) *np*
Also: conditioned orientation reflex audiometry
A type of pediatric audiometry in which a correct response to presentations of sound is reinforced by a visual reward,

e.g., a lighted toy or a pleasing digital image.

vitiligo *n* vĭt'ĭ'līgō [Lat *vitiligo* skin disease] An autoimmune, usually progressive, skin condition in which smooth white areas appear on the skin due to depigmentation. The entire pigmentary system is affected, including the melanocytes in the inner ear, which may interfere with the conduction of action potentials, causing hearing loss.

vocal cords/folds *np* [Lat *vox* voice] Two folds of membrane that project across the larynx and that vibrate to produce voiced speech sounds and other vocal noises.

vocalization (vocalisation) *n* A sound made with vibration of the vocal cords and modified by the vocal tract.

vocal tract *np* [Lat *vox* voice; Lat *tractum* passage] The system for the production of speech. It begins with air from the lungs that pass through the open or closed vocal folds to the mouth. This is modified by the cavities in the throat, mouth, and nose that act as resonators in the production of the required sounds.

vocoder *n* A voice operated decoder for the analysis and synthesis of speech based on the spectral characteristics of the input signal.

Vogt-Koyanagi-Harada syndrome (VKH) *np* fōkt-'kŏyănăgē-'hahrhada Named after Alfred Vogt (1879–1943), a Swiss ophthalmologist, who first described the syndrome in 1906, and Einosuke Harada (1892–1946) and Yoshizo Koyanagi (1880–1954), Japanese ophthalmologists, who further described cases in 1926 and 1929, respectively.
Also: uveoencephalitis
A rare autoimmune condition of possible viral origin that results in depigmentation of the skin and hair. Other character-

istics are neurologic, visual, and auditory abnormalities that may include eye pain, photophobia and loss of vision, dysacusis (a distortion of hearing), tinnitus, and vertigo.

voice box *n colloq*
Also: larynx
The cavity in the throat that connects the pharynx to the trachea and houses the vocal folds, which are vibrated to produce voiced sounds.

voiced *adj*
A speech sound produced with vibration of the vocal folds.

voice onset time (VOT) *np*
The interval between the release of closure, e.g., in a plosive sound such as /p/, and the onset of the following voicing.

Voit nerve *np* Named after Max Voit (1876–1949), a German physician and professor of anatomy at the University of Gottingen, who first described this nerve. The branch of the vestibular nerve that serves the saccule.

volley theory *np*
The theory that information relating to frequency is conveyed in the auditory nerve as successive bursts or volleys of nerve impulses.

volt (V) *n* Named after Count Alessandro Volta (1745–1827), the Italian inventor of the battery.
The International System (SI) unit of voltage. One volt is the potential difference across a conductor when a current of one ampere dissipates one watt of power.

voltage *n* Named after Count Alessandro Volta (1745–1827), the Italian inventor of the battery.
A measure of the force in an electric circuit, i.e., the strength of the current. Voltage = energy per charge, i.e., the amount of energy that a charge has at any point in the circuit.

Voltolini disease *np* Named after Fridericus Eduardus Rudolfus Voltolini (1819–1889), a German physician and pioneer in otorhinolaryngology.
A painful inflammation of the inner ear, leading to meningitis and deafness.

volumetric measurement *np*
A volumetric analysis by structural magnetic resonance imaging that is used to measure tumor growth.

volume unit meter (VU) *np*
A sound-level meter used in audio equipment and speech audiometers.

vomer *n* ˈvōme [Lat *vomer* ploughshare]
The thin flat bone that forms part of the septum separating the two nasal passages.

von Meyenburg disease *np* fŏn ˈmīyĕnberg Named after Hans von Meyenburg (1887–1971), a German pathologist and professor of pathology at the University of Zurich, who first described the disease.
Also: relapsing perichondritis
A degenerative disease of the cartilage producing an unusual form of arthritis in which the cartilage of the body collapses, e.g., in the ear, nose, trachea, etc.

von Recklinghausen neurofibromatosis *np* fŏn ˈrĕklĭnghowzen Named after Friedrich Daniel von Recklinghausen (1833–1910), a German pathologist and professor of pathological anatomy at the University of Strasbourg, who first documented the disorder.
Also: neurofibromatosis type 1 (NF-1)
The most common form of neurofibromatosis. An autosomal dominant disorder caused by a gene mutation on the chromosome responsible for cell division. Characteristics of the condition may include musculoskeletal abnormalities, café au lait spots, multiple fibromas of the skin and the peripheral nerves, nodules in the iris of the eyes, learning disability, and speech and language delay. Loss of vision and hearing occur if the optic and auditory nerves are involved. Hearing loss may be bilateral. Although normally benign, the fibromas may develop into cancer.

vowel *n* [Fr *vouel* vowel (from Lat *vocalis* voiced)]
A voiced speech sound that is the most prominent sound in a syllable.

Waardenburg syndrome *np* vahdɛnberg
Named after Petrus Johannes Waardenburg (1886–1979), a Dutch ophthalmologist and geneticist and professor of genetics at the Institute of Preventative Medicine in Leiden, who presented a detailed review of the condition in 1951.
A hereditary pigmentary condition characterized by a white forelock, vitiligo, different colored eyes, broad nasal root, cupid bow lips, prominent lower jaw, and congenital mild to profound hearing loss.

Waldenstrom macrogloblinemia *np* ˈvahldĕnstrŏm [Gk *makros* long, large + Lat *globulus* a little sphere + Gk *haima* blood]
Named after Jan G. Waldenstrom (1906–1996), a Swedish oncologist, who identified the condition in 1944.
A rare cancer that starts in the white blood cells, which are part of the body's immune system. It is marked by an abnormally high concentration of macroglobulin antibodies in the blood and may affect blood viscosity, making it thick and leading to visual and neurologic problems, e.g., headaches and vertigo.

Waldeyer ring *np* ˈvăldāɛrz Named after Heinrich Wilhelm Gottfried von Waldeyer-Hartz (1836–1921), a German anatomist and professor of pathology at the University of Strasbourg, who published the first description of this ring in 1884.
A ring of lymphoid tissue in the pharynx formed mainly by the two palatine tonsils, the lingual tonsil, and the adenoid that acts as a barrier against infection.

warble tone *np* [Gk *tonos* tone]
A frequency-modulated tone, i.e., a sound whose frequency varies rapidly around a mean value expressed in percent, often used in sound field audiometry to reduce the risk of standing waves affecting test results.

watt (W) *n* Named in honor of James Watt (1736–1819), a Scottish engineer, who developed the concept of horse-power and whose steam engine played a large part in the Industrial Revolution.
A unit of power equal to work done at a rate of one joule per second or produced by a current of one ampere across a potential difference of one volt.

wave *n*
A disturbance that travels, as a series of compressions and rarefactions, through a medium, usually air.

waveform *n*
A graph that shows features of an acoustic signal, i.e., its amplitude or pressure at any moment in time.

wavelength *n*
The distance between one peak of a wave or crest and the next peak.

wave, longitudinal *np*
A wave in which the oscillations are in the direction of travel.

wave, progressive *np*
A traveling wave.

wave, sound *np*
Propagation of a disturbance through a medium; when molecules are compressed, the pressure rises and when molecules are rarefied, the pressure falls.

wave, standing *np*
A wave that appears to be stationary that is caused by two identical trains of simple harmonic waves following the same path in a medium, but going in the opposite direction. It occurs when a reflected wave and an incident wave interact, such that there are points of increased intensity and other points where there are dead spots or areas of decreased intensity.

wave train *np*
A series of waves traveling in the same direction and spaced at regular intervals.

wave, transverse *np*
A wave in which the oscillations are at right angles to the direction of travel.

wax *n*
A waxy substance secreted by the glands in the ear canal that consists of cerumen from the ceruminous glands, sweat from the apocrine glands and oil from the sebaceous glands.

wax, dry *np*
A recessive inherited type of ear wax, common in Asians and native Americans, that is dry and flaky and contains about 20–30% lipid (fat).

wax guard *np*
A small cover or other device at the sound outlet of a hearing aid to protect it from wax ingression.

wax, wet *np*
A dominant inherited type of ear wax, common in West Europe, which contains about 50% lipid (fat).

Weber test *np* 'vēbe Named after Ernest H. Weber (1795–1878), a German otologist and professor of anatomy and physiology at the University of Leipzig, who first described this test. He is also considered a pioneer of psychophysics.
A bone conduction test of lateralization, performed with a tuning fork or bone vibrator placed to the center of the forehead. The tone will lateralize to the ear with the better hearing cochlea, or to the ear with the largest conductive component in cases of equal bilateral cochlear hearing.

Wegener granulomatosis *np* vēgĕne [Lat *granulum* a little grain + Gk –*oma* denoting tumor, swelling + Gk -*osis* denoting a diseased state] Named after Friedrich Wegener (1907–1990), a German pathologist, who described the disease in 1936.
An inflammatory process that affects the blood vessels, causing the walls to scar and thicken, which can affect the blood flow. Characteristics may include headache, sinusitis, rhinorrhea, otitis media, fever, and joint pain. It can also be a cause of sudden hearing loss.

weighted *adj*
To adjust to reflect a value or proportion, e.g., to vary numbers or variables to reflect relative importance.

weighting scale *np*
One of a family of filtering networks, e.g., A weighting, in sound-level meters that provides a frequency response for measuring noise as specified by international standards.

Wernicke aphasia *np* vernĭka [Gk *aphasia* speechlessness] Named after Karl Wernicke (1848–1905), a German neurologist, who is known for his study of aphasia.
A form of aphasia characterized by fluent, but meaningless speech and lack of comprehension.

Wernicke area *np* Named after Karl Wernicke (1848–1905), a German neurologist, who is known for his study of aphasia.
An area in the cerebral cortex associated with the comprehension of words and the production of meaningful speech.

whisper test *np*
A test of whispered speech at varying distances from the listener to determine hearing ability, but not considered a reliable test due to the variability in the intensity of the signal.

white forelock *np*
A white patch of hair over the forehead.

white matter *np*
The part of the brain that appears white in color because it contains nerve fibers that are covered with white myelin.

white noise *np* Named by analogy to light, which appears white when all the frequencies are combined.
1. Noise in which all frequencies within a specified range are present without regard to phase, and the average power over the frequency range is constant. 2. Noise that contains equal power per unit of bandwidth, i.e., equal sound energy at all frequencies.

wick *n*
A taper of cotton or similar material that absorbs and draws up fluid.

wideband noise *np*
Any complex noise that is contained within a wide frequency range.

wide dynamic range compression *np*
A compression circuit that compresses a wide range of acoustic signals to within the listener's residual dynamic range.

Wildervanck syndrome *np* ˈvĭlderfahnk
Named after Lambertus Sophius Wildervanck (1915–1976), a Dutch geneticist, who first described the condition in 1952.
Also: otofaciocervical dysmorphia; cervicooculoacoustic syndrome
A syndrome, similar to Klippel-Feil syndrome, where two or more cervical vertebrae are fused. Characteristics include narrow elongated face, short webbed neck, poorly developed neck muscles, facial asymmetry, deafness that may be total, prominent ears, preauricular fistulas, eyeball retraction, and nystagmus.

Williams syndrome *np* Named after John Cyprian Phipps Williams (1922–1978), a New Zealand cardiologist, who first identified the syndrome in 1961.
A rare congential disorder caused by missing genes. characterized by narrowed blood vessels, short stature, sunken chest, unusual elfin facial appearance, and high verbal ability but mild to moderate learning difficulties.

wind noise *np*
Sound produced in a hearing aid system from wind turbulence around and across the microphone.

window *n*
Also: fenestra
A membrane-covered opening in the bone, e.g., the oval and round windows in the cochlea.

Wolfram syndrome *np* Named after Don J. Wolfram, an American physician, who described the syndrome in 1938.
Also: diabetes insipidus, diabetes mellitus, optic atrophy, and deafness (DIDMOAD)
A progressive neurodegenerative syndrome that includes sensorineural hearing loss and visual impairment with diabetes mellitus and diabetes insipidus. There may also be other features, e.g., limited joint mobility and heart malformations. Onset is in late childhood or early adulthood

woofer *n*
A large loudspeaker that operates over the lower frequencies.

word deafness, pure *np*
The inability to comprehend the meaning of speech due to damage to the Wernicke area.

X

Xanthoma *n* zăn'thōma [Gk *xanthos* yellow + Gk *–oma* denoting tumor, swelling]
A skin disorder, in which fat deposits build up under the skin or the mucous membranes, that appears as flat soft yellowish nodules. It can develop anywhere on the body or systemically in any organs, but most often seen on the elbows, knees, hands and feet. It may affect hearing, e.g., xanthoma of the ear canal may cause narrowing and conductive hearing loss or there may be central nervous system involvement that can cause sensorineural deafness.

x-axis *n*
The horizontal axis of a graph.

X chromosome *np* [Gk *khroma* color + Gk *soma* body]
The chromosome that, together with the Y chromosome, carries genetic information that determines gender. Males have an X and a Y chromosome; females have two X chromosomes.

xeroderma pigmentosa *np* zerō'derma pĭgmĕn'tōsĭs [Gk *xeros* dry + Gk *derma* skin; Lat *pigmentosus* colored]
A rare genetic condition characterized by severe sunburn when exposed to sunlight.

X-linked *adj*
Pertaining to having only one X chromosome. X-linked inherited conditions occur mainly in males.

XO syndrome *np*
Also: Turner syndrome; gonadal dysgenesis
A chromosomal disorder in which there is not the usual pair of X chromosomes. It affects only females and is characterized by small stature, broad flat chest, absent or incomplete puberty, infertility, webbing of the neck, kidney and heart defects, and hearing loss that may be conductive and/or sensorineural

x-ray *n*
Short wavelength electromagnetic radiation that produces an image on photographic film. It is used in medical diagnosis to provide detail of solid areas of the body.

XX gonadal dysgenesis with sensorineural hearing loss *np* gō'nădal dĭs'jĕnēsĭs [Gk *gonades* gonads; Gk *dus-* bad + Gk *genesis* generation]
Also: Perrault syndrome
An autosomal recessive disorder characterized by ovarian dysgenesis in females and associated with severe or profound sensorineural hearing loss.

XXY syndrome *np*
Also: Klinefelter syndrome
A syndrome in which males are born with an extra X chromosome. Characteristics include abnormal body proportions, female characteristics, underdeveloped male genitalia and infertility, and possible hearing loss.

XYY syndrome *np*
A syndrome in which males are born with three sex chromosomes instead of the normal two. Characteristics include above average height and low levels of fertility and there may be a language impairment.

Y chromosome *np* [Gk *khroma* color + Gk *soma* body]
The chromosome that, together with the X chromosome, carries genetic information that determines gender. Females have two X chromosomes; males have an X and a Y chromosome.

Yes-no audiometry *np* [Lat *audire* to hear + Gk *metron* measure]
A form of audiometry where the verbal response "Yes" is given when a tone is claimed to be heard and "No" when nothing is claimed to be heard. This is an attention raising technique often used in pediatric testing in cases of suspected nonorganic hearing loss.

Y-lead *n*
A single cable from a body-worn hearing aid that divides in two to deliver identical split signals to two receivers.

Z

zero *n* [Fr *zéro* (from Old Spanish from Arabic *şifr* cipher)]
Arithmetic nought (0).

zero, audiometric *np* [Lat *audire* to hear + Gk *metron* measure]
The normal average hearing threshold, i.e., 0 dB HL.

zero level *n*
The reference level used for comparing sound intensities.

zinc-air battery *np*
A primary battery that uses oxygen as the cathode and zinc as the anode. Zinc-air button cells are used in hearing aids.

zona arcuata *np* ˈzōnₐ ahkyū̆ˈahtₐ [Lat *zona arcuata* curved area]
The thin inner part of the basilar membrane on which the the organ of Corti is supported.

zona pectinata *np* [Lat *zona pectinata* striated (combed) area (from Lat *pecten* a comb)]
The outer striated part of the basilar membrane that supports the structures from the outer rods of Corti to the spiral ligament.

Zwislocki coupler *np* Named after Jozef J. Zwislocki (b 1922), a Polish American acoustic engineer and professor of neuroscience at Syracuse University, who invented the occluded ear simulator in 1970.
An adjustable artificial ear used mainly for research. It can be adjusted to replicate different acoustic properties of the ear canal.

Z-weighting scale *np*
A flat-frequency response over the range 10 Hz to 20 kHz, which replaces older linear or unweighted scales that did not define the frequency range of operation.

zygote *n* [Gk *zugotos* yoked]
The cell formed from the joining of the ovum and sperm during sexual reproduction.